COMPARATIVE HEALTH POLICY AND THE NEW RIGHT

Also by Christa Altenstetter

DER FÖDERALISMUS IN ÖSTERREICH: 1945–1968
FEDERAL-STATE HEALTH POLICIES AND IMPACTS: The Politics of
    Implementation (*with James Warner Björkman*)
HEALTH POLICY MAKING AND ADMINISTRATION IN WEST GERMANY
    AND THE UNITED STATES
INNOVATION IN HEALTH POLICY AND SERVICE DELIVERY: A Cross-
    National Perspective (*editor*)
KRANKENHAUSBEDARFSPLANUNG: Was brachte sie wirklich?
NATIONAL-SUBNATIONAL RELATIONS IN HEALTH: Opportunities and
    Constraints (*editor*)

Also by Stuart C. Haywood

CRISIS IN THE NATIONAL HEALTH SERVICE (*with Andy Alaszewski*)
MANAGING THE HEALTH SERVICE

Comparative Health Policy and the New Right

From Rhetoric to Reality

Edited by
Christa Altenstetter
Professor of Political Science
The City University of New York's
Graduate School and Queens College

and

Stuart C. Haywood
Senior Lecturer, Health Services Management Centre
University of Birmingham

St. Martin's Press   New York

All rights reserved. For information, write:
Scholarly and Reference Division,
St. Martin's Press, Inc., 175 Fifth Avenue,
New York, N.Y. 10010

First published in the United States of America in 1991

Printed in Hong Kong

ISBN 0–312–05343–6

Library of Congress Cataloging-in-Publication Data
Comparative health policy and the new right: from rhetoric to reality
edited by Christa Altenstetter and Stuart C. Haywood.
p. cm.
Includes index.
ISBN 0–312–05343–6
1. Medical policy—Political aspects, 2. Conservatism.
I. Altenstetter, Christa.   II. Haywood, Stuart Collingwood.
RA393.C57   1991
362.1—dc20   90–44165
                                                   CIP

362.1
C737

TP

Contents

List of Tables and Figures

Tables

Figures

Acknowledgements

We would like to thank Ruth Liss, Arlene Diamond and Eugenie Pagano of the City University of New York's Queens College who aided in the typing of the manuscript. We would also like to express our appreciation to Gallya Lahav and Jennifer Holdaway for their help in the editing of the manuscript.

CHRISTA ALTENSTETTER
STUART C. HAYWOOD

Notes on the Contributors

Christa Altenstetter is Professor of Political Science at the City University of New York's Graduate School and Queens College. She received her Dr. phil. in Political Science, History, and Public Law from the University of Heidelberg, Germany. She holds a Master of Arts Degree from Duke University and received postdoctoral training at the Kennedy School of Government at Harvard University. Dr. Altenstetter has taught and–or researched at a number of universities and institutions in Europe and the United States. She has been a temporary advisor to the Regional Office for Europe of the World Health Organization in Copenhagen since 1976. Her interests are in comparative politics and comparative health and social policy and her current research is on the impacts of the Single European Market on health, health policies and delivery systems. She has published widely, including a recent publication 'An End to a Consensus on Health Care in the Federal Republic of Germany?'. She is the founder of the IPSA Study Group Comparative Health Policy.

James W. Björkman is Professor of Public Policy and Administration at the Institute of Social Studies, The Hague, as well as Professor of Public Administration at Leiden University, The Netherlands. He is also Executive Director of the International Institute of Comparative Government in Lausanne, Switzerland; Clinical Professor of Preventive Medicine at the University of Wisconsin-Madison, USA; and was Director of the American Studies Research Centre, Hyderabad Institute from 1987 to 1990. His many publications include *Federal-State Health Policies and Impacts* (co-author, 1978), *The Politics of Administrative Alienation in India's Rural Development Programs* (1979), Changing Division of Labor in South-Asia: Women and Men in Society, Economy and Politics (editor, 1987), and *Controlling Medical Professionals: The Comparative Politics of Health Governance* (co-editor, 1988).

William P. Brandon is Professor of Political Science at Seton Hall University in South Orange, New Jersey. He received his first degree from the Johns Hopkins University, where he was elected to Phi Beta

Kappa, and postgraduate degrees from the University of London, Duke University and the School of Public Health of the University of North Carolina at Chapel Hill. He has been a Robert Wood Johnson Faculty Fellow in Health Care Finance at the Johns Hopkins University Medical Institutions and a National Endowment for the Humanities Fellow at the Hastings Center Institute of Society, Ethics and the Life Sciences. His current research is on health politics and finance.

Paul Godt received his bachelor's degree from Bowdoin College (Maine) and Master of Arts and Doctorate from the Graduate Faculty of the New School for Social Research in New York. He is Associate Professor of Political Science at The American University of Paris, where he has taught since 1972, and Research Associate at the Centre de Recherches en Sciences Sociales du Travail, at the University of Paris-Sud. He has also been Visiting Professor at the Universities of Grenoble and Nice, France.

His research has focused on the political economy of health care policy in France and Western Europe and the reform of center–periphery relations in France. He edited and was a contributor to *Policy-Making in France: From de Gaulle to Mitterrand* (London: Frances Pinter, 1989), and has written several articles for professional journals. He is currently writing a book, with two co-authors, on public policy in France.

Stuart C. Haywood is a Senior Lecturer at the Health Services Management Centre, University of Birmingham, England. Previous publications have focused on management of the National Health Service, power, the management of conflicts, and funding issues. His writings draw on research and field experience as a consultant and board member of health authorities and voluntary organisations. He was trained as a hospital administrator before joining the staff at the University of Hull where he initially specialised in Social Security. Subsequently, he has moved into health care research and management, training and consultancies in the United Kingdom and overseas. He has been a member of the IPSA comparative health policy group since its foundation in 1982.

Pranlal Manga is a Professor in the Faculty of Administration at the University of Ottawa, Ontario, Canada. He was educated at McMaster University and the University of Toronto. For many years he was a National Health Research Scholar. He is a health economist who has published extensively in several health policy fields.

Wendy Ranade is a Senior Lecturer in the Department of Economics and Government, Newcastle-upon-Tyne Polytechnic, specialising in Health Policy and Management. She graduated in politics and sociology in 1972 from Newcastle University and after undertaking post-graduate work in political sociology joined Newcastle Polytechnic as a lecturer in 1974. From 1983–87 she was also a Research Associate at the Health Services Management Centre, University of Birmingham, and has researched and written on health policy as well as carrying out training and consultancy work with health authorities. Present research interests include monitoring the implementation of an 'internal market' in the National Health Service. As a member of a District Health Authority for the last four years, she has specific interests in health promotion and mental health.

Richard B. Saltman is Associate Professor in the Program in Health Policy and Management of the School of Public Health at the University of Massachusetts/Amherst. He holds a doctorate in political science from Stanford University. His research focuses on comparative health system behaviour among developed countries, particularly in Northern Europe. In 1987–88 he was a German Marshall Fund Research Fellow based at the Swedish Center for Working Life in Stockholm, studying emerging health policy strategies in the Nordic region.

William E. Steslicke is an Associate Professor in the Department of Health Policy and Management, College of Public Health, University of South Florida at Tampa. During 1989–90, he was a Fulbright Research Fellow and Visiting Associate Professor in the Department of Health Sociology, School of Health Sciences, Faculty of Medicine, University of Tokyo. He has published numerous articles on health care organisations, policies and politics in Japan and the United States.

Sonia Maria Fleury Teixeira is coordinator of a research centre on health policies at the National School of Public Health, Oswaldo Cruz Foundation, Rio de Janeiro, Brazil. In addition she is Head of the Department of Research and Publications, Adjunct Professor at the Brazilian School of Public Administration, Getulio Vargas

Foundation. She has published widely on social policy in Latin America. Sonia Maria Fleury Teixeira has a master's degree in sociology, and is currently finishing her doctorate in political science at the University Research Institute of Rio de Janeiro, Candido Mendes University.

Douglas Webber is a professor on the teaching staff of the Institute of Business Administration (INSEAD), Fontainebleau, France. Previously he was a research fellow at the Max-Planck-Institut für Gesellschaftsforschung at Cologne, Federal Republic of Germany, the author of various articles on the politics of the German health system and, with Bernd Rosewitz, the co-author of *Reformversuche und Reformblockade im deutschen Gesundheitswesen* (Reform Bids and Reform Blockades in the German Health System) (Frankfurt–New York: Campus, 1990). Dr. Webber is currently working on a study of the German private-practising doctors' associations.

Geoffrey R. Weller is President of the University of Northern British Columbia and Professor of Political Science at the same institution. He was a Vice-President (Academic) and Professor of Political Studies at Lakehead University in Thunder Bay, Ontario, Canada. He has written numerous articles on health policy, politics, and politics in the circumpolar north, and security and intelligence services.

Yael Yishai is a Professor in the Department of Political Science of the University of Haifa, Israel. Her major academic interest is in public policy-making and interest groups in Israeli politics. She has published numerous articles and books on these subjects, including *Land or Peace, Whither Israel* (Stanford, 1987), *Interest Groups in Israeli Politics* (Tel Aviv, 1988) and *The Israeli Medical Association: The Power of Expertise* (Jerusalem: forthcoming).

1 Introduction

Christa Altenstetter and Stuart C. Haywood

This book examines the impact of the New Right on health policy and health care in the last decade. With the provision of health care being the core of the welfare state, health policy has not escaped the intellectual challenge to the premises on which welfare states are founded. The advantages are manifest in markets and choice in the allocation of resources and the moral superiority of individual responsibility.

However intentions do not always find full expression in practice because of problems of implementation. Radical change is always difficult because of intra-organisational resistances, and rhetoric is as likely to provide post-hoc rationalisations and glosses on events so as to shape them. In the case of health care, there are also players, such as the medical profession and public sentiment, who hold considerable weight and must be contended with. Both groups have been unlikely to support changes which threatened long established privileges – assured jobs and positions, and access to health care irrespective of income. The theme of the book is accordingly an exploration of the links between rhetoric and reality in health care policy and provision, drawing on the experience of countries in Europe, Israel, Asia, and North and Latin America in the 1980s.

The book is a product of studies undertaken by a small group of interested scholars and researchers working under the auspices of the International Political Science Association (IPSA). The group first met at the XIIth World Congress of IPSA in 1982, receiving official recognition as a study group on comparative health policy in 1985. Since then there have been several meetings, initially concerned with developing a common analytical framework for the case studies of individual or groups of countries. Unlike many other studies, the book is not arbitrarily limited to advanced capitalist countries, but also deals with developing countries and many different kinds of health systems.

This book has been written with the interests of a number of audiences in mind: practitioners and scholars in a variety of disciplines. At the simplest level, comparisons remind practitioners that their problems are not unique and health policy cannot be looked at in isolation from other societal trends. More substantially, they should gain from analyses of the experiences of others. For scholars, structured comparisons have considerable potential for offering a more refined understanding of policy-making institutions, processes and outcomes. The book will thus be of value to scholars in comparative public policy and administration, comparative politics, social policy, health and social services administration, social work, and the political economy of the welfare state, management and business.

Comparative Policy Studies

This book is a contribution to the literature on comparative health policy and the capability of governments to effect change. It is therefore as much about governance as health policy. The studies shed light on the political nature of the policy-making process and its variability, according to issue and circumstance (Heidenheimer *et al.*, 1990; Heclo, 1978; Kingdon, 1984; Jordan and Richardson, 1982). They also contribute to the importance of organisations in the process (March and Olsen, 1984, 1989; Ashford, 1978).

They address another issue of central importance to students of policy-making and government relationships with interest groups. Three patterns of interaction have been generally identified: pluralism, societal corporatism and state corporatism (Lehmbruch and Schmitter, 1982; Lane and Ersson, 1987, pp. 210–51). In the case of health care and policy-making, boundaries between public and private sector and state-group relations have typically been fluid (Starr and Immergut, 1987). The papers point up the more durable links between them.

The studies also confirm and outline specific cultural attributes bearing on the policy process. The durability of some features of the process are well illustrated, particularly in the cases of Japan, the United States of America and the Federal Republic of Germany. Their tenacity in the face of short-term political and economic changes (Inglehart, 1987, 1989, 1990; Dalton, 1986; Eckstein, 1988) is explained by Eisenstadt (1987, p. 303). He identifies two types of control in each society. The first relates to the 'formulation, articulation and continual reinterpretation' of what he calls 'the basic semantic map of society or its basic ideological premises and their institutional symbolization and legitimation'. The second 'most enduring "structured" control' which demonstrates persistence is over 'the flow of resources in social interaction. Control of resources is exercised through access to major institutional markets (economic, political, cultural) through conversion of resources across these markets' (p. 303). The persistence of established control mechanisms in each country is striking but not surprising.

Rules and norms, at least in democratic societies, are about bargaining, negotiating and contractual arrangements which are influenced by legal cultures, administrative traditions and judicial practices (that is to say the extent of legalism, codification, or precedents). In addition the dialectic nature of society and law, the contradictory sources of the origin of law, and the dual role of law as 'medium' and law as 'institution' are evident in most cases (Habermas, 1988; Teubner, 1988; Zacher, 1988; Smith, 1988). The American case stands out for the use of judicial policy-making in health.

Why Health Policy?

Health policy is an important issue in its own right, irrespective of the light it sheds on political, economic and social processes. It touches every aspect of human experience from the cradle to the grave and health is a precondition of human happiness. Health care is recognised as an issue which all governments are expected to promote in some way. Its importance has advantages for our purposes because health policy provides a key indicator of the impact of the intellectual critique of state welfare.

Factors intrinsic to health care make it a particularly interesting and timely area of study. Many changes are combining to challenge taken-for-granted assumptions and ways of doing things and create a new situation for health care. Until now health services have been regarded largely as the province of professionals with increasing governmental involvement to protect the public, ensure resources are available to widen access to services, and regulate or provide services. The dominance of doctors and elite government personnel in health policy-making has been demonstrated countless times, as has the pre-eminence of the so-called medical model (Freddi and Björkman, 1989). The biological and medical paradigm which has dominated thinking about health services has defined the problem for attention (how to provide the means for the diagnosis and treatment of ill-health?) and determined the nature of services and roles of participants and their relative positions.

The preoccupation with the diagnosis and cure of ill-health is now increasingly challenged by a social–ecological paradigm which questions the theoretical basis of Western medicine (Abelin *et al.*, 1987). The new paradigm defines problems differently (how best to promote health?) and prompts much more emphasis on prevention, health promotion and protection from the causes of ill-health. Another implication is a holistic approach to the care of individuals, which also challenges the dominance of clinicians and their ways of thinking.

The range and scope of health issues has also widened, only partly as a consequence of the challenge to the medical model of health care. The 1970s and 80s have witnessed a new epidemic (AIDS/ HIV), an escalating social problem (drug taking) with significant implications for health care, and growing demands from increasing numbers of the elderly. There have been similar transformations on the supply side of health, particularly in pharmacology, bio-technology and the use of artificial intelligence. While the nature and scale of change on both the demand and supply sides of health (neither closely related to factors which determine resource availability) is well established, policy responses are still embryonic or partial. In many places the issues have yet to be addressed.

The emergence of an alternative, socio-ecological, paradigm for health care, together with claims for major changes in demand and supply, clearly represent major challenges for policy makers. An additional complicating factor is the rise of 'single issue' groups in health policy. There are now more potential players in the game to supplement those drawn from the medical–administrative elites who have largely determined the policy agenda. The success of some, for example women's groups and breast screening programmes, has breached closed networks for consultation, bringing in representatives of external interests. A changing pattern of policy networks is likely to emerge, partly as a response to the 'rediscovery' of the consumer. One problem remains the source of advocacy for the marginalised and stigmatised groups, for whom health indices are so poor. In Third World countries these groups represent the majority of the population in urban and rural areas.

The last two decades have also seen an end to illusions about health care, which have not everywhere been reflected in either rhetoric or policies. The idea that the volume of health care provided within a society should reflect 'need' is still widely held. However the illusory nature of the ideal of comprehensive health care for all became increasingly evident during the economic difficulties of the 1970s (Kervasdoué *et al.*, 1984). While economic growth has resumed in the Western industrialised nations and expenditure on health care has increased, the gap between what is provided and what is possible continues to grow (Maxwell, 1989). The latter is not governed by economic laws but by the application of a rapidly expanding technology and body of knowledge to medicine. Frequently these applications make treatment possible for a wider range of illnesses (for example surgery for older and older people), and existing treatment more expensive (for example pharmaceuticals for HIV infection). Health policies will need to respond increasingly and explicitly to issues of rationing, whereby the ethical issues involved will become sharper and more difficult.

Health Policy and the New Right

The studies in this volume examine the responses of governments and health systems to the ideas which we (with the others) subsume under the title of the New Right, rather than the intra–health care issues. The reasons for the choice were the sharper focus for comparisons and links with the wider issue of the impact of the New Right on welfare policy. Additionally their policy prescriptions are held to be relevant to intra-health system problems, which are put into the context of demand and supply.

The comparisons of health policy assume that national interpretations and perceptions are the independent variable. The relevance and persuasiveness of the ideas associated with the New Right will differ between countries and over time. They depend on and reflect national definitions of the problems of government and health care, themselves the product of perceptions of the major players, different arrangements and policy-making processes.

An increased acceptance of the case for adopting some element of privatisation and increased competition is an obvious broad test of the impact of the New Right on national policies. Comparisons of impact in different countries have to be based on broad rather than strict, universal, definitions of 'liberal' economic policies and basic concepts. For example, public or private ownership of assets remains an insufficient tool for establishing the nature of organisations when some private companies are totally or virtually dependent on public revenues to operate them.

Another reason for avoiding tight definitions of the policies of the New Right is that practical application will differ within countries as well as between them. For example, Young (1986) identified four 'elements' in policies in the United Kingdom in 1986. They are:

1. Reducing the size, scope and role of the public sector and attracting private resources into the resulting vacuum.
2. Creating opportunities for the private sector to grow.
3. Using private resources to help carry out tasks and solve problems facing government.
4. Bringing increased market pressures to bear on the use of public sector assets.

Within this context, Young has recognised seven different *forms* of privatisation. Only one involves selling off public assets.

Dunsire *et al.* (1988) have suggested a two-dimensional grid as a conceptual framework for testing these theories. One axis measures the *degree* of publicness and privateness, on the basis that differences in the nature of organisations are better captured by a continuum rather than a simplistic, sharp division. The second axis is market position. Organisations are again located on a continuum from monopoly to perfect market situations. This provides a useful way to proceed, with the caveat that definitions of privateness and publicness differ within and between countries. However this book is more concerned with the development and refinement of those definitions, their application and the insights the experience offers for policy making.

ANALYTICAL FRAMEWORK

The chapters describe the experience of different countries, each faced with New Right critiques and alternative strategies. Some analyse the macro cultural and macro political contexts, others are issue specific. All were written in the context of a brief which highlighted particular issues and broad concepts, each discussed below. The theme is the relationship between the rhetoric of liberal economics and the reality of health policies. A useful pointer to the general impact might be 'policy discontinuity'.

The approach also took account of criticisms of health-policy research. Wilensky *et al.* (1985), for example, have criticised those who claim an element of 'distinctiveness of the health sector' and the few attempts to examine policy 'in relation to other policies or social policy as a whole' (p. 49). Lisle (1987) has countered these criticisms and suggested that '(D)isaggregation or systems analysis may be necessary for meaningful cross-national comparisons' (p. 480). There is some force to Wilensky's argument. Health policy research can be parochial. Although the focus of this book is health policy, changes are related to a wider set of socio-economic imperatives which influence thinking about all areas of public policy, not just the welfare state.

Another critic (McKinlay, 1988) has argued that health services research also 'overlooks the political and economic setting in which the medical game is currently played'. He feels that 'the current preoccupation with . . . managerial changes and the management of efficiency . . . is likely to yield little . . . that could result in political action, effective social policy and change aimed at fulfilling collective needs' (p. 7). The voluminous literature on policy failure underlines the importance of attention to the details of administration for effective social policy. Otherwise good intentions so often remain nothing or little more. Collective action embraces implementation as well as policy formulation and therefore should draw on relevant literature and experience. Consequently the analyses of the processes of policy formulation and implementation in this book draw on, illustrate and develop ideas drawn from public administration and management as well as those of political science (Palumbo and Calista, 1987; Barrett and Fudge, 1981; Pressman and Wildavsky, 1984; Chase, 1979; Williams, 1980).

Ideas and Values

The starting point for the comparative studies was ideas and their integral values which inform the definition and consideration of problems. The intention was to establish the extent to which ideas associated with the New Right became more influential in the 1980s. In so doing there was no assumption that ideas and values necessarily drive changes. They are as likely to be used to justify and rationalise changes which are happening anyway. 'Ideology lags behind reality. Though Karl Marx died in 1883, his analysis of political conflict continued to fascinate, and sometimes mesmerise, social critics and social scientists for much of the following century' (Inglehart, 1987, p. 1289).

Conservative parties (and others) became increasingly interested in the connection between social policies and economic growth from the late 1960s, and this interest was sharpened by the economic dislocations of the 1970s. Earlier challenges to the assumption underpinning conceptions of government responsibility, particularly for welfare, had made little progress. However the combination of economic difficulties in Europe and North America, a developing critique of the impact of government spending, evidence of welfare policy failure, and increasingly confident assertion of the benefits of markets, quickened interest in the ideas of the New Right. This was true independent of the definition and shade of conservativism, official ideology and continent.

Nevertheless 'interpretations', selection, adaptation and development of ideas from the New Right on how to respond to these changes reflect different economic arrangements. Obviously privatisation of ownership is of less importance to countries with only small public sectors. The brief directed attention to other probably more important factors: the ideas and values of governments, civil servants, and interest groups; their relative power; and arrangements for policy-making and the organisation of health care services.

Alford (1975) has pointed to three structural interests in health care: professional monopolists, corporate rationalisers and community population. The IPSA group also added the state (Evans *et al.*, 1985; von Beyme, 1985) on the basis that it is more than a collection or reflection of constituent interests or 'statism', as Almond later argued (1988). In so doing there is no acceptance of the tenet of the public choice theories that bureaucrats and politicians inevitably act to increase budgets. Dunleavy (1986) has convincingly argued that the interests of senior bureaucrats may be served by extending control of policy areas rather than service departments. The comparative studies were expected to elaborate on this conception of these interests in health care and how the ideology and power of each influenced perception of problems and the relevance of New Right thinking. A key issue for health policy is which of these groups or others produce – manufacture – create – manipulate reality and how?

Another manifestation of dominant ideas and values are those embedded in the culture, history and religious, philosophical, political, social, economic, administrative and legal traditions. These are assumed to impact both on the substance of policies which incorporate New Right thinking, and on the rules and norms which govern process. The American and the Japanese cases are good examples of the persistence of these influences.

Socio-economic Imperatives

The interest here was to identify the circumstances which sparked the perceived need for new directions in health care policies and informed the new definitions of problems and what might be done to tackle them.

Two types of circumstances immediately suggested themselves. The first was changing economic realities, particularly the slow-down in the rates of growth in the 1970s. One inference from the studies is that macro-resource constraints offer insufficient explanation for the intensive and widespread re-examination of health care systems. Cost-containment measures and other policies to reduce and stabilise the rate of growth have continued in a period when economic growth has resumed in the Western world. Also governments have continued to be comparatively generous to health care in the developed world. In contrast health care enjoys very little priority in national development plans in developing countries.

Other economic realities are the intra-health-system ones to which we referred earlier. All the countries included in the study had been concerned with the rising percentage of the Gross National Product allocated to health, increasing costs per unit of services, rising demand and supply, diversification of medical practice, new technologies and diseases (OECD, 1985, 1987, 1990; WHO, 1988). Yet these pressures were not new, although the pace of change may have quickened. All were present in the 1960s.

The most convincing explanation for pressure to change was always likely to be social: the general change in ideas and values about the role of government and welfare. The general propositions of the New Right are applied to health care because government is so involved. This requires a redefinition of problems to fit the new beliefs. Difficulties are related to individuals, rather than to the problems of defining effectiveness and allocating resources accordingly. Another likely indicator of a change in beliefs is attitudes towards professional independance and autonomy, once seen as strong points of health systems. The alternative formulation, based on liberal economists' preference for competition, is unacceptable dominance linked to productive inefficiency and neglect of consumer interests.

The key issue remains the circumstances which relate ideas to practice and turn them into pressures for change. Why and how do those involved in the policy process change? The case studies serve to remind us that more liberal economic policies for health care are not necessarily fostered by the electoral fortunes of political parties, normally categorised as 'right' or conservative. There are many different meanings of conservative, and non-conservatives have taken some aspects of New Right thinking on board, for example in Scandinavia. The case studies illustrate well some of the different strands of conservativism, even within one country (United States), including fledgling attempts at democratic conservativism in Brazil, the links with race and religion in Israel, and the social conservativism of parties in Canada and the Federal Republic of Germany.

Policy Networks

One factor in the translation of ideas and response to environmental changes is the arrangements for policy-making and implementation. The well established and stable 'networks' of actors and groups, the pattern of relationships and shared perceptions of those involved in a policy area, are a mediating factor between intentions and outcomes. The particular dynamics of a network of actors influence and shape definitions of problems and situations, appropriate issues and policy outcomes. They also embody values about appropriate process, embedded in routines and taken-for-granted ways of handling policy problems. The latter both exhibit and reinforce pre-eminent values about due process of those in the network. The work of March and Olsen, among others, is a reminder that institutions matter (1984, 1989).

References to the concept of networks were intended to direct attention to the relationship between their characteristics and policy outcomes, specifically the level of incorporation of New Right thinking. The literature points to administrative and professional elites as the key actors. Politicians are less important. The structural explanations for this state of affairs – permanence, expertise, seniority, authority and responsibility for recommendations – are only part of the story. Additional factors are the commitment to established definitions of problems, and ways of working which reinforce the position and location of key actors in the process.

Kingdon (1984) argues for three separate 'streams' in policy-making which involve separate players. They are:

1. The policy stream, which includes actors from the bureaucracy, political arena and individual scientists or advisory committees who work on a particular solution.
2. The political stream which embraces the established decision-making structures, rules and norms.
3. The problem stream.

The streams become coupled occasionally on an opportunistic basis in the context of stronger connections between 1 and 3 than between 2 and 3.

In health policy, challenges to the policy stream are coming from technocratic managers (for example in the United Kingdom), health advocates and interest groups. However it is not easy to see the incorporation of these groups effecting a change in the nature of the networks which will facilitate the adoption of liberal economic policies. The more likely outcome is policies and services which promote the interests of a group (for example women's groups and breast cancer screening, the grey panthers and others).

The adoption of more radical policies may require the injection of stronger transitional forces (personnel, processes, circumstances) or an exercise of will by the political stream in policy-making and unfamiliar machinery through which analysis and recommendations are processed. Recent developments in the United Kingdom (which post-date the case study in the book) are a good example of how the pattern can change. Previous reforms and policy initiatives were developed by the professional and administrative elites in a reasonably open and consensual fashion (Haywood and Hunter, 1982). However the latest (and probably the most radical) proposals for reform were developed by a group of ministers, led by the Prime Minister, supported by selected civil servants and policy advisors. It was essentially a closed system with an influential contribution from an economist in the United States.

An important aspect of these comparative studies has therefore been the relationships between the policy networks and policy change. The network has to be set in a policy universe in which other forces operate.

The case studies make it plain that key institutions are country specific: there is no common, key institution. This was true even in 'democratic' countries where national parliaments were not among

the key institutions. Nevertheless policy networks have been relatively open (that is to say more pliable, more open to incorporation
and change) in the democratic countries. In Brazil for example, they
have unsurprisingly been closed, described by the concept of
'bureaucratic rings'.

There is little evidence of changes in the nature of continuing
policy networks in the European, Israeli and Japanese cases. They
remain complex, particularly so in decentralised systems such as the
one in Sweden, where county councils provide services and have
considerable autonomy. Authority is dispersed among bureaucratic
and professional institutions, government and social insurance, and
provider organisations. Predictably the chapters also illustrate the
conflicts over priorities and preferences within the networks and the
absence of clear policy goals. There is little consensus and relationships are essentially political. The dynamics are characterised by
bargaining and negotiated solutions. The outcome in Sweden is said
to be a 'policy vacuum'. A possible exception to this generalisation is
Brazil.

Strategies

The comparative studies were also concerned with the strategies and
policy instruments used by governments pressured by the need to
change; in this case to apply New Right policy prescriptions. An issue
of particular interest was the means available to government to
promote and implement different definitions of problems and
appropriate behaviour. How do governments successfully transform
the values and ideas into concrete measures, activities and programmes? The literature on policy failure (Barrett and Fudge, 1981) offers
countless examples of difficulties of effecting meaningful and lasting
change.

Central to the New Right prescriptions is 'privatisation' which,
with a competitive market, is predicted to produce less rule-bound
and more entrepreneurial behaviour. A shift in ownership from
public to private sectors is therefore an obvious policy instrument to
effect the changes. The chapters demonstrate the many faces of
privatisation, many of which do not however impact on ownership. It
becomes a generic title for associated changes and a description of
supposedly hidden motives for incremental organisational changes
(Scandinavia, Canada). The American case is unusual in that the
motives for changes were open and direct.

The many faces of privatisation include contracting out, largely funded from the public purse (Scandinavia, Brazil), cost shunting from central to local government (Federal Republic of Germany) and from federal to state governments (United States), and cost-sharing (Federal Republic of Germany again). In the United Kingdom it took the form of a reorganisation of the management of a national service. The Nordic case is a little different, in spite of the contracting out of services at the margin. The author states, 'there is of course no certainty that the policy and structural conditions . . . will remain indefinitely'. There is no threat of significant privatisation of ownership, except perhaps in the minds of those who wish to defend the *status quo* and at the level of rhetoric.

Another key element in New Right thinking is more responsibility (and choice) for individuals. There have been shifts of responsibility mainly between agencies, but no clear pattern has emerged. In any event, boundaries between government, local authorities, funding agencies and consumers have never been sharp and unchanging. Nor are the shifts consistent; in some cases there is more decentralisation to lower level governments (Scandinavia), in others more centralisation (United Kingdom). The American case indicates simultaneous shifts in both directions.

The chapters underline the obvious and expected: there was no new beginning. The welfare temple was not brought crashing down. Rather policy change was incremental and focused on particular aspects of the health care systems. The possible exception is the United Kingdom. The British government is trying to introduce another factor of liberal economics, competition, into the National Health Service. An 'internal market' has been proposed, which will separate responsibility for buying and providing services and encourage more competition for shares of a cash-limited allocation from the national exchequer. It remains to be seen how potent a policy instrument internal competition will prove to be in inducing less rule-bound and more entrepreneurial behaviour.

Constraints

Major constraints on successful policy change are the perceptions of problems and appropriate solutions, rooted in long standing commitments and incremental developments. These are reinforced by:

–   Inherited structures, programmes, routines and institutions.

- Inertia, routine behaviour of participants in the policy process.
- Legacy of policies, priorities and values.
- Unresolved conflicts in current arrangements.

The analysis is familiar and further reinforced by the case studies. For example, the radical proposals of the policy commission in the Federal Republic of Germany were considerably watered down before final legislation was passed. The resurfacing of 'moral-agenda conservativism' and its coexistence with 'economic conservativism' in America provides another powerful example of systemic and established value constraints.

The case studies also point to constraints other than those associated with intraorganisational and governmental factors and the control of policy networks by powerful interests. The potential for change of the policies themselves is limited. Marginal shifts in responsibility are unlikely to transform organisations; nor is contracting out for esoteric or very specialised services for a small number of people a solution. Third World countries experience all these constraints, in addition to severe resource constraints.

Public opinion is more likely, in normal times, to be a constraint on the introduction of radical change in the nature of health care provision than a facilitating factor. The Brazil case study suggests that it may remain so even in the context of a change from authoritarian rule to a democratic system when 'public opinion' might be expected to be more malleable and influential. Public perceptions of appropriate systems and arrangements still reflect those of current providers, particularly doctors.

Outputs

The last concept, essential to a comparison of rhetoric and reality, was the policy outputs. The interest was in changes in policy and practice, which could not have been predicted from recent history, and their links with ideas from the New Right.

The concept of output goes beyond intention, policy pronouncement and the content of legislation, although all are included. It embraces changes in practice. Examples are observed changes in the pattern of resource allocation, rapid growth of primary care or performance related payments. It also embraces changes in the process of policy-making, as for example in the nature and make-up of policy networks' policy-making fora and the incorporation of epidemiological analyses in decision-making.

In the context of New Right policies, actual shifts in responsibility for welfare to the individual, larger roles for private suppliers, and competition between providers of care are policy outputs which would indicate substantive changes, rather than rhetoric.

There are examples of such shifts, with not always desirable side effects. Numerous commentators have linked the rise of the New Right in Germany in 1989 to cuts in benefits which affected those least able to pay larger out-of-pocket expenses. Nor have the actual changes been in a consistent direction. Increased centralisation within government is evident in France, the United Kingdom and the United States, in spite of assumptions of the benefits of decentralisation in New Right rhetoric. More expectedly, the legitimacy of the private sector is enhanced in Scandinavia and the United Kingdom although it remains small; there are attempts to reduce the power of doctors in France and transfer more costs to consumers (France, Federal Republic of Germany, United States).

However policy discontinuity is limited when the analysis is confined to policy outputs. There are changes at the margin, no radical reforms in prospect (except perhaps in the United Kingdom) and old priorities are reinforced.

Assessment

These studies were based on the likelihood of an imbalance between rhetoric, potential, considered changes and policy outputs. The chapters suggest that the expectation was sound, even for the United Kingdom where government has explicitly supported the continuation of a publicly provided service, financed from taxation. There have been few changes in the elements of policy and provision central to the critique of the New Right:

– Ownership.
– Funding.
– Competition.

There are similarly few indications of changes in the policy-making process. It is very much business as usual in most cases, with the possible exception of the United Kingdom. Here the most effective use of New Right thinking was in management arrangements which had the effect of enhancing the relative positions of ministers, civil servants and managers. The representatives of the medical profession have been noticeably uninfluential on subsequent changes intended to introduce more market features within the National Health Service.

Nevertheless this should not necessarily be taken as evidence of a paradox; a centrally planned and controlled system is best suited to implement changes intended to reduce its power. The effect of the reforms of the National Health Service will not be any diminution of central government power, even if promises of decentralisation (not devolution) are to be implemented. The main change is intended for more market type behaviour among National Health Service *managers*.

Rhetoric and Reality

There are many explanations for the limited (so-far) impact of New Right thinking on health policies, even when 'friendly' governments have been in power. An obvious one is the inappropriateness – or unacceptability – of the ideas even when the economic philosophy is publicly accepted. This is evident in the failure of New Right ideas to inform and supplant existing definitions of problems. Nowhere has health policy been centred only on the use of markets to balance demand and supply. Indeed in the Nordic countries it was seemingly never an issue. Wherever health care is seen as a right (very evident in the Nordic chapter), this will remain the case. The paradoxes between rhetoric and reality are even more severe in the Third World, as the concluding chapter serves to remind us.

The flirtation with ideas from the New Right (developing into a courtship in the United Kingdom), nevertheless owed something to their relevance to second order questions. They have something to offer on the efficiency of delivery systems, linking volume and distribution more to consumer preferences than to decisions by 'pointy-heads' (George Wallace of Alabama fame). However even in this respect they have serious limitations, offering few or no solutions to problems of over-employment of expensive technology and unnecessary medical intervention.

There are other attractions. The ideas of the New Right might help government avoid getting into impossible and spuriously scientific calculations about priorities which would guarantee the greatest good for the greatest number. The political and intellectual impossibility of directing resources to services which will produce the greatest good is seemingly by-passed by leaving all to consumer choice. They also have the advantage of a seeming consistency with the paradigm which dominates health policy. The presumption of health care as a normal consumer good, tradeable in the market place, focuses attention on discrete services for which individual consumers will pay. The view of health care as essentially the application of scientific methods to the diagnosis, cure and limiting the damage of ill-health, also directs attention to transactions between individuals, rather than the collective good of better community health.

The agenda of the New Right may have had attractions for governments in addition to its coincidence with philosophies. It has been attractive because of its seeming relevance to more immediate problems; its role has been more like that of the garage mechanic than the salesman persuading the customer to change a make of car.

However the conclusion is that perspectives which have influenced economic policy profoundly have not been applied rigorously to health policy, at least not in the cases included in the book. Connections between New Right perceptions of the problems of health care and the utility of more individual responsibility, private ownership and supply and competition have not been made. They were relevant but not central to the preoccupation of policy makers, even national treasuries whose ministers usually outrank those of health departments. The failure of the New Right to capture the high ground of thinking about health policy suggests that their ideas also may have not been sufficiently persuasive even to those usually identified with prudence in public spending and economy. For them the experience of the United States, with the most liberal system of health care, would hardly be encouraging.

Consequently, health policy remains governed by a social welfare perspective. The key issues remain access to a valued service (with as much cost-containment as possible) and how to respond to professional definitions of need.

Health Policy and Needs

The ideas of the New Right do not challenge the paradigm which currently governs thinking about health, health care policy and practice. So it was unlikely to be seen to relate to the concerns of critics of that paradigm, from whom an alternative is beginning to take shape. This paradigm is discernable in the increasing interest in primary care, particularly in the developing world, public and individual actions independent of health care systems to prevent illness and promote health, and holistic approaches to care.

Some of these features would commend themselves to those who see solutions in reducing health care spending by governments: primary care falls into this category. However the mainspring is epidemiology and social medicine rather than economics and it is from this source that the main challenge to the dominant paradigm comes.

However there is little evidence that the alternative paradigm is as yet very influential in the policy process. The Brazil case describes a reaction to it and a reaffirmation of commitment to the old one. The Israeli case also demonstrates nicely that even in issues about life and death the rules of the administrative–professional–political games are set by the old rules. Ischaemic heart disease in Israel is noticeably higher than in Europe and prevention (as elsewhere) offers a promising alternative or complementary service to the curative one. Yet the latter continues to attract more investment, with lip service paid to prevention. Curative services 'benefit' from shorter term benefits which have higher political pay-offs. There are also fewer constraints which are assisted by the present structure of the policy universe and the superior skills of the personnel involved in the policy process. The chapters on the developing world make the same familiar point, even in countries which would benefit disproportionately from greater priority to primary care, prevention and health promotion. Health policy is still not orientated to maximise the impact of services on the health status of groups and populations.

A shift in paradigms which govern health policy will manifest itself in changing definitions of need, an obscure concept which nevertheless symbolises the non-economic perspective which informs health policy-making. There are (at least) two dimensions: evidence of individual need and the health status of groups or populations. The former, as we have repeatedly asserted, is still paramount in policy making and practice. An indication of a growing influence for the latter would be investment decisions increasingly based on benefits to the health status of groups, something largely absent in all the case studies. Another indication will be changes in the relative status of clinicians and epidemiologists and those involved in social care. A greater recognition of the latter should also flow from a paradigm which leads to collective action to remove environmental causes of ill-health and recognises the increasingly blurred dividing lines between health and social care.

The alternative paradigm is being supported by governments, albeit largely in a complementary and rhetorical fashion. There is increased emphasis on prevention, health promotion and primary health care in health policy pronouncements. The chapters point to a considerable gap between this rhetoric and policy reality, as with the commitment to New Right economic prescriptions for health care. However its roots in health care, support from some of its practitioners, and its emergence on agendas make it a likelier candidate to influence policy in the future. This alternative also has another potential attraction. It could attract the enthusiastic support of national treasuries since it offers the possibility of reigning in spending on health care. Prevention, health promotion and primary care are likely to be cheaper and more cost-effective than endlessly increasing investments in curative medicine.

The American experience merits separate mention. By giving priorities to New Right values – economic conservativism and moral-agenda conservativism – Washington policy-makers have managed to weaken the fragile consensus about health care as public responsibility and to reduce health protection for many groups. Regulatory measures during the Reagan administration imposed many and far-reaching restrictions on all health care providers, thereby endangering quality care. Experiments with diverse forms of financing, delivering and managing health care and control costs have been unproductive. As a result the average American citizen, unlike his or her counterpart in other industrialised nations, risks financial disaster when severe illness strikes.

HEALTH POLICY MAKING: THE FUTURE?

Comparative studies furnish baseline knowledge, valuable even in political change. They provide essential inventories of established patterns of political behaviour and social and political organisation bearing on health care, health-policy and practice. Such studies also provide a reminder of continuities as well as discontinuities. In the case of health-policy-making in the developed world (and Brazil), established means of control and definition of problems, appropriate processes for their considerations and acceptable solutions proved very robust. This is also true of the poorest countries where health care is given a low priority.

Economic circumstances in each country in the 1980s explain the particular pressures placed on policy-makers for developing solutions to old and new problems. Their responses have been political solutions and compromises. The primacy of political forces over economics and over 'scientific' knowledge and research shaping policy content and practical solutions, as all the cases demonstrate, remains unabated. There is a need for political science to record, assess and explain the tensions between competing influences and forces. This function is a legitimate task and remains critical in any society.

References

Abelin, T., Z.J. Brzezinski and V.D.L. Carstairs (eds) (1987) *Measurement in Health Promotion and Protection* (Copenhagen: World Health Organization Regional Office for Europe. WHO Regional Publications, European Series No. 22).

Alford, R. R. (1975) *Health Care Politics: Ideological and Interest Group Barriers to Reform* (Chicago University Press).

Almond, G. A. (1988) 'The Return to the State', *American Political Science Review*, no. 82, pp. 853–74.

Ashford, D. A. (ed.) (1978) *Comparing Public Policies: New Concepts and Methods* (Beverly Hills: Sage Publications).

Barrett, S. and C. Fudge (1981) *Policy and Action: Essays on the Implementation of Public Policy* (London and New York: Methuen).

Chase, G. (1979) 'Implementing a Human Services Program: How Hard Will It Be?', *Public Policy*, no. 27, pp. 385–435.

Dalton, R. J. (1988) *Citizen Politics in Western Democracies* (Chatham, NJ: Chatham House Publishers).

Dunleavy, P. (1986) 'Explaining the Privatization Boom: Public Choice versus Radical Approaches', *Public Administration* no. 64, pp. 13–34.

Dunsire, A. *et al.* (1988) 'Organizational Status and Performance. A Conceptual Framework for Testing Public Choice Theories, *Public Administration*, no. 66, p. 4.

Eckstein, H. (1988) 'A Culturalist Theory of Political Change', *American Political Science Review*, no. 82, pp. 789–804.

Eisenstadt, S.N. (1987) 'Cultural Premises, Political Structures and Dynamics', *International Political Science Review*, no. 8, pp. 291–306.

Evans, P., D. Rueschemeyer and T. Skocpol (eds) (1985) *Bringing the State Back In* (Cambridge University Press).

Freddi, G. and J. W. Björkman (eds) (1989) *Controlling Medical Professionals: The Comparative Politics of Health Governance* (London and Berkeley: Sage Publications).

Habermas, J. (1988) 'Law as Medium and Law as Institution', in G. Teubner (ed.), *Dilemmas of Law in the Welfare State* (Berlin and New York: de Gruyter, pp. 203–20).

Haywood, S. C. and D. Hunter (1982) 'Consultative Processes in Health Policy in the United Kingdom: A View from the Centre', *Public Administration*, no. 69, pp. 143–62.

Heidenheimer, A. J., Hugh Heclo and Carolyn Teich Adams (eds) (1990) *Comparative Public Policy. The Politics of Social Choice in Europe and America* (New York: St. Martin's Press, Third Edition).
Heclo, H. (1978) 'Issue Networks and the Executive Establishment', in Anthony King (ed.) *The New American Political System* (Washington, DC: American Enterprise Institute, pp. 87–124).
Inglehart, R. (1987) 'Value Change in Industrial Societies', *American Political Science Review*, no. 81, pp. 1289–303.
Inglehart, R. (1989) 'The Renaissance of Political Culture', *American Political Science Review* no. 82, pp. 1203–30.
Inglehart, R. (1990) *Culture Shift in Advanced Industrial Society* (Princeton University Press).
Jenson, U. J. (1987) *Practice and Progress. A Theory for the Modern Health Care System* (Oxford: Blackwell Scientific Publications).
Jordan, A. G. and J. J. Richardson (1982) 'Policy Communities: The British and European Policy Style', *Policy Studies Journal*, no. 11, pp. 603–15.
de Kervasdoué, J., J. R. Kimberly and V. G. Rodwin (eds) (1984) *The End of an Illusion: The Future of Health Policy in Western Industrialized Nations* (Berkeley: University of California Press).
Kingdon, J. W. (1984) *Agendas, Alternatives, and Public Policy* (Boston: Little, Brown).
Lane, J. E. and S. O. Ersson (1987) *Politics and Society in Western Europe* (London: Sage Publications).
Lehmbruch, G. and P. Schmitter (eds) (1982) *Patterns of Corporatist Policy-making* (London: Sage Publications).
Lisle, E. (1987) 'Perspectives and Challenges for Crossnational Research', in M. Dierkes, H. M. Weiler and A. B. Antal (eds) *Comparative Policy Research. Learning From Experience* (London: WZB Publications and Gower Publishing House, pp. 473–97).
March, J. G. and J. P. Olsen (1984) 'The New Institutionalism: Organizational Factors in Political Life', *American Political Science Review*, no. 78, pp. 734–49.
March, J. G. and J. P. Olsen (1989) *Rediscovering Institutions. The Organizational Basis of Politics* (New York: The Free Press).
Maxwell, R. (1989) 'The National Health Service: A Future Agenda', *Public Money and Management*, no. 9, p. 2 (Summer).
McKinlay, J. B. (1988) 'Introduction to The Changing Character of the Medical Profession', *The Milbank Memorial Fund Quarterly*, no. 66, supplement 2, pp. 1–9.
Newton, S. (1986) 'The Nature of Privatization in Britain: 1979–85,' *West European Politics*, no. 9, pp. 235–52 (April).
Organization for Economic Co-Operation and Development (1985) *Measuring Health Care: 1960–1983* (Paris: OECD).
Organization for Economic Co-operation and Development (1987) *Financing and Delivering Health Care. A Comparative Analysis of OECD Countries* (Paris:OECD).
Organization for Economic Co-Operation and Development, (1990) *Health Care Systems in Transition. The Search for Efficiency* (Paris: OECD).

Palumbo, D. J. and D. J. Calista (1987) 'Symposium: Implementation: What Have We Learned and Still Need to Know', *Policy Studies Review*, no. 7, pp. 91–216.

Pressman, J. L. and A. Wildavsky (1984) *Implementation* (Berkeley: University of California Press, Third Ed.).

Smith, R. (1988) 'Political Jurisprudence, the "New Institutionalism", and the Future of Public Law', *American Political Science Review*, no. 82, pp. 89–108.

Starr, P. and E. Immergut (1987) 'Health care and the boundaries of politics', in C. S. Maier (ed.) *Changing Boundaries of the Political* (Cambridge University Press, pp. 221–254).

Teubner, G. (ed.) (1988) *Dilemmas of Law in the Welfare State* (New York and Berlin: W. de Gruyter).

von Beyme, K. (1985) 'The Role of the State and the Growth of Government', *International Political Science Review* no. 6, pp. 11–34.

Wilensky, H. L., G. M. Luebbert, S. R. Reed Hahn and A. M. Jamieson (1985) *Comparative Social Policy. Theories, Methods, Findings* (Berkeley: Institute of International Studies, University of California).

Williams, W. (1980) *The Implementation Perspective. A Guide for Managing Social Service Delivery Programs* (Berkeley: University of California Press).

World Health Organization Regional Office for Europe (1988) 'Monitoring of the Strategy for Health for All by the Year 2000'. Thirty-eighth Session, Copenhagen, 12–17 September.

Young, S. (1986) 'The Nature of Privatization in Britain 1979–85', *West European Politics*, no. 9: pp. 235–52.

Zacher, H. F. (1988) 'Law, Social Welfare, Social Development', *Basic Document*, (24th International Conference on Social Welfare (ICSW), Berlin, 31 July – 5 August, pp. 1–18.

2 Liberalism in the *Dirigiste* State: A Changing Public – Private Mix in French Medical Care*

Paul Godt

INTRODUCTION

Liberalism and pluralism – basic assumptions posited on the autonomy of individuals and groups in society – have always been distinctly minority views held by dissenters from the statist tradition in French political culture. Instead, from Richelieu to the revolutionaries, from the Bonapartes to de Gaulle, the centralised, unitary Jacobin state has been considered the only legitimate advocate of the public good, while private interests remained suspicious. Although the industrial age brought new cleavages between Right and Left, both agreed that the strong state was needed to achieve their aims, either to preserve the political order or nationalist goals, or to mobilise collective power in the marketplace to combat social inequities.

Two World Wars and the Depression only increased state activism, and the postwar period saw the state's role expand through the nationalisation of basic industries and most of the banking sector, and extended controls over prices, credit and exchange rates, with the national planning process coordinating public and private action (Zysman, 1983; Hayward, 1986). By arming the executive with additional powers to act in the national interest, the Fifth Republic gave renewed vigour to bureaucratic *dirigisme*.

* Portions of this chapter have been adapted from my 'Health Care: The Political Economy of Social Policy', in Paul Godt (ed.), *Policy-making in France: From de Gaulle to Mitterrand* (London: Frances Pinter, 1989), and are reprinted with permission from the publisher.

The extended economic crisis of the 1970s, however, began to engender new attitudes in the industrial democracies concerning the role of the state. In the 1980s, for the first time under the Fifth Republic, coherent party coalitions of Right and Left alternated in power: first a Socialist–Communist alliance behind François Mitterrand ended 23 years of government by the Right in 1981, and then a conservative coalition led by Jacques Chirac, explicitly committed to liberalism, won the legislative elections of 1986.

These changes provide an opportunity to assess the rhetoric and the reality of the new liberalism in French politics. This chapter will examine the Chirac government during its two years in office, 1986–8, focusing on its policies in health care, a key sector of public policy, with definable constituencies and a measurable impact on the economy. It argues that the rise of liberal discourse is due in large part to the changing configuration of partisan competition and to the economic constraints imposed by international economic competition. It seeks to demonstrate that the achievements of a government committed to liberalism failed to match the promises of liberal rhetoric because of the singular features of the French health care delivery system.

The Political Constraints

Confronted in the 1970s with international market restructuring and financial turbulence, the major industrial democracies faced high inflation and unemployment levels and sought new and often radical policy approaches. In the most notable examples, Margaret Thatcher and Ronald Reagan rode to power on a wave of anti-statism and moral regeneration; hoping to liberate 'natural' market forces by removing state interference, they proceeded to reduce their governments' commitments to both inherited social policies and established practices of macro-economic management. Although the contrast is less marked, West Germany also witnessed a shift to less interventionism.

In France, on the other hand, the movement was in the opposite direction. François Mitterrand's reflationary programme promised to use state authority to redirect the economy, involving nationalisation of major industrial concerns, increased public expenditure, and a broad array of redistributive social measures. When 'Socialism in one country' (Hall, 1985) proved impossible, his government switched to a deflationary approach barely a year later. 'Socialist rigour', more suited to adjust France to the rapidly changing international market situation, nevertheless undermined the government's political support and led to its defeat in 1986.

By returning the conservatives to power after five years of Socialist rule, France finally seemed to be catching up with the anti-statist mood prevailing elsewhere. The French Right itself however had only recently been converted to the values of free-market capitalism. De Gaulle had asserted the pre-eminence of national over private interests, and his success with economic modernisation had been achieved through the traditional instruments of *dirigisme*. After crushing the political centre, de Gaulle and his successor, Pompidou, incorporated its modernising, liberal elements into the governing coalition. However Pompidou's death in 1974 opened up a contest for control of the conservative majority between the liberal centre, led by newly elected President Valéry Giscard d'Estaing, and the Gaullist movement led by his Prime Minister, Jacques Chirac. In the background of this rivalry was the economic crisis, and the challenge from a united Left coalition of Socialists and Communists.

As the heart of his political strategy to ward off the double challenge of the Left and the Gaullists, Giscard d'Estaing defined a new liberalism (his 'advanced liberal democratic society') behind which he sought to rally the centrist parties in an electoral alliance, the Union for French Democracy (UDF) (Giscard d'Estaing, 1976). The tensions between the UDF and Chirac's Rally for the Republic (RPR) were exacerbated by the political jousting of their leaders in the 1981 presidential campaign. When François Mitterrand's victory placed them in the opposition, the liberals and Gaullists not only gained time to bind old wounds, but also found a common target in the leftist orientation of the Socialist–Communist Government.

The rival movements stressed their unity, supporting combined slates of candidates in the municipal (1983) and European parliamentary (1984) elections. Nonetheless competing ambitions dictated political strategies: at stake were the presidential elections of 1988, which Chirac could not win without the support of the centrist electorate. Chirac thus quietly broke with traditional Gaullism and discovered the virtues of the free market and the vices of bureaucratic *dirigisme*. With Giscard side-lined by his defeat in 1981, Chirac's principal centrist rival became former Prime Minister Raymond Barre, who had already staked out the territory with his rigorous monetarism. Competing for the same electorate, the RPR and the UDF leaders both espoused the themes of liberalism, increasingly popular in the wake of the Socialists' difficulties, and a conveniently vague slogan behind which both movements could rally. 'Liberalism', an emulation of British and American models became an antidote to Socialism and the coalition's unifying cement.

The Economic Constraints

The economy was in much better condition in March 1986 than it had been when the conservatives left office five years earlier. 'Socialist rigour' had succeeded in reducing inflation to three per cent annually (the February 1986 price index actually declined for the first time in 20 years). Still unemployment was up to 12 per cent of the workforce, and the budget deficit was just over three per cent of a Gross Domestic Product which was growing, if at only 1.3 per cent during 1985. The trade balance had been restored, but foreign debt was high (469 billion francs). More significantly, direct and indirect tax revenues (the *prélèvements obligatoires*) had risen to more than 45 per cent of GDP, a figure even Mitterrand had sought to reduce because of its dampening effects on the competitiveness of French firms (Hall, 1986; Belassa, 1987).

Health care expenditures accounted for more than nine per cent of GDP and, although the sector is labour intensive, the continued acceleration of medical consumption threatened government efforts to control inflation, reduce public spending, and stimulate economic growth. Over the period 1950–80, health care expenditures had advanced at an average annual rate of more than 15 per cent. Growth in the 1975–80 period was particularly strong, principally in the hospital sector, due to increased coverage of the population, ageing of the population,[1] and the increasingly technical nature of hospital care, among other factors. A record high was reached in 1982, with an 18.4 per cent rate of growth. Expenditure was also taking an ever larger share of the GDP: three per cent in 1950, 4.3 per cent in 1960, 6.1 per cent in 1970, 8.5 per cent in 1980, and 9.2 per cent in 1982 (Sandier, 1983).

Most disturbing was the changing relationship between health care expenditure and GDP growth. In the 1960–75 period, elasticity (in constant prices) in France was 1.8 (nearly the same as the average for all OECD countries), meaning that health care expenditure increased 1.8 times faster than overall economic growth. From 1975 to 1982 however, as the OECD average rate declined to 1.5 (1.4 in the US; 0.8 in West Germany!), elasticity in France increased to 2.6 (OECD,

1985 and 1987). Measured in constant francs, per capita medical consumption (care and goods) doubled between 1970 and 1986 (CNAMTS, 1988b). In short it was evident that features particular to the French health care delivery system were generating increased consumption. Expenditure increases did begin to decelerate thereafter: +13.1 per cent in 1983, +11 per cent in 1984, and +6.5 per cent in 1985. These figures are misleading however because the inflation rate was also declining. Regardless of the cost-containment measures adopted since the late 1970s, the annual growth rate of final medical care consumption continued to be roughly four per cent above the growth rate of the GDP (Jolly and Majnoni d'Intignano, 1985).

The financial dilemma of health expenditures outstripping economic growth was of course compounded by the economic crisis, when unemployment slowed down the source of revenue for the payroll-based financing of the health insurance system, without proportionally decreasing demands upon it. Bringing the costs under control has become a permanent preoccupation of policy-makers since the mid-1970s, although major measures to respond to the disturbing trends were not introduced until 1979.

Given these trends and circumstances, French governments (Conservative and Socialist alike) have chosen to act on supply by restricting the number of hospital beds and the number of doctors graduating from the medical schools, imposing capped budgets on the hospitals, and controlling physician fees through the system of contracts (*conventions*) negotiated between the sickness funds and the medical unions. In addition successive governments have sought to enhance parafiscal revenues by periodic increases in payroll tax rates and expansion of the taxable wage base. Other measures acted on demand increased patient co-payments on certain pharmaceuticals, physician fees, and hospital charges. These measures have had an important impact, as suggested by the figures above, in slowing down the growth rate of medical care expenditures in the 1980s. But all the actors in the health system have come to recognise that major additional reductions in expenditures require addressing the fundamental structural problems.

THE LIBERAL AGENDA IN FRANCE

The fundamental thrust of the RPR-UDF alliance's domestic programme was anti-statist, drawing on the classic liberal themes of monetarism, tax reform, deregulation, privatisation, competition, and emphasis on individual choice, initiative and responsibility. Specifically the joint platform signed in January 1986 promised to privatise a number of state-owned industries, banks, financial institutions and insurance companies; to eliminate state subsidies to private industry; to end the extensive post-war barrage of state controls over prices, credit, interest rates and currency exchange; to abolish administrative control of private-sector lay-offs; to reduce public debt and budget deficits; and to reduce personal, corporate and parafiscal taxes.

The conservatives recognised that a completely private system was not politically feasible, and would be found socially unjust by many. The broad support that the Social Security system enjoys in public opinion precludes any measures that might appear to threaten its egalitarian nature (Duhamel, 1986). Moreover the system has traditionally blended liberal and statist features, an elaborate interpenetration of public and private. National legislation, for example, makes participation in the Social Security scheme compulsory, and the government sets the rates and wage base for the payroll taxes to finance it. Yet it is semi-private boards controlled by labour and employer representatives which manage and disburse the funds. Concerning medical care, the state operates the hospitals and medical schools but the ambulatory sector is overwhelmingly private, independent and office-based; patients pay their physicians directly and are subsequently reimbursed by their local Social Security agency.

Some liberal critics hoped to inject more liberalism into the existing system by introducing competition between public and private provision of medical services. Several experts have devised a proposal called Coordinated Health Care Networks, modelled after American Health Maintenance Organisations (HMOs), in which the insured may choose among competing pre-paid health protection programmes, a base uniform annual premium being paid by the collectively-financed sickness funds. Patients can opt for more extensive coverage if they are willing to pay extra (Launois *et al.*, 1985). One observer refers to HMOs as 'a liberal solution to the crisis of the Welfare State' (Sorman, 1984, 1985).

On the whole though, given the existing political constraints and economic imperatives, the conservative alliance in power in 1986 had few truly liberal elements in their medical care agenda: the emphasis was more on reducing the state's presence than on eliminating it. They promised to devolve greater responsibility to health professionals, hospital managers, and the sickness funds, to grant greater managerial and budget autonomy to hospitals and private clinics, and to re-establish in the hospitals the order that the Socialists had purportedly destroyed. Their programme also hinted vaguely about instituting greater competition among private complementary insurers. Public sentiment therefore seemed to dictate the path of least resistance: restored economic growth, by reducing unemployment and increasing parafiscal revenues, would enable the government to safeguard the system from its perennial financial difficulties without having to consider restructuring along liberal lines.

THE POLICY COMMUNITY

Health care policy-making in France is quite complex (see Godt, 1989). Financing is collective, mandatory and wage-based, while expenditures are open-ended (that is to say, determined by the individual decisions of patients and doctors), creating a structural separation with insidious effects (Rodwin, 1984a, 1984b, 1987). Indeed control of the various parameters of health care is fragmented among a number of actors: the central state, local governments, the medical profession, and the para-public sickness funds, not one of which is in fact a single entity with a single will. Within the state for example, authority concerning health care is divided among the Ministry of Social Affairs (and within it between junior ministries for Social Security and for Health), the Ministry of Finance and, for curricular matters, the Ministry of Education.

The state's role is pivotal: in addition to educating and licensing all health professionals, it owns and operates the public hospital sector with more than a thousand hospitals, a half a million beds, and some 700 000 employees (Ministry of Social Affairs, 1987). Hospitals are managed by state-appointed directors, under the supervision of boards of administration presided by local mayors; physicians are represented on these boards and on hospital medical committees with decision-making authority in certain areas. The departmental and regional field services of the Ministry of Health exercise oversight functions, even if they are generally underequipped in qualified personnel to do so (Commissariat Général du Plan, 1986).

The state also has legislative authority to determine the means and levels of financing for the health care system, and many of the elements of expenditure as well. The government sets the rates and wage bases for the payroll taxes which are the source of revenue for the sickness funds, must approve fee increases for office-based physicians, decides the method of financing for both public and private hospitals, establishes guidelines for annual hospital budget increases and capital investment, fixes salaries for public hospital personnel, and controls the prices of pharmaceuticals and laboratory tests. Since the 1950s the Ministry of Finance has increasingly extended its involvement in these matters, and since the 1970s the formerly independent Health Ministry has been under a broad Ministry of Social Affairs. Evidently certain policy issues also concern the ministries of labour and industry, but they are not principal actors.

Among the more than 150 000 active physicians, any common corporatist interests are outweighed by cleavages between general practitioners and specialists, between the salaried hospital doctors (part-time and full-time) and the independent office-based, between those practicing in urban and in rural settings, and so on. In addition to this partitioning by practice, the French suffer from a multiplicity of professional organisations divided further along political–ideological axes. Most of these are grouped within one of the two major national peak organisations, the CSMF (the *Confédération des Syndicats Médicaux Français*) and the FMF (the *Fédération des Médecins de France*). Recently a third union specifically devoted to defending the interests of general practitioners, MG-France, succeeded in gaining recognition to participate in national bargaining.

Completing the complex policy network are the sickness funds. The 1945 statutes and subsequent legislation sought to insulate these from the state by having them chosen by and responsible to the payers and the beneficiaries of the Social Security system. Insofar as these were to be represented by their officially recognised professional associations (the employers' CNPF and the three main labour unions, the CGT, CFDT, and FO), partisan politics is never far below the surface in the relations between the government and the sickness funds. The largest fund, the CNAMTS *Caisse Nationale d'Assurance-Maladie des Travailleurs Salariés*, is the principal spokesman (covering more than 80 per cent of the population) and policy leader in this area, but special funds for a number of professional groups[2] exist independently, with separate accounting procedures and a similar but different array of benefits for their members. The CNAMTS itself is organised on the national level, responsible for research, policy-making, and coordination. There are 16 regional funds responsible for relations with hospitals and financing and 129 local funds which reimburse patients for their outlays on insured risks. The funds employ well over 100 000 people.

The policy-making process varies according to the issue in question. In ambulatory care the basic pattern is one of dialogue between the sickness funds and the doctors' unions, but is more accurately understood as a *ménage à trois*, in which the sickness funds alternate between supporting the state's cost-containment strategies to keep its costs in line with its revenues, and protecting the providers of beneficiary services against the incursions of an excessively interventionist state (Godt, 1985).

The sickness funds have since 1971 negotiated a series of national agreements (*conventions*) with the physicians' peak associations, establishing the nature of the contractual relations between the participating doctors and the funds. Associated with these contracts are complex fee schedules which set the relative prices of the various medical procedures. Since these schedules are the result of negotiations, not carefully refined assessments of relative worth, they are approximate and rigid at the same time, and give greater weight to technical procedures; nonetheless the fee schedules are the basis for determining the sickness funds' expenditures in ambulatory care.

The 1980 agreement created a new category of participating physicians (Sector II), who were free to set fees above those of the schedule; patients would be reimbursed on the basis of the schedule, paying the difference out-of-pocket. In exchange for this right, doctors forfeit having the sickness funds pay most of the premiums toward their own health and pension coverage, as well as certain tax deductions afforded those in Sector I who aligned their fees with the schedule's. Sector II was meant to be a safety valve, allowing the state to clamp down on fees while leaving an alternative for those physicians who object. Sector II is also evidently a 'liberal' element, insofar as it subjects those opting for it to the competitive market formed by their colleagues. Initially both the government and the CNAMTS expected that few physicians would be so daring, but the proportion of those choosing Sector II has gone from eight per cent to nearly 28 per cent since 1980 (CNAMTS, 1988a).

Increasingly, because of the dynamic relationship between the Social Security budget as a whole and the economy, the state has been more closely involved in designing and imposing policies which affect not only the incomes but also the clinical behaviour of physicians; the cost containment strategy has gone beyond controlling fees to trying to influence prescriptive patterns, employing statistical profiles and review procedures, which unite the profession against the state. Similarly it has sought to remodel the delivery system by acting on the training of physicians and the administration of hospitals.

On purely medical questions, such as public health campaigns, an extensive network of ministerial committees bring government and medical experts together and few problems emerge. Occasionally controversial social issues, such as abortion, euthanasia, genetic engineering or AIDS, divide the medical community and breach the usual pattern of in-house consensus-building on technical policy matters.

In the hospital sector, the Ministry of Health's Hospitals Division is responsible for determining the practices within the public hospitals and the more than 400 not-for-profit private hospitals which accept participation in the public service. The Division was at the core of the hospital reforms in the 1980s, which profoundly modified internal administrative practice. It designed and tested, for example, new financing procedures, and adaptations of Fetter's Diagnostic Related Groups, and it proposed the re-organisation of the hospitals' clinical services.

For a long time the sickness funds were excluded from hospital policy-making, although they provide roughly 90 per cent of the hospitals' budgets, accounting for half of the funds' expenditures. More recently however the funds have been seeking to influence how their monies are spent, especially in long-term planning and management. As of 1968 for example, the CNAMTS began making substantial long-term interest-free loans (averaging a billion francs a year) to subsidise hospital capital investment; although this aid was suspended by the government in 1983 (and re-established in 1986), the funds assumed a new role thereafter in advising the Health Ministry's field services in the preparation of hospital budgets (Delanoë, 1987; Catrice-Lorey, 1987). Similarly the local funds' medical consultant has acquired the right to comment on hospitals' clinical practices. Given the enormous effort the sickness funds have made in computerising their data-gathering since the 1970s, and the trend toward applying statistical analyses to hospital accounting methods, it is likely that the funds' role and influence will grow.

There is also a rapidly developing private sector in French health care, which currently represents some seven per cent of expenditures. On the one hand, private 'for-profit' clinics are blossoming, expanding their segment of the market for institutional care. Until the 1987 Hospital Law, growth was restrained by legislation which prevented proprietors from owning more than one clinic, and by the *Carte Sanitaire* a national mechanism for allocating beds and equipment. Some 27 000 surgeons and others work in 1400 private acute-care clinics (for-profit clinics account for 14 per cent of beds – non-profit clinics 15 per cent). The former do mostly minor operations, such as tonsillectomies and obstetrics, while the latter are mainly mental institutions, geriatric or physical therapy centres. Private clinics are a growth industry: finance companies are investing in them, and several have already begun following the American model by constituting chains.

On the other hand, insurance companies and mutual societies are increasingly concerned about the rising co-payments left to the consumer, since they cover them for all but 5 per cent; their share of national health expenditure has grown from 3.2 per cent in 1970 to 4.4 per cent in 1987. The National Federation of Mutual Societies, by far France's largest association, claims well over 25 million members and accounts for 80 per cent of the complementary insurance reimbursements; when it speaks out, as it did recently to criticise the growing number of doctors in Sector II, it has a powerful voice (*Le Monde*, 16 June 1988).

REFORM STRATEGIES

On coming to power in 1986, the new conservative government was pressed for time, bound by economic constraints, political competition and popular attitudes, and had to deal with an incumbent Socialist president who had two more years in his term. Although the president had limited power to interfere with the parliamentary majority's legislative programme, the office gave him the opportunity to focus public attention on issues of his choice, amplifying the criticisms voiced in parliament by his partisan supporters. In addition to the Socialist and Communist opposition, the government faced criticism from the far-right National Front, ultra-liberal on health care issues, which urged complete state disengagement.[3]

By 1986 the public was inured to the too-often repeated dire warnings of the imminent collapse of the Social Security system. Popular attachment to the health system in particular precluded major reductions in benefits, or any radical systemic changes. An IFOP poll showed that 85 per cent of the French are deeply attached to their 'Sécu' as they refer to it; more than half those polled preferred that additional revenues be raised from the employer contributions, not their own (*L'Humanité Dimanche*, 25 May 1986). However Finance Minister Balladur was personally committed to reducing the share of taxes in the GDP and resisted proposals to raise parafiscal taxes yet again.

Given these constraints the government had to navigate carefully. While maintaining the cost-containment priority to reassure the public, demonstrate its responsible and effective governance, and quiet its critics, it also needed to regain the support of the medical community, not only for electoral reasons, but also to gain its acquiescence and cooperation in the efforts to control health expenditures. Consequently the government promised fee increases in ambulatory care, but only if the volume of medical procedures and prescriptions was kept in line. Gaining the hospital physicians' good will would require reversing the Socialist measures with the most symbolic value.

The first objective was to finance the immediate Social Security deficit for 1986 (variously estimated between six billion and 25 billion francs). The only solutions available, pending more extensive consultations and consensus-building, were fiscal. Social Affairs Minister Séguin prevailed upon the Prime Minister to overcome the opposition of the Finance Minister; in July 1986 he announced increased payroll deductions and reestablished the one per cent special income surtax the Socialists had applied in 1983–4 and lifted in 1985 before the elections. The even larger 1987 deficit, predicted to be between 15 and 40 billion francs, necessitated more radical measures.

The second element of the strategy thus strove to build legitimacy for these measures – rumours suggested that the Social Affairs Ministry was studying ways to reduce the mandatory health coverage and to introduce competition between the sickness funds and private insurance (*Le Monde*, 2 July 1986) – while gaining time. In early 1987 the government created a Committee of 'Wise Men', six widely-respected experts who would examine the whole of the Social Security system and first propose some immediate steps. Then, following a 1967 precedent which led to major reform, the 'Wise Men' organised a nationwide consultation process, consisting of hearings in which any and all interested citizens or groups could present their views. At the end a final National Roundtable allowed more than a hundred unions, professional associations and prominent individuals to give their official comments. The Six then drew up a complete report, containing its suggestions for reform (*Comité des Sages*, 1987). Although the report was clearly the result of many compromises and avoided proposing major change,[4] it permitted the government to demonstrate that there were no miraculous solutions.

POLICY OUTPUTS

Looking back over her two years as Chirac's Minister of Health, Michèle Barzach characterised her approach to health issues as pragmatic and non-ideological. She had managed to re-establish a cooperative relationship between government and the medical profession. On public health issues she had mounted major campaigns against drugs, tobacco and alcohol consumption, and AIDS. But the most important achievements, within her jurisdiction, concerned the hospitals (*Le Quotidien du Médecin*, 4 March 1988).

The hospital reforms were high in symbolic value, because they were designed to roll back the 'collectivist' measures of Health Minister Jacques Ralite, one of the four Communists in Mitterrand's first cabinet. But in a real sense they demonstrated the pragmatism of bureaucratic policy-making in France. The hospital reforms had been either under study or in initial stages before the Socialists came to power, reflected the lessons of the Socialists' difficulties in implementing them, and resulted in more broadly accepted and effective change. Although the Socialists criticised the Barzach hospital reforms, when they returned to power in May 1988 Claude Evin, the new Minister responsible for health policy, made clear they would not reform the reforms (*Le Généraliste*, 31 May 1988).

The Private Sector in the Public Hospital

The creation of a private sector in the public hospitals was a critical element of the momentous 1958 Debré Law, which aimed to transform the public hospitals from charitable institutions into the technologically advanced centerpieces of modern French medicine. In order to attract top specialists from the private sector into full-time positions as salaried consultants, the law allowed them, in addition to their public clinical service, research and university teaching, to continue consulting and hospitalising their private patients, often with the right to charge significantly higher fees. They could devote only two half-days a week to private consultations, and use no more than eight per cent of the ward beds for their private patients. Although conceived as a transitional measure the privilege soon became an inviolable right.

The practice was widely criticised on ethical grounds. A report by the Social Affairs Inspectorate in 1978 denounced abuses by some physicians, including some who did not declare (to the hospital or the tax authorities) all their income from private fees, while others, often renowned specialists, failed to perform their required public service; the report proposed phasing out the practice. The 1980 Report of the Court of Accounts also noted significant 'anomalies' and urged reform, suggesting that government consider abolishing the privilege. Faced with growing debate and not anxious to create a crisis with the hospital élite by abolishing the practice, then Health Minister Barrot tried to get the message across by suspending two surgeons for abuse of privilege (inciting their patients to consult them privately, instead of publicly).

As there appeared to be no behavioural change, the government announced plans to impose ceilings on private sector earnings, but quietly abandoned them in view of the physicians' vigorous reaction. Instead its December 1980 decree required that hospitals collect the fees, deduct their share of the payment (a portion of what the doctor actually received), and pay the doctor. Although only 3763 full-time hospital physicians were concerned, when several hundred of them denounced the decree as a discredit of the profession the government postponed its application until after the presidential elections of 1981.

In his campaign for the presidency, Mitterrand criticised the practice because it distinguished among patients on the basis of their ability to pay, and was an unethical privilege granted to a hospital élite who used public facilities for private gain. Fulfilling Mitterrand's commitment to abolish the private sector, Health Minister Ralite issued a decree to eliminate private beds as of 1 July 1982;[5] private consultations were to be phased out by 31 December 1986. University Hospital physicians (led by Bernard Debré, son of the former Prime Minister and grandson of the architect of the 1958 Hospital Reform) constituted an opposition front called 'Medical Solidarity'[6] to denounce the reform for restricting patients' access to the hospital physicians, maligning physicians' motives and making them entirely dependent on their salaries.

The conservatives' platform of 1986 promised to restore the private sector, an 'indispensable' element, giving the patient the 'freedom of choice' while opening the public hospital to the outside world, presumably improving the articulation between ambulatory and hospital care. In her maiden speech in the National Assembly, Health Minister Barzach – a physician herself – denounced the flight of competent physicians from the public service and the inability to fill vacancies due, in her view, to the elimination of the private sector.[7] In fact the real issue was the relatively low public salaries: in gynecology, radiology and anaesthesiology, where the vacancies existed, doctors in the private sector earned considerably more than their colleagues in the public hospitals.

Implicitly admitting there had been some abuses, Barzach promised to establish 'transparency', by which she meant a rigorous control of ethics (*Le Monde*, 7 May 1986). After a decree revoked the deadline for phasing out private consultations, new legislation in 1987 conditioned the right to private practice in the public hospitals on a contract negotiated between physician and hospital management, subject to state approval. In addition the privilege was not transferable: when appointed to another hospital, a physician would have to seek a contract with his new employer. Private activity would be limited to 20 per cent of the physician's public obligations (that is to say, two half-days a week); the hospital would collect 30 per cent of the schedule fee plus a fixed percentage of whatever the doctor charged over that. Control committees were set up at local and national levels, with power to sanction abuse.

The Hospital Services

Approximately half of all health care expenditures in France occur in the hospitals, a tribute to the success of the modernisation of the public hospital sector undertaken with the 1958 and 1970 Hospital Reforms. Since 1943 hospitals have been organised by medical service units, under the authority of a Service Director who was granted a life appointment at the peak of his career by the Minister of Health. With this distinguished rank came the responsibility of directing junior doctors, as well as para-medical and non-medical staff. As more physicians attained this status over the years, hospital organisation fragmented into water-tight units (Services), with considerable duplication of tasks, restricted career mobility and no oversight. Since patronage power and influence grew directly with the number of beds, personnel and equipment these 'mandarins' controlled, they were impervious to appeals to control costs.

Hospital financing was also inflationary. Rates were determined retrospectively on the basis of the number of patient-days, thus motivating longer stays than were perhaps necessary in order to increase the hospital's revenues. Giscard d'Estaing's Health Minister, Simone Veil, had initiated studies of alternative means of financing, seeking ways to dissociate increasing revenues from increasing activity; she also had a report drawn up (May 1976) on ways to improve coordination and reduce duplication between the services.

It was the Socialists however who instituted what was probably the hospitals' most important and most durable reform. A January 1983 law replaced the patient-day financing with 'global budgets', an innovative if somewhat rigid process whereby the public hospitals would henceforth receive a monthly Block Grant from the local sickness funds. The grants were first determined annually from the previous year's expenditures, augmented by a national guideline rate. They were not really budgets however in the sense of a distributional mechanism; they were clearly expenditure ceilings, setting finite limits (with an adjustment procedure) to the hospital's resources. Introduced into the public hospital network progressively, the annual increase of hospital expenditures declined from 18.1 per cent in 1982 to 8.5 per cent in 1985 (Séguéla, 1987).

In connection with this reform, the Socialist government sought to remodel the internal organisational structure of the hospitals, to improve efficiency and accountability and curb the spending incentives. Because the Services linked management function and rank, the Socialists determined to replace them with discipline-defined *Départements*, administered by a Council composed of both medical and non-medical staff, which would elect its director for a four-year term, renewable once (Demichel, 1983; Clément, 1985). In this way physicians' status and career patterns were to be dissociated from the functional administration of the hospitals, while the junior consultants could participate in management. The Report of the 'Mediators', a blue-ribbon panel commissioned by the Prime Minister in April 1983 to examine the public hospitals and the hospital career patterns, had criticised the failure of the excessively specialised Services to consider the *patient*, not just his organs and pathologies. It envisaged the departmental organisation as an instrument of more rational functioning and management of the public hospitals, and as the focal point for implementing the 'global budgets' (Mediators, 1983).

Although the departmental reform reduced state power by transferring responsibility for administrative organisation to the hospitals and ending the Health Ministry's appointment power, it was met by hostile criticism from the conservatives and was never fully implemented; the texts were ready in July 1984, but when the Mauroy government resigned the new Social Affairs Minister, Georgina Dufoix, ordered a reassessment of the proposals and new negotiations. From the issuance of the first circulars in December 1984, the hospital physicians boycotted the departmentalisation process; new circulars were delayed for a year, by which time it was clear the conservatives would soon be back in power. The Services had been abolished by law in January 1984, but departments were set up in only three hospitals and a few psychiatric institutions, leaving the rest of the public hospitals without a legal structure.

The July 1987 Hospital Reform Law re-established the hospital Services, but under new conditions designed to correct the defects of the old system. The new Service Directors continued to be appointed by the Minister of Health, but for five-year renewable terms. The Minister was obliged to seek the formal opinions of the hospital's board of trustees and the Director's colleagues on the Medical Committee. Although some (like Debré) doubt that Health Ministers can ignore the political sympathies of the candidates, the selection process does offer a recourse which, even if rarely used, would allow the Service's team of doctors to dispose of a poor administrator without destroying his career.

In the same pragmatic vein, the Barzach hospital reform recognised the need to introduce greater managerial flexibility into the hospital structures. On the one hand, within each Service the Director can delegate certain responsibilities to some of the junior physicians by creating 'activity centres', sorts of mini-Services organised by discipline, pathology or medical technique for example. On the other hand, the law admits the utility of the Departments, and authorises their creation as 'voluntary' groups of Services, to insure the coordination of hospital care sought by the 1984 Law. By bringing together related medical activities, the Department can help reduce duplication of diagnostic examinations, encourage common usage of costly technical equipment, and encourage pluridisciplinary research. Each Department is to be managed by a 'coordinator', chosen according to internally determined procedures, not by statute.

Rationalisation of Benefits: the Séguin Plan

The other major element of conservative reform in health care was handled by Barzach's hierarchical superior, Social Affairs Minister Philippe Séguin, whose portfolio included the Social Security system as a whole. The 'Séguin Plan' was more than just another set of cost-saving measures: it merits examination because it put into practice liberal values of individual responsibility, rationalised management and efficiency.

The national sickness fund had for a long time been reviewing the practice of granting exemptions from the customary co-payment (25–35 per cent of fees and other outlays) for those patients suffering from long and costly afflictions. Over the years a list of 25 diseases had been drawn up defining those illnesses (for example active tuberculosis, degenerative cancer, haemophilia, muscular dystrophy, acute psychological disorders, severe cardiac conditions, and so on) which once diagnosed gave patients the right to 100 per cent coverage by exonerating them from co-payments. A statistical 26th 'disease', defined as any affliction whose treatment left the patient with co-payments of more than 80 francs a month for at least six months, was created to cover miscellaneous cases. By 1987 the co-payment exemption (meaning virtually free health care) concerned more than three million patients and took up three-quarters of health insurance expenditure, compared to 36 per cent only thirty years earlier. In 1985 alone some 170 000 new patients were given exemptions for the twenty-sixth 'disease', whose annual cost for the sickness fund was estimated at over one billion francs a year. Most of the beneficiaries were the elderly, who suffered from numerous interconnected afflictions. The difficulty arose from the fact that prescriptions made no distinction between the illness for which the exempt status was granted and other unrelated illnesses.

Introducing the reforms in November 1986, Séguin announced that the list of 25 diseases would be revised, and that henceforth 100 per cent coverage would be granted only for those illnesses on the new list; no more patients would be admitted under the twenty-sixth 'disease', while the cases of those previously admitted would be re-examined. Henceforth a heart patient treated for a common cold, for example, would have to pay the normal co-payment for medical and pharmaceutical care for the cold. Physicians did not like having the responsibility for determining whether their patients had to pay something, but most recognised the need for reform.[8] At the same time the 'rationalisation' plan required that these patients, like the rest of the insured population, bear the increased co-payment (60 per cent) for the so-called 'convenience' drugs (for example, vitamins or aspirin) unless their physician stipulated they were part of the treatment for the qualifying illness.

After a year's implementation, the sickness fund claimed the measures saved 6 billion francs directly and an estimated 5.8 billion as a result of induced behavioural changes, but these figures are difficult to prove.[9] The number of exempted patients had been reduced by some 400 000, although more cases remained to be re-examined (CNAMTS, 1988a, b). Whereas prior to the reform some 567 000 people were admitted annually to the exonerated status, the number was expected to drop to 490 000. Of the 373 000 new cases admitted in the first nine months of 1987, two-thirds concerned chronic heart illness, malignant tumors, neuroses–psychoses and diabetes; 60 per cent of the new admissions were over 60 years old. The plan also included abolishing the postal franchise granted all letters mailed to the sickness funds, a saving of some 675 million francs in 1987 alone.

The Rocard government announced shortly after taking office in 1988 that, in keeping with President Mitterrand's campaign commitments, it would reestablish 100 per cent coverage for the elderly suffering from long and costly afflictions. It also announced that the Chirac government's fiscal measures (discussed above) would be prolonged. After further study the government found little to amend. It was estimated that if the sickness fund reimbursed the 'convenience' prescriptions at 100 per cent instead of 40 per cent, it would cost 1.2 billion francs; if the coverage were applied only to those below the standard minimum income level, the cost would be only 60 million francs. The issue illustrates the dilemma facing the government: while recognising the cost-containment logic of the Séguin reforms it had to find something distinctive to do, a set of measures that would be 'socially effective, politically significant. . . and inexpensive' (*Le Monde*, 22 June 1988).

CONCLUSION

The Socialists' hospital reforms – abolishing private beds and consultations, departmentalisation, prospective budgeting, the daily hotel charge – were not incompatible with a liberal agenda, partisan rhetoric notwithstanding. Having adopted the cost-containment strategy of their predecessors, the Socialists went on to transform it into a managerial strategy, emphasising more efficient allocation of resources by designing and implementing new organisational and accounting procedures borrowed from the corporate world. The deceleration of health care expenditures began to appear in 1983 and continued throughout the Socialists' term in office. The Chirac government easily accommodated most of these reforms, with relatively few adjustments, when it took office.

The French Health Care System in the 1980s

The 1980s have thus witnessed much more than continuity with the fiscal imperative which emerged in the late 1970s. Although there has not been any sharp break with the past, the subtle, pragmatic, and qualitative changes which have taken place combine to make the health care system today substantially *different* from what it was just 10 years ago. A public enterprise mentality has begun to replace the public service concept, with consequences in authority patterns, management techniques, the reimbursement mechanisms and the configuration of the delivery system.

There has been a sifting out of roles and powers between the managers of the system, the state and the sickness funds. In its domain the state has applied a firm grip on supply: cutting in half the number of medical students admitted into the second year, reducing hospital capacity, capping both hospital expenditures and physicians' fees in ambulatory care. The public hospital system is being redesigned to focus on the highly technical medical procedures, while ambulatory care is being made more flexible and adaptable to the cultural and demographic changes taking place in French society. Alternatives are being developed to hospitalisation for non-medical social cases (the elderly and the mentally disturbed for example), placing them where feasible in appropriate centres, or in home care with para-medical assistance.[10] The medical community has been exploring French versions of HMOs, multidisciplinary public care clinics, day hospitals, and so on.

Modern managerial and accounting techniques are being progressively refined and gradually introduced into the hospitals. In financing the prospective budgeting procedure has already created incentives to improve efficiency; in addition analytical accounting was introduced in 1985 to give hospital administrators a means of examining their expenditures by cost centres (administrative, hotel charges, clinical, medico-technical). A comparable budgeting instrument must still be developed for private clinics, where the global budget procedure is not suitable. Reliable, sophisticated means of determining hospital costs are also being developed. To make the hospital budgets real tools for forecasting needs, the Ministry's Hospital Division has worked out a French version of the Diagnostic Related Groups (*Groupes Homogènes de Malades*) (Hatchuel *et al.*, 1985), and is currently collecting standardised exit data on patients.

This strategy of flexibility in health care delivery requires a more sophisticated gatekeeper role for the family doctor, directing his patients to the appropriate diagnostic and therapeutic centres when necessary. In order to enhance the pivotal role of the general practitioner, the government began revamping the medical school curriculum to make general medicine a different kind of specialisation. In addition it has also begun closing the gap between the fees of GPs and specialists.[11]

In the course of this reshaping of the health care delivery system, the sickness funds have also diversified and extended the scope of their role in the public hospitals and in ambulatory care (Catrice-Lorey, 1987). As the intermediaries between the state and the medical profession, it was the CNAMTS which redesigned the *convention* in 1980 to defuse conflict over the fee schedule by opening up Sector II. Since then the focus of negotiations has shifted to finding acceptable ways to get physicians to reexamine how they practice their art. They have urged them to identify not only the best remedy for a given affliction, but the best remedy at the lowest cost, a perspective foreign to most doctors' training. Tripartite discussions are currently under way to set up professional review procedures which, while respecting professional confidentiality, should provide qualitative, not just quantitative analyses of medical behaviour and its financial consequences, to help in this pursuit.[12]

The CNAMTS also was responsible for drawing up the 'Séguin Plan', which rationalised reimbursement practices, helped to dampen demand for pharmaceuticals and produced significant savings for the health insurance system. The increased co-payments have helped to make consumers more aware that health care does indeed have costs, although experts are dubious about the length of the effect.

Liberalism in Medical Care?

The French health care system has for centuries been characterised by a shifting public and private balance; in the nineteenth century the state was called upon to help the profession regulate the medical market by controlling supply (to eliminate quacks) and creating demand (through public health campaigns and medical care for the poor). The public role in private care has been so extensive that some authorities even question whether France's sacred *médecine libérale* has ever really existed (Launois, 1987; Steffen, 1987). The public–private mix today seems nonetheless to satisfy most French – patients and physicians alike – who find that their system is an excellent compromise between the egalitarian but financially strapped British NHS and the technologically advanced but profligate American way. Consumers receive high quality care, accessible to all at not too great a cost, while preserving a certain measure of individual choice. This consensus has served over the past three decades as a formidable constraint in policy-making, precluding radical change and guiding both Left and Right toward consensual policies.

Given the direction of change during the 1980s, it seems likely that the next decade will focus on increasing the efficiency and reducing the scope of the public sector, assigning greater roles to the private sector, whether private insurance, private clinics, or consumer responsibility. Although the sickness funds are not likely to have to compete with private insurance, further rationalisation is possible, such as limiting mandatory coverage to 'major risks', leaving complementary insurance to the consumer, with income supplements to protect the less well-off.[13]

The conservative coalition that came to power in 1986 began with a relatively modest reform programme in medical care, despite its liberal rhetoric. Although some of its achievements were of 'liberal' inspiration, it is fair to say that the measures adopted were largely those initiated before the 1980s, imposed by economic circumstances that also constrained the Socialists between 1981 and 1986. Clearly, despite the shift in public opinion away from statism, the Chirac government faced a public attached to a familiar policy of social benefits, and thus was limited in its ability to mobilise the political support necessary for introducing reforms of a more liberal nature.

Notes

1. More than 14 per cent of the population is over 65 (6.3 per cent are 75 or older); they account for twice the average consumption of medical care.

2. For example, miners, farmers, civil servants, rail transport employees, unsalaried professionals, Bank of France employees, and so on. See *Le Monde*, 30 June 1987. The CNAMTS subsidised the special funds for 37 billion francs in 1986, *Le Monde*, 9 March 1987.

3. For his government's first budget bill on May 1986, for example, Chirac had to employ extraordinary procedures to avoid passage of a National Front amendment abolishing insurance reimbursement for abortions. Later the National Front's medical spokesman carried on a major campaign to isolate AIDS victims from society, criticising the government's lax attitude.

4. Such as moving toward a completely state-administered system, modeled on the British, or evolving more or less rapidly toward complete budgetisation of any or all of the risks (especially health or pensions), or reviving the 1979 proposal of Committee member Simon Nora to separate major risks (publicly insured) and minor risks (privately insured).

5. Private beds were actually a constraint for the consultants. Since private patients could not occupy more than 8 per cent of the total number of beds, they could not be transferred following surgery to 'public' beds to recuperate, thereby freeing beds for more private patients. Abolishing private *beds*, while private *consultations* were still in effect, meant that physicians could hospitalise more private patients.

6. The name suggested a parallel with the oppressed Polish workers' movement, *Solidarnosc*.

7. On TV in January 1987, Health Minister Barzach complained that two-thirds of the 18 000 vacant hospital posts remained unfulfilled.

8. SOFRES-Médical poll in June 1987 showed that 66 per cent of GPs found the measures necessary, and 76 per cent expected difficulties in getting patients to accept.

9. Not that the CNAMTS did not try; it produced several brochures filled with sometimes conflicting statistics on the numbers of cases reconsidered, excluded, reclassified, and the 'direct' and 'induced' effects of the measures.

10. Jean de Kervasdoué, former Director of Hospitals in the Ministry of Health, estimated that at least 30 per cent of a given day's hospital admissions should not be there at all. (See de Kervasdoué, 1987).

11. The steady growth in the number of doctors over the past decade brought about an oversaturation in the most desirable locations for setting up practices. Combined with the slow evolution of the fee schedules since 1980, this high density resulted in stagnating incomes for most doctors, declining incomes for GPs. See CREDES, 1986. The market for specialists, however, is not so Malthusian. Overall,

doctors' purchasing power showed modest (1–2 per cent) real increases since 1984, according to CERC (*Centre détudes des revenues et des coâts) study* (*Le Monde* 13 July 1988).

12. See, for example, *Le Monde*, 24 February 1988. Evaluation techniques were initially sponsored by Professor Emile Papiernek, a Socialist consultant; Health Minister Barzach chose to set up her own committee, but the objectives were not modified.

13. This was the essence of Simon Nora's 1979 proposal. It is still being discussed within the CNAMTS and the medical profession.

References

Belassa, B. (1986) 'Five Years of Socialist Economic Policy in France: A Balance Sheet', *The Tocqueville Review*, no. 7, pp. 269–83.

Belassa, B. (1987) 'French Economic Policy since March 1986', *The Tocqueville Review*, no. 8 pp. 311–23.

Catrice-Lorey, A. (1987) 'L'Assurance Maladie et le Système de Sante', *Revye Française d'Administration Publique*, no. 43, pp. 71–89.

Clément, J.-M. (1985) *Les Réformes hospitalières, 1981–1984* (Berger-Levrault).

CNAMTS (1987) 'Un an après: bilan du Plan de Rationalisation des dépenses de l'Assurance Maladie'.

CNAMTS, (1988a) 'Le Secteur Libéral des professions de Santé en 1987', *Bloc-notes Statistiques*, no. 35.

CNAMTS (1988b) 'Contribution de l'Assurance Maladie aux Dépenses de Santé en France: 1970–1986; *Bloc-notes Statistiques*, no. 36.

Comité des Sages (1987) *Rapport* (Les Etats-Généraux de la Santé).

Commissariat Général du Plan (1986) *Une Décentralisation du système de santé* (Paris: La Documentation Française).

CREDES (1987) 'Géographie Economique de la Santé', *Revue de Socio-Economie de la Santé*, pp. 43–59.

de Kervasdoué, J. (1987) 'Prescrire l'hôpital', in *Prospective et Santé*, no. 43 pp. 18–27.

Delanoë, J.-Y. (1987) 'Grandes Orientations de la Politique de la Santé de 1981 à 1986', *Revue Française des Affaires Sociales*, no. 1 pp. 87–106.

Demichel, D. (1983) 'La Réforme Hospitalière: Eléments pour une Problématique', *Revue Française de Finances Publiques*, no. 2 pp. 107–15.

Duhamel, O. et al. (eds) (1986) *SOFRES: Opinion Publique 1986* (Paris: Gallimard).

Giscard d'Estaing, V. (1976) *Démocratie Française*, (Paris: Fayard).

Godt, P. (1985) 'Doctors and Deficits: Regulating the Medical Profession in France', *Public Administration*, vol. 63:2, (1985) pp. 151–63.

Godt, P. (1989) 'Health Care: The Political Economy of Social Policy', in Paul Godt (ed.), *Policy-Making in France: From de Gaulle to Mitterrand* (London and New York: Frances Pinter) pp. 191–208.

Hall, P. A. (1985) 'Socialism in One Country: Mitterrand and the Struggle to Define a New Economic Policy for France', in Philip G. Cerny and Martin A. Schain (eds), *Socialism, the State Public Policy in France* (London and New York: Frances Pinter) pp. 81–107.

Hall, P. A. (1986) *Governing the Economy: The Politics of State Intervention in France and Britain* (Oxford: Polity Press).

Hatchuel, A., J.-C. Moisdon, and Hu Molet (1985) 'Budget Robal Hospitalier et Groupes Homogènes de Malades', *Politiques et Management Public*, vol. 3:4, pp. 99–114.

Hayward, J. E. S. (1986) *The State and the Market Economy: Industrial Patriotism and Economic Intervention in France* (Brighton: Wheatsheaf).

Jolly, D. and B. Majnoni d'Intignano (1985) 'La Gestion du Système de Santé en France: Vers des Innovations Libérales?', *Politiques et Management Public*, vol. 3:4, pp. 17–37.

Launois, R. (1977) 'Le Médecine Libérale a-t-elle Jamais Existe?', *Politiques et Management Public*, no. 53, pp. 87–97.

Launois, B. Majnoni d'Intignano, V. Rodwin, and J.-C. Stéphan (1985) 'Les Réseaux de Soins donnés: Proposition pour une Réforme Profonde du Système de Santé', *Revue Française des Affaires Sociales*, no. 1 pp. 37–61.

Mediators (1983) *Le Système de Santé Française Réflexions et Propositions: Rapport au Premier Ministre* (Paris: La Documentation Française).

Ministry of Social Affairs (1987) *Annuaire des Statistiques Sanitaires et Sociales* (Paris).

OECD (1985) *Measuring Health Care* (Paris: OECD).

OECD (1987) *Financing and Delivering Health Care: A Comparative Analysis of OECD Countries* (Paris: OECD).

Rodwin, V. (1984a) 'Quand le Payeur Séveillera', *Le Monde Diplomatique* (1984a).

Rodwin, V. (1084b) *The National Health Planning Predicament* (Berkeley: University of California Press).

Rodwin, V. (1987) 'Le Contrôle des Pouvoirs Publics et des Payeurs: (comparaisons Internationales', Commissariat Général du Plan, *Systèmes de Santé, Pouvoirs Publics et Financeurs: Qui Contrôle Quoi?* (Paris La Documentation Française pp. 55–68.

Sandier, S. (1983) 'Les Dépenses de Soins Médicaux en France Depuis 1950', *Reveue Française de Finances Publiques*, no. 2 pp. 5–30.

Séguéla, J.-P. (1987) *Report on the Hospital Reform Bill (#689) of the Cultural Family and Social Affairs Committee of the French National Assembly* (Paris: Assemblée Nationale).

Sorman, G. (1984) *La Solution Libérale* (Paris: Fayard, 1984).

Sorman, G. (1985) *L'Etat Minimum* (Paris: Fayard).

Steffen, M. (1987) 'Les Médecins et l'Etaten France', *Politiques et Management Public, vol. 5:3 pp. 19–39*.

Zysman, J. (1983) *Governments, Markets and Growth: Financial Systems and the Politics of Industrial Change* (Ithaca: Cornell University Press).

3 Health Policy and the Christian–Liberal Coalition in West Germany: The Conflicts over the Health Insurance Reform, 1987–8

Douglas Webber

INTRODUCTION

Even before the parliamentary deliberations over the Christian–Liberal federal government's health insurance reform bill had begun in May 1988, most commentators agreed that it did not amount to the major reform which the government had promised. In one view, nothing was going to be done to get to grips with such critical problems as the oversupply of doctors and hospital beds or change the existing (fees-for-service) method of payment for private-practising doctors. The so-called 'health reform' boiled down to nothing more than a 'muddled tangle of a hundred compromises' (Gehrmann, 1988).

The Christian Democratic and Liberal coalition endeavours to reform the German health system seemed to have been a little more successful than those of its predecessors in the Federal Republic (FRG). To be sure the coverage of the statutory health insurance had been widened in the post-Second World War period to include more and more occupational groups, so that nowadays roughly 90 per cent of West Germans are insured in the statutory scheme. But this membership expansion occurred on top of essentially unchanged system structures. Health care is overwhelmingly *collectively-financed*, with most citizens belonging compulsorily to either local or, in the case of white-collar workers (*Angestellte*), 'substitute' insurance funds (*Ersatzkassen*). It is predominantly *privately-provided* ambulatory care by private-practising general practitioners and specialists and other independent professions. Institutional care, on the other hand, is offered in hospitals owned mainly by local government or by charitable, non-profit-making organisations. It is *regulated* procedurally by law, but substantively also by *collective bargaining* between the organisations of the health-care financers and health-care deliverers (described in Germany as the *gemeinsame Selbstverwaltung* (Webber, 1988, pp. 5–9). In contrast to the other social insurance schemes in the FRG, and to the health systems in most other advanced industrial democracies, West German health insurance has not been thoroughly overhauled in the post-war period (Jung, 1987, p. 190).

The apparent lack of radical changes in the West German health system cannot be attributed to the existence of a consensus that none were necessary. Rather, perceived deficiencies in the system and its functioning have regularly prompted attempts to reform it, but such attempts have more often failed than succeeded, and when they have succeeded, the reform ultimately implemented usually no longer bore very much resemblance to the project initially proposed by the government. The aim of this chapter is to trace the course of the conflicts over the Christian–Liberal health reform and to investigate the extent to which its *substantive* outcome parallels or differs from that of earlier such conflicts and can be attributed to the same determinants.

A RECAPITULATION

In a previous paper, the present author tried to account for the comparatively high resistance of the German health system to radical *structural* reform roughly up until the 1982 change of the federal government in the FRG. Structural *reforms* were defined as those changes in health system structures brought about by purposeful government intervention. It was assumed that a health system is composed of three kinds of structures: a financing structure (who pays?), a delivery structure (who provides?), and a regulatory structure (who decides?). *Structural* (as opposed to other kinds of) reforms were conceived as being those which redistributed responsibilities or competences with regard to funding, providing or regulating health care. It was argued that the last very radical structural reforms of the German health system occurred in the closing years of the Weimar Republic and the early phase of the Nazi dictatorship in the 1930s (Webber, 1988).

It was argued that conjunctural factors – the macro-economic situation, the acuteness of the problem-constellation in the health system and the *Zeitgeist*, the 'climate' of public opinion – facilitate or militate against the conception and implementation of health system reforms. However even when the economic and political-economic conjunctures were reform-friendly – that is to say, when there was a strong *will* within the government to reform the system, or at least the widely-perceived perception that such reforms were (politically) urgently necessary – the obstacles to radical structural reforms generally proved insurmountable. The high degree of political difficulty of health system reforms in the FRG was attributed essentially to three variables:

1. **The wide range and heterogeneity of the health system interests or clienteles represented in the (almost always multiparty) federal government.** As a consequence of the proportional-representation electoral system, the federal government always rests on, and to be re-elected must mobilise, the support of more than 50 per cent of the electorate. It therefore has a broad, heterogeneous socio-economic clientele. Normally most of the collective actors in the health system – the trade unions, the employers' organisations, the health insurance funds, the doctors, and so on – will have a bridgehead or advocate in the government. In coalition governments, majoritarian decision-making typically gives way to decision-making negotiation and compromise. In the FRG the big parties, the Social Democratic Party (SPD) and the Christian Democratic Union–Christian Social Union (CDU–CSU), have normally only been able to form a federal government with the liberal Free Democratic Party (FDP), which consequently has spent more time in federal office than any other party. The FDP has its social roots in the (Protestant) middle classes, and on health policy issues represents more purely than the big parties the goals of the professional health-service providers and good producers. The FDP plays an important role in preventing the adoption of structural reforms adversely affecting their health system 'clientele'. But also the Christian Democrats, with their very broad and heterogeneous voting constituency ranging from the Catholic manual working class across the free professions, farmers and small business people to big business, have experienced great difficulties trying to agree on health reform issues. Conflicts within governing

coalitions had a major role in preventing structural reforms of the health system not only in the late 1950s and early 60s and during the Social-Liberal coalition, but also during the period of Allied military occupation (1945–9).

2. **The constitutionally-entrenched veto power possessed by the state governments.** This applies most of all to the hospital sector, where reforms require the consent of the upper chamber of the Federal Parliament, the *Bundesrat*, in which the state governments are represented. Even when the same parties had a majority in the two houses of Parliament, hospital reforms often failed, since the federal and state governments were confronted with different expectations by different electorates. Since the federation is responsible for social insurance legislation, the federal government is expected to act to contain health expenditure. Since the states are responsible for hospital policy, they are the 'scapegoats if a hospital somewhere is closed or the number of beds cut back' (state government minister quoted in Webber, 1988, p. 165). They have a positive incentive to maximise the provision of hospital care and none to curb its cost, since the hospital's running costs are financed by the health insurance funds. In the early 1970s, the mid-1970s and again in 1984, the state governments had succeeded in defeating or in extensively 'watering down' structural reform affecting the hospital sector.

3. **The specific, strongly corporatist mode of interest-organisation of the private-practising doctors (*Kassenärzte*).** This was said to have contributed to the prevention or absence of major reforms in so far as it afforded the doctors' organisations a high capacity to mobilise compliance (or non-compliance) with the government. This capacity in turn enabled the doctors to offer the government deals whereby the latter forewent structural reforms at the doctors' expense in return for the public-law doctors' associations (*Kassenärztliche Vereinigungen*) enforcing a policy of voluntary incomes restraint vis-à-vis their members. Such a policy was facilitated by these associations' monopoly of the provision of ambulatory care, by the fact that private-practising doctors are compelled to belong to them, and by the legal powers which they possess to negotiate, calculate and distribute doctors' fees. 'We are strong in our external relations because we have a strong position vis-à-vis our members' (interview statement by a doctors' association official). Such deals offered the government, for its part, the chance of finding at least a temporary solution to the recurring problem of rising costs and avoiding a potentially damaging conflict with a well-organised profession, which

in the past was allocated an important opinion-forming function. It was 'exceptionally difficult' to make a law against the opposition of '70 000 doctors, each of whom sees 30 patients a day', said Chancellor Adenauer as he abandoned plans for a comprehensive reform of the health insurance in 1960 (quoted in Schwarz, 1983, p. 162).

THE BACKGROUND TO THE REFORM

For all the rhetoric at the time about a fundamental 'change of direction' (*Wende*) in public policy, the Christian–Liberal coalition government which came into office in October 1982 had no concrete or detailed programme to reduce the role of the state and increase the scope for the operation of market forces in the health system. Like that of the Social-Liberal coalition, Christian–Liberal policy aimed first and foremost at stabilising health insurance contributions. This reflected the *Wende* credo that the high level of social security contributions undermined the competitiveness of German industry and the work incentive and had a negative impact on employment. In terms of policy instruments, the new government arguably placed a stronger emphasis than its predecessor on steering collective bargaining between the insurance funds and organised service providers rather than by state intervention. This corresponded to the expectations – and hopes – of the service providers, such as most of the doctors' organisations, which had greeted the change of government in 1982 (Deppe, 1987, p. 72).

Cost-containment measures implemented or agreed by the old coalition helped to restrain the rise in health-care costs in the new government's first two years in office. By 1985 however, resurgent cost and contribution increases had rekindled the debate about the need for a thoroughgoing reform of the health insurance. However policy disagreements within the coalition and the political calendar – the fact that a number of important state elections were imminent, as well as, in 1987, federal elections – persuaded the government to postpone any such reform until the next parliamentary period. In return for the government rewarding them with some legislative concessions, the doctors' associations and the pharmaceuticals industry promised to exercise voluntary fees and price restraint. The major provider and producer groups in the health system wanted to avoid drawing attention to themselves at the wrong time (Forster,

1985). All such efforts notwithstanding, expenditure in all major budget titles of the health insurance, except those for ambulatory care and dentures rose in 1986 more than twice as rapidly as wages and salaries (see table 3.1).

THE CONCEPTION OF THE REFORM

Expenditure trends and the concomitant increases in contributions in 1986 and early 1987 made a reform of the statutory health insurance seem more rather than less urgent after the reelection of the Christian–Liberal coalition in January 1987. Apart from their feared negative impact on industrial competitiveness and employment it was thought that rising contributions would negate the impact of the proposed tax reform, which formed the centrepiece of the new government's legislative programme and should guarantee its reelection in 1990. The rising contributions no doubt also conditioned the widespread popular acceptance that a health insurance reform was necessary. Together with a pensions reform, the health insurance and tax reforms were the government's main legislative projects.

The new coalition agreement between CDU–CSU and FDP was relatively vague as to the concrete shape of the proposed reform. The signs were however, that the government would refrain from proposing radical reform measures. The Labour Minister had pledged that market principles would not be introduced *holus bolus* into the health insurance and even that the existing division of responsibilities between state and the *gemeinsame Selbstverwaltung* would be maintained (*FAZ*, 8 December 1986). The reform would be drafted in 'intensive talks' with the interest groups in the health system – on whose expertise the ministry, he said, was dependent.

The interest groups in turn did not show very much interest in a radical reform of the health insurance. The thrust of the insurance funds' demands was that their regulatory competence vis-à-vis the service providers, especially the hospitals and producers, the pharmaceuticals and medical aids manufacturers, should be strengthened (*Handelsblatt*, 24 October 1986). The local insurance funds explicitly rejected the need for fundamental reforms (*ibid.*, 17 December 1986). The Federal Insurance Doctors' Association (*Kassenärztliche Bundesvereinigung*) opposed the transformation of the health insurance according to market principles and the abandonment of the principle of services being rendered in kind (*Sachleistungs-*

Table 3.1 Expenditure trends in German statutory health insurance (percentage change compared with the previous year)

Year	Ambulatory Care	Dental Care	Drugs	Medical Aids	Dentures	Hospital Treatment	Total Spending	Average Salary	Average Contribution
1980	+8.7	+5.7	+10.6	+12.1	+13.6	+9.5	+11.0	+5.4	11.38
1981	+7.4	+7.6	+8.4	+8.0	+10.3	+7.3	+7.3	+5.0	11.79
1982	+2.6	+2.3	+1.1	−4.3	−13.8	+8.3	+0.5	+4.4	12.00
1983	+5.0	+3.4	+4.9	+3.7	−4.6	+4.6	+3.5	+3.8	11.83
1984	+6.5	+4.5	+7.6	+15.9	+10.1	+7.3	+8.0	+4.7	11.44
1985	+3.9	+1.4	+6.8	+7.4	+4.5	+5.5	+5.0	+3.1	11.80
1986	+3.0	+7.0	+6.3	+10.4	−10.1	+6.9	+4.8	+3.1	12.19
1987	+3.5	+3.2	+7.1	+8.8	+9.0	+4.9	+4.4	+2.2	12.47

Source Kassenärztliche Bundesvereinigung: *Grunddaten zur kassenärztlichen Versorgung in der Bundesrepublik Deutschland 1988.*

prinzip) in favour of consumers being billed and their being re-
funded for the costs of medical treatment by the insurance funds
(*Kostenerstattung*) (*FAZ*, 8 December 1986). Thus it was evident that
a radical reform of the health insurance could be implemented only
over the heads of the Labour Ministry, the health insurance funds
and the organised private-practising doctors (*FAZ*, 18 November
1986). However this did not rule out the possibility that these actors
could agree on far-reaching reform measures affecting the hospital,
pharmaceutical, dental care and medical aids sectors – the ones
which the Labour Minister in fact diagnosed as being most ripe for
reform (*SDZ*, 18–19 November 1986).

The guiding idea behind the reform package on which the coalition
eventually agreed, was that the health insurance funds could not be
responsible for financing everything that is desirable in terms of
health policy. They should only fund what was 'medically necessary'
(BMASO, 1988a, p. 2). The money saved by the planned economy
measures was not only to be used to lower contributions however. A
half of the savings was intended to be put to this purpose, the other
half to expanding preventative health care and home care for the
elderly disabled. In addition more competition was to be introduced
into the statutory health insurance, and waste and the exploitation or
abuse of the system to be combated (*ibid.*).

The Labour Minister and his bureaucracy's strategy for the reform
and its implementation suggested that they had indeed studied the
'lessons from the history of the statutory health insurance' and were
especially at pains to avoid the pitfalls into which Blüm's Christian
Democratic predecessor, Blank, had fallen when trying to reform the
health insurance in the late 1950s and early 1960s (Jung, 1987, p. 190;
Webber, 1988, pp. 45–8). Firstly they had to have the support of the
private-practising doctors for the reform, or at least ensure that they
did not oppose the reform outright. Through 1986 and 1987 the
Labour Minister seemed to use every opportunity to praise the
doctors for their fees policy moderation. As early as May 1987,
before coalition negotiations on the details of the reform had begun,
the head of the health insurance division in the ministry assured the
doctors that, given the contributions the doctors had already made to
containing costs, it would be unjust to demand sacrifices from them:
'A reform against the doctors is neither desired nor necessary and will
therefore not take place' (quoted in KBV, 1987, p. 52).

Secondly, sacrifices had to be exacted not only from consumers,
but also from service-provider and producer groups – the reform

should not be seen to be socially too inequitable.[1] This thread ran through all the Minister's and his civil servants' pronouncements on health reform issues from 1985 onwards (*FAZ*, 28 March 1985) and resurfaced in the post-election coalition agreement. This component of the implementation strategy may be attributed to their wanting to ensure that the reform would be supported by the CDU's labour wing, and above all to avoid offering the opposition parties and the trade unions ammunition for a campaign accusing the government of trying to dismantle the German welfare-state. The allegation that the government's austerity policies were socially inequitable was widely believed to have contributed to a decline in the CDU–CSU's voting support in the coalition's first years in office.

Thirdly the Labour Minister and Ministry had to ensure that the reform was backed by the social policy experts in the coalition Parliamentary parties and by the Chancellor. The task of securing the latter's (erstwhile) backing for the reform was facilitated by the crisis in the North Rhine–Westphalian CDU in May 1987. The Labour Minister agreed to take over the leadership of the state party in return for the Chancellor's pledge of support for him on the health reform and other major social policy projects (*Der Spiegel*, no. 20, 11 May 1987; *Wirtschaftswoche*, no. 21, 15 May 1987).

The Parliamentary parties' social policy experts' backing for the reform was to be secured by their close integration in its formulation. In spring 1987, a coalition commission consisting of two representatives from each of the three parties (CDU, CSU and FDP) was formed to draft the details of the reform in collaboration with Labour Ministry staff. The commission's deliberations carried on into autumn 1987, but it could not agree on numerous aspects of the reform. The original target of autumn 1987 for the publication of a draft Labour Ministry bill could not be kept. The outstanding issues on which the coalition's social policy experts had not been able to compromise were passed up for resolution by the party chairmen, managers and Parliamentary party chairmen. Their agreement over some aspects of the reform in December 1987 was followed in January 1988 by consultations between the Labour Ministry and the organised interests, and the ministry's publication of a draft bill.

Press leaks concerning the first reform proposals, said to have been agreed by the coalition commission, sufficed to generate a 'broad front' of opposition (*FR*, 9 October 1987). Following the coalition agreement of December and the publication of the Labour Ministry's draft bill, the opposition of the 'health care lobby' (*Der Spiegel*) to the proposed reform broadened further and intensified. Protest campaigns were initiated by voluntary doctors' and dentists' pressure groups and the pharmaceuticals industry association (BPI – *Bundesverband der Pharmazeutischen Industrie*). Chemists and taxi-proprietors (the latter affected by a proposal to restrict the insurance funds' funding trips to doctors and hospitals) demonstrated against the government's plans. Pharmaceuticals firms prophesied cuts in research and development expenditure, export order and job losses and investment flight. Funeral proprietors protested that the proposed abolition of the death grant would lead to the 'devastation of the Western cemetery culture' in the FRG. An indignant Labour Minister claimed that the campaign against the reform far exceeded anything he had previously experienced (*FR*, 23 March 1988). He defended the proposed reform as a 'last-minute attempt' to save the statutory health insurance from collapse, vilified the use of doctors' waiting-rooms as a forum of political protest, warned of an impending usurpation of political power by the 'pressure groups' and vowed that the government would not bow to 'political blackmail' (Blüm, 1988, p. 23).

THE MUTILATION OF THE REFORM

Well before the Labour Minister made this pledge, the coalition had already agreed to put off any comprehensive attempts to reform the hospital sector and the health insurance funds or propose new legislation to curb the number of doctors. Numerous other components of the original reform package had also been weakened or were in the process of being diluted. The process by which the mutilation of the health insurance reform occurred is described and analysed according to issue-area in the following setions.

The Consumers (Benefits and Services)

The progressive dilution of those elements of the reform relating to insurance fund services and benefits were less marked than those aimed directly at service providers and medical goods producers. Whereas one or the other measure was moderated in response to interest-group and intra-coalition pressures, other proposals for cutting health insurance expenditure were actually *toughened*. According to the established pattern, the implementation of benefit and service cuts and consumer charges proved politically less difficult than curtailing the acquired privileges of service providers and producers (cf. Webber, 1988, pp. 20–21).

There was a broad consensus within the Christian–Liberal coalition that the reform had to cut back the range of services financed by the statutory funds and increase consumer charges. Common to almost all the health reform programmes formulated by business organisations and pro-business lobbies in the governing coalition, such as the CDU's association for small and medium sized enterprise (*Mittelstandsvereinigung*), and that of the FDP were demands for (1) the transformation of the existing flat-rate charge for prescription drugs into a (higher) percentage one, (2) billing patients for a (higher) proportion of the 'accommodation costs' in hospital and (3) the introduction of direct payment of doctors by patients (see above) (*Mittelstandsvereinigung der CDU–CSU*, 1987, pp. 57–8; *Dienst für Gesellschaftspolitik*, no. 43, 29 October 1987, pp. 8–10 and no. 46, 19 November 1987, pp. 5–7; *Handelsblatt*, 3 February 1987). Limits on how far the government could go in cutting services and increasing patients' charges were set by the CDU's labour wing, which did not oppose benefit cuts and consumer charges in principle, but made their acquiescence conditional on their being accompanied by measures to ease any possible social hardship (*Soziale Ordnung*, nos. 11–12, 3 December 1987, pp. 8–9; Limbach and Arentz, 1987). Also the Social Committees wanted austerity measures to be accompanied by the introduction of new benefits for the nursing of the severely disabled at the cost of service providers and producers (*Handelsblatt*, 25 March 1987; *FR*, 19 September 1987 and 16 October 1987; Fink, 1987). The financing of nursing care for the disabled by the health insurance funds was in turn opposed by the business organisations and their allies in the coalition – as well as by the funds themselves.

When the Social Committees got wind of the proposals being considered and likely to be made by the coalition commission, they found them alarming. One such proposal was that 20 per cent consumers' charges be introduced for all prescription drugs and medical aids (glasses, hearing-aids, and so on.) The Labour Minister was warned that such a reform, aimed at appeasing the clientele of the FDP, would unleash a 'storm of indignation' in the Christian Democratic parties (*FR*, 16 October 1987 and 9 October 1987; *Handelsblatt*, 4 October 1987).[2] This warning shot across the minister's bows obviously achieved its intended effect. Shortly afterwards the idea of compelling the pharmaceuticals industry to make a DM1.7 billion 'solidarity contribution' to the reform was conceived in the Labour Ministry. The December reform package agreed by the coalition leaders contained no reference to percentage consumer charges for prescription drugs and medical aids, but instead foresaw the introduction of a system of fixed prices (*Festbeträge*) or subsidies (see below).

The December coalition agreement also envisaged the abolition of death grants, increases in consumers' charges for dentures and orthodontic dental treatment, restrictions on fund financing of taxi trips to doctors and hospitals and various other, in financial terms less significant, measures restricting the range of products and services financed by the insurance funds and increasing consumer charges. However in exchange for the other planned measures affecting service providers and producer groups, and the proposed introduction of fund-financed nursing care for the disabled, the labour wing of the CDU was evidently prepared to acquiesce in these cuts and support the bill as a whole. Its social policy spokesman rated it as a big success that the demands from the doctors, the pharmaceuticals industry and from within the coalition for the introduction of percentage consumer charges for prescription drugs had been resisted and saw a close correspondence between the social committees' reform proposals and the Labour Ministry's draft bill (Kudella, 1988, p. 6).

The health insurance funds' and trade unions' responses to the benefit and service cuts proposed in the December coalition agreement were relatively moderate. It was noticeable that the insurance funds, although they expressed their opposition to the death grant and denture charge provisions, were less perturbed by these proposals than by the absence of complementary measures to reduce overcapacities in the health system – on which they laid the primary blame for rising costs. The sickness funds were not opposed in principle to benefit and service cuts, but wanted them to fulfil the same criteria stipulated by the labour wing of the CDU (*Kölner Stadt-Anzeiger*, 5 February 1987). By adopting the latter's line on benefit and service cuts issues, the funds may have wanted to try to strengthen their position in the coalition negotiations. The restrained reaction of the local insurance funds to the proposals may also have been influenced by the employers represented in their supervisory organs – they did not view higher consumer charges as constituting the right approach to solving the problems of the statutory health insurance, but regarded them as acceptable components of a 'balanced' reform (*Handelsblatt*, 9 November 1987). The main trade union federation (DGB – *Deutscher Gewerkschaftsbund*) spoke of a 'massive shift' towards privatised health care if the Labour Ministry's January bill was to become law, but nonetheless stopped short of opposing the bill in its entirety. This may have been because the unions welcomed some proposals, such as those aimed at cutting prescription drugs spending. The latter measures however were strongly opposed by the Chemical Industry Employees' Union (*IG Chemie*), which feared they would bring about job losses in the pharmaceuticals industry (*Handelsblatt*, 20 January 1988). Compared with those of providers' and producer groups' organisations, union and insurance funds' reactions to the coalition's initial reform plans remained mild.

The different strength of the consumers and producers lobbies' protests against the proposed reform may help to explain what then happened to the Labour Minister's bill on its way to the Cabinet. The bill itself had contained an important amendment to the December coalition agreement – hospital patient charges which, according to the December agreement were to be abolished, were now to be retained: As late as October 1987, the Labour Minister had rejected these charges as having no cost-dampening impact and promised their abolition (*Soziale Ordnung*, nos. 11–12, 3 December 1987, pp. 13–14). In coalition negotiations over his reform bill, and despite his insistence that the bill was already a coalition compromise whose main elements could no longer be changed, the minister conceded to the FDP the introduction of percentage consumer charges for prescription drugs on which no fixed price (see above) could be agreed by 1991 (*Handelsblatt*, 9 March 1988; *Der Spiegel*, no. 15, 11 April 1988 and no. 16, 18 April 1988).

This was a most significant change in the original bill, not least because the amount of prescription drugs that would be subject to fixed prices was uncertain (see below). The CDU's labour wing had prematurely celebrated the Labour Minister's victory over the pharmaceuticals industry lobby, the doctors, and the advocates of consumer charges in the coalition. Its response to the revised bill was correspondingly much more cool than it had been to the original Labour Ministry version – while the Christian Democrats' small and medium-sized businesses' association, which shared the FDP's stance on the prescription drugs issue and had been a co-sponsor of the abolition of death grants, professed to be well satisfied with it (*FR*, 2

May 1988; *Ärztezeitung*, 2 May 1988 and *Handelsblatt*, 14 July 1988). Now fears grew in the CDU–CSU that the reform could be widely seen as socially too inequitable; the coalition's plans were in fact unpopular in the electorate (*Der Spiegel*, no. 18, 2 May 1988; *Die Welt*, 1 June 1988). The CDU–CSU Parliamentary party indicated that the Christian Democrats wanted to moderate both the proposed abolition of the death grant, which was considered to be a potentially highly emotive issue, and the increased patients' charges for dentures (*FAZ*, 26 July 1988). In their final talks on reform, the coalition leaders agreed to retain death grants for existing members of the health insurance funds, but eliminate them for newcomers. However, to buy these concessions from the FDP, the Labour Minister had to acquiesce in the doubling of hospital patients' charges (those which he had initially wanted to abolish completely (*SDZ* and *FR*, 14 October 1988).

The reform's saving grace for the labour wing of the CDU was undoubtedly the introduction of health insurance fund-financed home nursing care for the most severely disabled (see above). This issue had been on the agenda since the previous Parliamentary period. The Bavarian and other state governments had wanted this service to be financed by the federal government (*Der Spiegel*, no. 42, 13 October 1986; *Handelsblatt*, 16 February 1987). The federal Finance Minister refused. Neither could the states force the federal government to foot the bill nor the federal government force the states, but both together could unload the costs of the new service on the health insurance funds. Despite the united protests of the funds, the employers' organisations (which feared the volume of the spending cuts yielded by the benefit and service cuts would be exceeded by the cost of the new scheme) and the organised health care suppliers (which saw in it a new competitor in the already intensifying conflict for health insurance resources), the coalition proposed to do precisely that. However the FDP wanted to acquiesce in this step only if, at the same time, some measures were agreed to cut hospital costs.

The Hospital Sector

The conflict lines within the coalition on hospital sector reforms ran in quite different directions to those on benefits and services issues. The main adversaries of the latter – the labour wing of the CDU and the Labour Minister on the one side, the FDP and the pro-business currents in the CDU–CSU on the other – were united, together with the health insurance funds and other supplier groups in the health system, in the goal of extracting savings from the hospital sector. The opposition to hospital reforms was led by the state governments which, through their veto rights in the *Bundesrat*, had hitherto managed to disembowel all federal legislation aimed at containing rising hospital costs, and above all by the CSU, which could represent the regional interests of Bavaria *in* the federal coalition. The conflict over reforms in the hospital sector was thus principally a central–local one.

The FDP's strategy of making its acquiescence in the introduction of home nursing care for the severely disabled conditional on the implementation of hospital sector economies, seems to have rested on the calculation that the (political) costs to the state governments of hospital reforms could be balanced out by the benefits which fund financed care for the disabled could yield in the form of lower local government supplementary benefits expenditure, a substantial portion of which is financed indirectly by the states (*Handelsblatt*, 8 October 1987). At the same time the Liberals may have hoped that the Chancellor and the Labour Minister could mobilise the acquiescence of the Christian Democratic-led state governments in hospital reforms with the threat that the reform as a whole might otherwise collapse. Right from the beginning of the coalition negotiations however, the CSU displayed little preparedness to accept any substantial reforms in the hospital sector.[3] As early as September 1987 it was reported that the state governments' opposition would stymie the FDP's efforts to include the hospitals in the reform project (*FAZ*, 23 September 1987). The party leaders quickly agreed to postpone any major hospital sector legislation until the Labour Ministry had received a report it had commissioned on the impact of the hospital financing and fees legislation which the government had enacted in 1984 and 1985 (Webber, 1988, pp. 55–6 and Döhler, 1987, pp. 34–7).

The few interim measures proposed to contain hospital costs were themselves controversial enough however. These envisaged the formulation of hospital price-lists, which assisted doctors who are now required to refer patients to the cheapest hospitals. They also tied hospital expenditure to the growth of the insurance funds' revenues, which would have undermined the principle that hospital fees should cover their costs. These price-lists also enabled health insurance funds to refuse to sign contracts with uneconomical or, in their view, superfluous hospitals, but only with the state governments' consent. The latter condition, on which the CSU insisted, was marketed by the Labour Ministry as a step in the right direction since it would shift the burden of proof that a hospital was efficient or necessary on to the states (BMASO, 1987, p. 13).

Whereas the insurance funds all regarded these proposals as likely to be completely ineffective, the state and local governments viewed them as unacceptable or even, as in the case of the rural local governments' association, 'appalling' (*Handelsblatt*, 8 March 1988). Equally, all the state health and labour ministers were united in rejecting any weakening of the states' planning competences in the hospital sector (*FR* and *FAZ*, 26 February 1988). The repeated threat of the FDP that it would withdraw its support for the introduction of home nursing care for the severely disabled if the CSU and the states did not acquiesce in cost-cutting hospital reforms proved to be of no avail (*FAZ*, 30 October 1987; *Handelsblatt*, 4 March 1988; *Kölner Stadt-Anzeiger*, 28–9 May 1988). The *Bundesrat* made major amendments to the government's bill in the hospital sector. The principle of cost-covering hospital fees was anchored in the reform law, and it was made more difficult for the health insurance funds to refuse contracts with hospitals which they regarded as uneconomical or superfluous, but which were included in the states' hospital plans (*FAZ*, 11 June 1988). The state governments acquiesced in the drawing-up of hospital price-lists, but no sanctions were foreseen for use against doctors who did not send their patients to the 'cheapest' hospital. The FDP declared that the preconditions for the introduction of insurance fund-financed home nursing care for the disabled which it had stipulated no longer prevailed (*Handelsblatt*, 13 June 1988). Rather than vetoing the new programme however, the FDP in the end insisted, as a *quid pro quo* for its introduction, on new and higher patients' charges, including for hospital stays.

The Pharmaceuticals Manufacturing and Retailing Sectors

In no other sector of the health system were such radical reform proposals made as in pharmaceuticals. In no other sector was the conflict between the reforms' proponents in the government – above all the Labour Minister – and the organised producers so intense. The lines of conflict in the coalition ran principally (as on the issue of benefit cuts and patients' charges) between, on the one hand, the left wing of the CDU and, on the other, the FDP, whose opposition to some proposed reforms was however shared by Christian Democratic-governed states with a strong pharmaceuticals industry. In this sector too, the Labour Minister, although he was partially successful in holding the line on fixed prices, had to accept a far-reaching dilution of his original reform proposals.

The voluntary price-restraint policy agreed by the BPI to ward off the threat of state intervention in 1985 (see above) had been successful in containing price rises, but not in restraining the health insurance funds' outlays for prescription drugs (see table 1). The BPI attributed the increase in spending in 1986, despite almost stable prices, to a rise in the number of prescriptions brought about by increased illness (*Handelsblatt*, 16 March 1987). To try and keep out of the political firing line, the association pledged that the industry would try to restrain price increases for a further year after the expiry of the initial agreement (*SDZ*, 7 June 1987). It opposed radical reforms of the health insurance and any regulation of pharmaceutical prices either by the state or the health insurance funds. The association had long demanded the legal power to negotiate with the funds directory over prices (*Handelsblatt*, 4 July 1987). The industry wanted to retain what it described as the 'last bastion of the market economy' in the health system and what its critics labelled the 'last paradise' of the pharmaceuticals multinationals (Münnich, 1987; *FAZ*, 31 March 1987). The BPI's own health reform proposals centred on percentage consumer charges for prescription drugs, increased price competition among chemists, and halving VAT on prescription drugs in accordance with practices in some other EEC states (*FAZ*, 30 September 1987).

The Labour Minister attributed the rise in prescription drug spending to the firms effectively undermining the price freeze by marketing drugs in larger packets. The first report of a council of experts set up to advise the Concerted Action for the Health System (Webber 1988, pp. 58–9) provided the minister with ample ammunition for a political conflict with the industry, pointing out as it did that pharmaceutical prices were much higher in the FRG than in most other European states, that there was little price competition on the German market and that if the industry could be forced to reduce its very high sales promotion expenditure by a quarter, the health insurance funds could save almost DM1.5 billion (Sachverständigen-rat für die Konzertierte Aktion im Gesundheitswesen 1987, pp. 86–92). Nonetheless, and despite the minister's frequent criticisms of the industry and doctors for rising prescription drugs expenditures during

1986 and 1987, the proposals initially discussed in the coalition reform commission – primarily, it seems, the introduction of percentage consumer charges – were positively industry friendly. Up until autumn 1987, according to the BPI chairman, there had been a consensus between the industry and the coalition, for example, that consumer charges should constitute the top reform priority (*Handelsblatt*, 19 May 1988).

The BPI chairman's remark that the industry had not reckoned with the Social Committees of the CDU, supports the conclusion that the Labour Minister was forced by the CDU's labour wing to make an abrupt change of course on this issue (*ibid.*) All at once the idea of introducing percentage consumer charges was dropped (as it turned out, temporarily) from the agenda and the talk was instead focused on the introduction of fixed prices for prescription drugs (see above). Since the introduction of the system was expected to take some years, the proposal was made that a (compulsory) DM1.7 billion 'solidarity contribution' be levied on the industry. These revenues were to flow to the health insurance funds.

The 'solidarity contribution' was explicitly designed to forestall the accusation that the health insurance reform was socially inequitable (*Der Spiegel*, no. 46, 9 November 1987 and no. 51, 14 December 1987; *Wirtschaftswoche*, no. 46, 6 November 1987 and no. 52, 18 December 1987). The BPI viewed it as no accident that the sum of DM1.7 billion was equivalent to the savings which had been calculated would be achieved by the imposition of a 20 per cent consumer charge on prescription drugs (*Handelsblatt*, 4 November 1987). The BPI and its members' reactions to the Labour Minister's new proposals were ferocious. In the following weeks and months, the BPI and the firms warned that the industry's turnover from sales to members of the statutory health insurance would be cut by the proposals by 40 per cent, that its research and development spending might have to be cut by a half, and that 10 000 (of 90 000) jobs in the industry might be lost as small and medium-sized firms went bankrupt and the big firms transferred their investments abroad. The 'solidarity contribution' demanded by the Labour Minister was described as a 'dramatic attack on the market economy' which, the BPI maintained, would be contested before the Federal Constitutional Court (*Handelsblatt*, 30 October 1987 and 4 November 1987; *FR*, 4 November 1987).

The possibility that the government would make such an attempt was however precluded from the outset by the FDP. For the Liberals, a legally-imposed drugs price freeze or cut was not negotiable (*FAZ*, 30 October 1987; *Handelsblatt*, 2 November 1987). Since the Labour Minister must have anticipated that the FDP would reject the proposal, at least in this form, it is conceivable that he saw in it a bargaining counter to secure the Liberals' acquiescence in the fixed drug prices regime and–or that of the pharmaceuticals industry in continued ('voluntary') price restraint (*Die Zeit*, no. 48, 20 November 1987; *Handelsblatt*, 7 December 1987).

As the conflict over the health insurance reform progressed, the likelihood that the pharmaceuticals industry would make any kind of short term 'contribution' to cost-containment became increasingly remote. In the December talks between the coalition leaders, the Christian Democratic parties supported their Labour Minister and a compromise was reached whereby he was empowered to *negotiate* a *'voluntary'* contribution from the industry. The Minister said that the industry was 'obliged' to share the burden of the reform and that if it refused to do so, the reform would collapse (*FAZ*, 4 December 1987). In January when the Labour Ministry's draft bill was published, it was announced that not the Labour Minister, but rather the Chancellor would negotiate with the industry over the contribution. However the (three) company executives with whom the Chancellor negotiated had no mandate from the BPI to make a deal with the government, and the Chancellor's engagement on behalf of the Labour Minister proved to be short-lived (*Der Spiegel,* 7 March 1988). By the time the Cabinet approved the revised reform bill in April, the pharmaceuticals industry's 'solidarity contribution' was no longer mentioned – although the Labour Minister claimed that he might revive the issue, depending on the development of prescription drug prices and the impact of the proposed flat-rate prices once they had been introduced (*FAZ*, 28 April 1988).

In contrast to the 'solidarity contribution', the fixed prices concept for prescription drugs was supported – initially – by all the members of the coalition commission, including those of the FDP, whose chief social policy expert regarded himself as its co-inventor (*Handelsblatt*, 2 November 1987 and 29 March 1988). According to this proposal, the federal committee of insurance doctors and health insurance funds would identify identical and comparable drugs, for which the funds would then determine a fixed price or subsidy. If the consumer wanted a drug which cost more, he would have to pay the difference between the fixed and the actual price. This method of price-determination was expected to lead to a substantial fall in average prices. The 'traditional' pharmaceuticals industry feared that this system would place it at a considerable competitive disadvantage vis-à-vis the generic product manufacturers, who were in any case capturing a growing share of the market.

According to the December coalition agreement, fixed prices were to be introduced first for drugs with identical ingredients and then extended to cover the entire (prescription) drugs market (BMASO, 1987, p. 12). But this consensus did not last very long. In early 1988 various FDP regional parties, including the biggest, the North Rhine–Westphalian, began to put the federal Parliamentary party under pressure to have the fixed-price provisions of the reform modified. In particular, fixed prices should be applied only to drugs with identical ingredients (roughly one-third of those on the market) (*Handelsblatt*, 9 March 1988; *FAZ*, 9 April 1988).

The Parliamentary party's chairman and its social policy experts defended the bill against its intra-party critics (*Handelsblatt*, 11 March 1988). The Liberals' social policy spokesman argued that if the pharmaceuticals industry prevented the introduction of the fixed prices, it would be harder for the FDP to resist future interventionist measures in the sector (*Handelsblatt*, 4 March 1988).

The party leadership did not hold this line very much longer. The party's economic policy spokesman soon changed sides on the fixed drug prices issue and was joined by the party chairman and Economics Minister – both had belonged to the FDP team which had negotiated and approved the original coalition agreement envisaging the determination of fixed prices for all prescription drugs (*Handelsblatt*, 25 March 1988). The change in their stance may be attributable to the outcome of the state election which had meanwhile taken place in Baden-Württemberg, where the CDU had defended its absolute majority with an 'anti-Bonn' campaign, and the FDP with a 'pro-Bonn' campaign had recorded its worst-ever result. Following the election, the FDP leadership had resolved to display greater loyalty to the party's clientele and less to the coalition, and to do more to try to implement traditional party policies in the health reform (*Wirtschaftswoche*, no. 13, 25 March 1988; *Handelsblatt*, 25 March 1988).

Conceivably the Labour Minister was saved from being confronted by a complete about-face of the FDP on the fixed-prices issue by the Liberals' social policy experts' continued support for the concept (Cronenberg, in Deutscher Bundestag 1988b, pp. 5291–2). However this support had become more limited and conditional. In the government bill agreed in April, it was stipulated that the pharmaceuticals manufacturers and the chemists should be incorporated in the process of determining the fixed prices, and that for drugs on which the patents had expired, such prices could first be set two years after the patents had lapsed. The latter constituted a conciliatory gesture towards the major pharmaceuticals firms, which had meanwhile expressed their willingness to accept the fixed-price model in return for improved patent protection (*Wirtschaftswoche*, no. 13, 25 March 1988).

The FDP social policy experts' support for fixed prices had become more limited or partial in so far as they wanted these prices to be set only for drugs with identical ingredients (Cronenberg in Deutscher Bundestag 1988b, p. 5191 and *FAZ*, 29 June 1988). On this issue the FDP could reckon with the support of the Christian Democratic state governments, especially those of Hesse (location of the chemicals and pharmaceuticals manufacturer, Hoechst) and Baden-Württemberg (location of numerous small and medium-sized pharmaceuticals firms). If this coalition were to have succeeded in having fixed drug prices limited to those with identical ingredients, the firms could have escaped them simply by making minor changes in the chemical composition of their products. The fixed prices would then have been rendered ineffective (*Der Spiegel*, no. 30, 25 July 1988). At the final coalition summit on the health reform, the Labour Minister held his ground on this issue. However the period within which fixed prices could not be agreed for drugs on which patents had expired was extended, and the coalition parties agreed that pharmaceutical manufacturers could contest decisions as to which fixed prices should apply to which prescription drugs in the courts. For those prescription drugs for which no fixed price had been agreed by 1992, a 15 per cent patients' charge was to be introduced. Past experience suggests that the process of setting fixed drug prices might be accompanied by protracted legal battles. The local health insurance funds expected fixed prices to be accepted for no more than 30 to 50 per cent of all prescription drugs (Ausschuß für Arbeit and Sozialordnung 1988, p. 133). The pharmaceuticals companies reacted to the first fixed prices by increasing the prices of their other drugs, so that the insurance funds lost most of what they gained on either one side or the other (*Der Spiegel*, no. 42, 16 October 1989).

Any weakening of the fixed drug-price component of the health insurance reform benefited not only the (traditional) pharmaceuticals industry, but also the chemists, since they received percentage mark-ups on producer prices. The December coalition agreement envisaged the replacement of percentage by fixed mark-ups. This step had been proposed by the Concerted Action's Council of Experts (see above) and was designed to ensure that chemists no longer had an incentive to sell the most expensive drugs (BMASO, 1987, p. 12). In addition, the price discounts which the pharmacies are obliged to grant the health insurance funds were to be differentiated by pharmacy size. Thus the net volume of the discount increased by some DM200 million.

The chemists' association argued that the introduction of fixed drug prices alone could lead to drops in chemists' turnovers of as much as 40 to 50 per cent (*Handelsblatt*, 10 February 1988). Objections to these provisions of the reform were raised in the FDP (*Handelsblatt*, 3 February 1988 and 9 March 1988). The party's chief social policy expert stated that he would acquiesce in the chemists' demands and ensure that the percentage mark-ups on drug prices were retained (*Handelsblatt*, 4 March 1988). The Labour Minister likewise intimated his preparedness to forego the introduction of fixed mark-ups, but wanted to stick to the provision that the value of the chemists' discounts to the insurance funds be increased (BMASO, 1988b, p. 2). However both these provisions of the original agreement were deleted from the bill in the last round of talks among the party leaders. The health insurance reform left the pharmaceuticals retailing sector untouched, except in so far as chemists' turnovers were affected by the introduction of fixed drug prices.

The Doctors and Dentists

The Christian–Liberal coalition's reform plans for the ambulatory sector were, for the most part, as limited as its original proposals for the pharmaceuticals sector had been radical. This reflected the concern of all forces in the coalition to avoid a confrontation with the private-practising doctors of the kind that had been instrumental in defeating Labour Minister Blank's reform efforts in the early 1960s (see above). However those proposals which did affect the doctors were exposed to strong attack from the voluntary private-practising doctors' pressure groups and more tempered criticism from the (public-law) insurance doctors' associations. The latter pursued a strategy of limited conflict vis-à-vis the government, insofar as they stopped short of rejecting the reform project outright and refrained from trying to mobilise the doctors against it. This strategy was conditioned by their dependence on the government to take action to limit the increase in the number of doctors. It was effective to the extent that the original reform proposals which most antagonised the doctors were all substantially diluted – primarily through the intervention of the FDP. However the reform contained no measures to combat the 'over-supply' of either. The proposed reforms in dental care were more radical than those foreseen in general ambulatory medical care, and the organised dentists' opposition to them more strident than that of the doctors. Since the dental care reforms actually corresponded closely to the dentists' associations' own demands, it is probable however that their objective was not to prevent their implementation, but rather to subject individual doctors' *and dentists'* fees claims to closer monitoring and scrutiny by the insurance funds (see below).

In 1983 and 1984, following the expiry of a prior fees self-restraint agreement, the growth of health insurance spending on ambulatory care (doctors' fees) had accelerated (see table 1). When in 1984–5 the expenditure trend in the statutory health insurance revived the threat of state intervention, the insurance doctors' federal association (KBV – *Kassenärztliche Bundesvereinigung*) reacted with a fresh offer of voluntary fees restraint, initially for the period up to the middle of 1986, coupling it with a plea for the government to do something to curb the number of doctors and–or medical students. The government obliged with a bill – enacted in 1986 – enabling the insurance doctors' associations and insurance funds to prevent doctors setting up new practices in districts where they diagnosed a surplus of doctors (see BMASO, 1985, pp. 7–9). The KBV hereupon consented to keep the growth in the overall budget for doctors' fees in line with that of wages and salaries for two more years, and indicated its willingness to reform the doctors' fees schedule to make the provision of personal services more lucrative, and that of technical services less so. Such a reform had been debated in the FRG since at least the mid-1970s and was to be claimed by the association subsequently as its 'advance contribution' to the health insurance reform, and was presented as proof that state intervention in the determination of doctors' fees was unnecessary. The Labour Minister pledged before the 1987 elections that – over and beyond its 1986 legislation – the government would take further steps to try to reduce the number of doctors (*FAZ*, 8 December 1986).

On this issue the insurance doctors' associations were also backed by the health insurance funds. However the Labour Minister's capacity to honour his side of the 'bargain' with the insurance doctors was extremely limited. In 1961 the Federal Constitutional Court had declared the hitherto existing absolute limits on the number of insurance doctors to be unconstitutional. Concrete proposals to limit the number of doctors revolved around cutting the capacity of the universities to accept medical students, and making it more difficult for qualified doctors to set up private practices – for example, by extending the period of practical training they must undergo before they could be authorised to treat insurance fund patients. This the Labour Ministry intended to do – contrary to the original intention and against the opposition of the federal Youth, Family, Health and Women's Ministries – by retaining a special probationary period for private-practising *insurance* doctors after the long-planned introduction in 1988 of a new practical traineeship for graduate medical students.

The latter measure might provide the insurance doctors with some temporary respite from new competitors, but could hardly be expected to stem the growth in the number of insurance doctors – other than in the short term. Given the constraints imposed by constitutional law, this goal would best be achieved by cutting the number of medical students, which had doubled in the decade up to the middle of the 1980s (*Der Spiegel*, no. 8, 17 February 1986).

The competence for policy-making on this issue lies however with the state educational and science ministries (whose priorities and client groups differ from those of the Federal Labour Ministry). Apart from securing the retention of the probationary period for insurance doctors, all that the Labour Minister could do to try to cut the number of medical students was to appeal to the state education ministers to reduce the capacity of the university medical schools (*FAZ*, 30 March 1988 and *Ärztezeitung*, 28 April 1988). It was thus little wonder that the critics of the KBV's allegedly too moderate stance vis-à-vis the proposed reform, claimed that the government had not honoured the doctors' fees policy restraint (*FAZ*, 10 May 1988).

The doctors' reactions to the December 1987 coalition agreement and the subsequent draft bill were conditioned not only by what they did not contain (the KBV also lamented the absence of radical reforms of the hospital sector), but also by a series of proposals which the association described as encroaching on doctors' professional autonomy and leading to an 'excessively bureaucratic' regulation of ambulatory treatment (*FR* and *FAZ*, 7 December 1987; *FAZ*, 13

January 1988). It objected in particular to (1) proposals to revamp the control doctors' service (VÄD – *Vertrauensärztlicher Dienst*) and turn it into a medical advisory organ for the health insurance funds; (2) making it possible for hospitals to diagnose and treat patients before and after hospitalisation; (3) setting prescription expenditure guidelines for doctors; (4) increasing and regulating by law the number of inspections of doctors' accounts. The latter provision was clearly aimed at combatting fraudulent claims by doctors for treatment never rendered; according to one source, state prosecutors had carried out over 5000 investigations of doctors on this count in the five-year period up to 1986 (*Der Spiegel*, no. 16, 18 April 1988).

Following the publication of the draft reform bill in January 1988, the federal insurance doctors' association's opposition to the reform stiffened. It threatened to suspend its erstwhile policy of collaborating with the Labour Ministry (*FAZ*, 13 January 1988). The hardening of the association's position on the reform may have been a response to pressures originating from the voluntary private-practising doctors' pressure-groups. The biggest of these, the *Hartmannbund*, had been much more unequivocal in its rejection of the proposed reform. In February 1988, together with the equivalent dentists' pressure group (see below), it launched a large-scale propaganda campaign against the reform which, it was suggested, would introduce a nationalised health service through the back door (*FR*, 11 February 1988).

The federal insurance doctors' association's threatened 'boycott' of the Labour Ministry did not however eventuate. Its chairman saw it as a success of this policy of collaborating with the Ministry on the reform that most of the proposals were substantially modified when the bill was approved by the Cabinet between January and April. Plans to strengthen the control-doctors' service were weakened by providing for the bulk of the service's work to be performed by doctors on a commission basis rather than by permanent medical staff. The provision of ambulatory care by the hospitals was no longer to be regulated in the reform law itself, but by collective agreements to be negotiated between the hospitals, the health insurance funds and the insurance doctors' associations. The original provisions concerning doctors' prescriptions were moderated so that the envisaged guidelines would not be so restrictive, and that the doctors would not have to be so fearful of having their prescription behaviour scrutinised if they did not stick within them (Zöllner, 1988, pp. 60–7). Moreover the original proposal, that random surveys of the accounts of five per cent of insurance doctors be carried out every three months by committees consisting of representatives of the insurance doctors' associations and the health insurance funds, was changed so that now only two per cent of the doctors would be investigated. At the annual German doctors' conference, the federal insurance doctors' association's chairman described the new bill as 'clearly more favourable' for the doctors than its predecessor (*Ärztezeitung*, 10 May 1988 and 11 May 1988; *FR*, 10 May 1988). Not the provisions of the health insurance reform, but rather the number of doctors seemed to be viewed as the main problem now confronting the medical profession (*Deutsches Ärzteblatt*, no. 23, 9 June 1988, pp. 1170–1).

The efforts within the coalition to modify the reform bill's provisions to make it more acceptable to the private-practising doctors had been spearheaded by the FDP. The Liberals' social policy specialist had already intervened in the early stages of the drafting of the bill in the Labour Ministry, and secured the abandonment of proposals to reduce the autonomy of the white-collar workers' insurance funds and that of the insurance doctors' associations vis-à-vis the health insurance funds and the Labour Ministry. These were measures on which the FDP, Cronenberg told the Labour Minister, was not prepared to entertain any compromises (*Dienst für Gesellschaftspolitik*, no. 1, p. 7 January 1988). He likewise took the credit for the modification of the proposed measures to reorganise the control doctors' service (Deutscher Bundestag, 1988b, p. 5290). Insurance doctors' leaders attributed the 'decisive improvements' in the proposed reform to the FDP (*Deutsches Ärzteblatt*, no. 39, 29 September 1988, p. 1838 and no. 23, 9 June 1988, p. 1170). These 'improvements' were so far-reaching that the insurance doctors' lobbying during the Parliamentary phase of the decision-making process concentrated largely on a single issue – that of the number of quarterly investigations of doctors' claims (*Deutsches Ärzteblatt*, no. 23, 9 June 1988, p. 1171 and no. 39, 29 September 1988, p. 1838; *FR*, 10 May 1988). Here too the FDP's main social policy spokesman pledged to try to persuade the Christian Democrats not to regulate the issue in the bill itself, but rather to leave this task to the doctors' associations and health insurance funds to work out amongst themselves (*Deutsches Ärzteblatt*, no. 39, 29 September 1988, p. 1838; Deutscher Bundestag, 1988b, p. 5290; *Handelsblatt*, 3 February 1988).

Compared with that of its doctors' counterpart, the Federal

Insurance Dentists' Association's (KZBV – *Kassenzahnärztliche Bundesvereinigung*) condemnation of the government's reform plans was much more unequivocal. The proposals relating to dental care were described as unsocial, or so interventionist as to undermine the free dental profession (*FAZ*, 21 January 1988). The main target of the former criticism was the proposal to increase patient charges for dentures and the related dental treatment. However this and other proposals in the Labour Ministry's bill actually corresponded quite closely to the association's own reform 'programme', which demanded the general introduction of patients' charges, coupled with the transition to a system whereby dentists would bill patients for dental treatment (*Handelsblatt*, 21 October 1986). Moreover the dentists could expect to compensate somewhat for loss of turnover through these measures by offering more prophylactic treatment, for which provisions in the reform bill were to provide stronger incentives. It is likely that the dentists' lobby was more disturbed by the proposals the association attacked as being too *dirigiste*. Apart from the proposals concerning the regular random sampling and investigation of claims, which affected insurance dentists as well as insurance doctors, the Labour Ministry's bill contained a provision which would have empowered the Ministry to set the fees for certain kinds of dental treatment negotiated between the dentists' associations and the health insurance funds (*FAZ*, 21 January 1988 and 20 May 1988; *Ärztezeitung*, 19 May 1988). The federal dentists' association clearly viewed this provision as constituting the thin end of a dangerous wedge (*FAZ*, 21 January 1988).

The greater (at least verbal) militancy of the KZBV, compared with that of the companion doctors' association, may be attributable to two factors. Firstly, owing to the restricted capacity of the universities to train dentists, there has been no growth in the number of dentists compared to that of doctors. There was hence no comparable pressure on the dentists to keep 'on-side' with the Labour Ministry in the hope that this would increase the likelihood of legislation being enacted to control entry to the professional labour market. Secondly, in elections in 1985–6, and after the introduction of a new fees schedule which had been negotiated with the health insurance funds and brought substantial cuts in fees for certain kinds of dental treatment, the insurance dentists had elected a new, more militant leadership, which had adopted a tougher bargaining position vis-à-vis both the funds and the federal government. Thus in 1987 the dentists had stymied a Concerted Action recommendation on the overall increase in dentists' fees, and staged what was in effect a one-day strike against a new government fees schedule for private dental patients.

To be sure, the more militant posturing and rhetoric of the dentists' (compared with the doctors') association had not secured the dentists' bigger increases in dental care budgets in the years immediately prior to the health insurance reform (see table 1). The moderate growth in the cost of dental care and dentures however had permitted the dentists, like the doctors, to argue that they had made their contributions to the health insurance reform, so to speak, 'in advance' (*Handelsblatt*, 23 September 1987). These sacrifices, in the dentists' view, had not been honoured by the government in the health insurance reform (*FAZ*, 18 May 1988). The only reform proposals in the Labour Ministry's January bill which could reasonably be described as radical however, went in the very direction which not much earlier the KZBV itself had demanded. The otherwise modest character of the dental care reform proposals reflected the Labour Minister's perception, shared by the health insurance funds, that the need for reforms in this sector was not as pressing as in the hospital and pharmaceuticals sectors (*SDZ*, 18–19 November 1986; *FR*, 23 October 1986; *Handelsblatt*, 5 December 1986).

The proposal to increase the number of random investigations of practitioners' claims was substantially modified before the Labour Ministry's bill reached the Cabinet (see above). The provision empowering the Ministry to set dentists' fees for certain services disappeared altogether. On this issue, as on the former two, the FDP rallied to the cause of the medical professions. The deletion of this proposal from the reform was one of the main changes demanded in the original bill by the party's main social policy spokesman and the North Rhine–Westphalian FDP (*Handelsblatt*, 3 February 1988 and 9 March 1988). In advertisements seeking donations in the professional press, the FDP had emphasised its role as a champion of dentists' interests (*Der Spiegel*, no. 10, 7 March 1988). But also the Bavarian CSU had objected to the Labour Ministry's usurping the regulatory powers of the 'joint self-administration' for dental care.

As in the case of the pharmaceuticals sector, the FDP (this was the view, at any rate, of the KBV leadership) was the driving force in the process by which the original proposals for reforms in the ambulatory medical (including dental) care sector were diluted. What is striking however, when one compares them with those relating to the pharmaceuticals (and medical aids) sectors or indeed the hospitals, is that even the *initial* proposals to reform ambulatory medical and dental care provision were for the most part quite marginal. Contrary to the case in the other sectors, hardly any reforms were proposed, for example, to strengthen the hand of the health insurance funds in the process of price (fees) determination and infrastructural planning. Certainly the FDP's preparedness to entertain 'anti-doctor' or anti-dentist' reforms was more limited than that of the Labour Minister and the CDU. However, for all the disagreements in the coalition over the details of the ambulatory care reform proposals, there was still a fairly broad consensus within the coalition that there should be no health insurance reform 'against the doctors'.

Why did the government eschew attempting to reform the health insurance 'against the doctors' from the outset? Conceivably the government's concern to steer clear of a confrontation with the insurance doctors was the product of a mixture of motives. One may be, and here the failure of the CDU Labour Minister Blank's attempts to reform the health insurance in the 1960s served as a forbidding example, that all three coalition parties feared that a major conflict with the doctors might incur heavy electoral costs, not so much through doctors striking or withdrawing their electoral support from the government as through their being able to mobilise public opinion against the government. In addition the coalition politicians involved in the decision-making process may have feared that if the government antagonised the doctors too greatly, this might lead to the formation of a united front of producer group opposition to the government and diminish their chances of being able to implement other central components of the proposed reform – some of which presupposed the doctors collaborating with the health insurance funds.

The coalition did however have one trump card it could play against the doctors: the power of whether or not to undertake or support measures to reduce the future number of (private-practising) doctors. Had it so wished, it presumably could have used this to try to secure the doctors' associations' acquiescence in reforms which they otherwise might have tried to resist, or to resist more strongly (although the doctors regarded the former measures as a reward for the fees restraint they had already exercised). Since the attempts to reform health insurance in the 1960s, the 'over-supply' of doctors had changed the 'strategic situation' of the organised medical profession

(Müller, 1985). The principal motive of the coalition's policy of refraining from attempting major reforms affecting the doctors and dentists may rather have been that, in the ambulatory care sector, it perceived no problems which made radical solutions (politically) necessary or at least no need for reforms which entailed incalculable political risks. For the coalition the major objective of the reform was to cut the level of health insurance contributions. Therefore the need for reform was most acute in those sectors in which costs had risen most rapidly. Compared with other spending titles, the cost of doctors' and dentists' fees to the health insurance funds had risen very moderately under the Christian-Liberal government (see table 1). Not just the coalition but also – and this indicates that the coalition's policy of not trying to reform the health insurance 'against the doctors' was not merely dictated by political opportunism – the local health insurance funds were satisfied with the existing institutional arrangement for the regulation of ambulatory medical care (Deutscher Bundestag, 1988a, pp. 134–5; Ausschuß für Arbeit und Sozialordnung, 1988, p. 132).

After the health reform debate gathered new momentum in the FRG in 1985, no producer group was as adept as the insurance doctors at 'not drawing (unfavourable) attention' to itself (see above). Despite the growing numbers of insurance doctors, their associations acquiesced most years in relatively low increases in the overall budget for doctors' fees – which implied reductions in doctors' per capita real incomes. Moreover the KBV had first agreed to, and then pushed through, a reform of the doctors' fees schedule which, in line with the Labour Minister's views, increased the value of personal services and decreased that of technical services, and implied relative cuts in incomes for some groups of specialists. This pattern of behaviour corresponded to the KBV's past tactic of offering 'voluntary' monetary sacrifices in order to stave off malevolent, or encourage benevolent, state intervention (Webber, 1988, pp. 15–16). But if all the supplier groups in the health system were aware of the political advantages of 'not drawing attention' to themselves during the reform debate, as Forster argues (1985), why were the insurance doctors able to pursue this strategy more effectively and successfully than the others?[4]

The most plausible explanation of the insurance doctors' greater capacity to pursue such a strategy relates to the peculiar structure of the insurance doctors' (and dentists') associations. In contrast to the interest-organisations of the pharmaceutical industry, the chemists, the hospitals and the manufacturers of medical aids and supplies, the insurance doctors' associations have compulsory members, can (must) bargain directly with the health insurance funds and – possessing as they do public-law status – can implement bargains reached at the centre (with the government or the health insurance funds) vis-à-vis their membership, if need be by reducing doctors' pay per service rendered. The hospitals' association (*Deutsche Krankenhausgesellschaft*) has neither compulsory members nor the capacity to implement centrally-negotiated bargains with the health insurance funds or the federal government vis-à-vis its members (Schwefel and Leidl, 1988). It in fact opposed proposals in the original reform bill which it claimed implied a stronger centralisation of bargaining between the hospitals and the funds (*Handelsblatt*, 25 February 1988).

Similarly, despite its adoption of successive 'voluntary' price restraint agreements, the BPI was effectively unable to dampen the growth of prescription drug expenditure. This is not so much a reflection of a failure by the association to influence the price policies of its member firms – although it does not possess any formal sanctions to discipline those which do not adhere to such agreements – as it is of the firms' refusal to allow the association to negotiate with the health insurance funds on 'new' products and drug packet sizes (the factor held responsible for the greater part of the increases in prescription drug spending). On these issues, on which the essence of entrepreneurial autonomy and the firms' capacity to circumvent price-restraint agreements were at stake, the (majority of the) industry was not prepared to give the association a mandate to negotiate with the health insurance funds (Groser, 1986, pp. 223–4; *Handelsblatt*, 24 July 1984; *FAZ*, 19 October 1984).[5]

There is of course no guarantee that the insurance doctors' associations can always reproduce this superior capacity to put their own house in order, and thus avert the danger of radical 'anti-doctor' reforms of ambulatory care through state intervention. The association's leadership must always obtain a mandate to negotiate the necessary bargains with the health insurance funds or the federal government and needs the approval of the association's congress. Furthermore the leadership must defend and justify such bargains to the 'grass-roots' when it is up for (re-)election. The combination of continuing intense competition for resources between different sectors of the health system, the growth in the number of private-practising insurance doctors, the moderate overall growth in the budget for doctors' fees, and the restructuring of the fees schedule for ambulatory care with its concomitant redistribution of income between different groups of doctors, could lead to a radicalisation of insurance doctors. Indeed in 1987 and 1988, with the increasing articulation of discontent with the fees policies of the associations and the formation of dissident doctors' groups campaigning for the adoption of a more aggressive stance vis-à-vis the health insurance funds and the government, there were signs that such a process might be beginning.

The Health Insurance Funds

The structure of the health insurance funds, in particular the issue of whether there should be a single health insurance fund or a multiplicity of (competing) funds, has often been at the heart of conflicts over the statutory health insurance in Germany. However, in the course of the postwar period, the traditional advocates of a unitary health insurance – the local insurance funds, the trade unions and the SPD – gradually reconciled themselves to the so-called 'stratified' (*gegliederte*) or occupationally-based system of statutory health insurance. By the 1980s it was no longer seriously contested. However even the CDU–CSU and the FDP, both traditional defenders of this structure, diagnosed problems arising from it which warranted state intervention.

The most significant of these problems was the big differences in the level of insurance contributions between different insurance funds. In some – economically weak or declining – districts, local fund contributions were almost twice as high as in others which benefited from strong local economies and low rates of unemployment. Such differences were described by the Labour Ministry's health insurance division head as 'intolerable' (*FR*, 12 May 1987). A second was the unequal legal treatment of manual and white-collar workers in the health insurance. Unlike white-collar workers, who may insure themselves with a 'substitute' fund, manual workers were compelled to belong to local or, where they exist, company insurance funds. In the reform debate there were growing demands that all compulsorily-insured persons should be free to choose which (statutory) fund they wished to join. This was an issue, according to one commentator in the early phases of the debate, with which the coalition could no longer put off dealing (Strack, 1987).[6]

The coalition could and did avoid dealing with it, and also

postponed introducing any sweeping measures to try to equalise the level of contributions between different local insurance funds, or between different types of funds. In November 1987 the coalition parties agreed to delay any major reform of the funds' organisation. According to the government, the scope of the changes which an equalisation of the legal status of manual and white-collar workers might bring about, and their potential consequences for the 'stratified' health insurance system, were too unpredictable for this issue to be dealt with for the moment (Deutscher Bundestag, 1988a, p. 143). The postponement of any major reform of the funds was also a reflection of the breadth of the opposition to such a reform. This opposition was located in two main quarters in respect of a financial redistribution between the funds; opposition in the employers' organisations, trade unions, health insurance funds and governments in the economically buoyant (and Christian Democratic-dominated) states; and all the white-collar workers' funds. In regard to the free choice of fund membership, opposition was found in all the various health insurance funds.

The reform bill passed by the Cabinet in April 1988 made it possible for funds of the same type (for example, the *local* funds) to take measures to try to equalise contributions at the *state* level. This proposal itself was weaker than that contained in the Labour Ministry's January draft, especially insofar as it defined more restrictively the circumstances under which such measures could be taken. It could help to moderate relatively large differences in contribution levels between local funds in those states in which economically 'booming' and economically declining areas co-exist, but not the (greater) differences associated with varying levels and trends of economic development between the states. The local health insurance funds had wanted the burden of insuring such 'bad-risk' groups as the unemployed, the disabled and recipients of supplementary benefits to be spread equally across the different kinds of funds, according to the model which had been introduced for pensioners by the Social-Liberal coalition in the 1970s (*Handelsblatt*, 18 August 1987, and 23–4 October 1987). The financially more robust white-collar workers' funds – in unison with the company funds – rejected this demand, arguing that there was little difference between the average contribution levels of the (federally-organised) white-collar and the (regionally-organised) local funds, and that the local funds did not insure proportionately very many more 'bad risks' than they did (*Handelsblatt*, 9 June 1987). The local funds' demand, in their view, was an alibi for their incapacity to reach a consensus on a fund-internal financial redistribution.

Irrespective of the possible merits of the local funds' case for an inter-fund-type equalisation of the burden of insuring 'bad-risk' groups, this latter claim was not far off the mark. At an early stage in the reform debate, it was reported that the Labour Ministry wanted to propose the introduction of an interregional financial redistribution for the local insurance funds (*Handelsblatt*, 6 August 1987). Among the states in relative economic decline, mostly in northern Germany, such an idea could be expected to be welcomed with open arms; the southern states were vehemently opposed (*Der Gelbe Dienst*, no. 25, 25 November 1987). This applied above all to the CDU administration in Baden-Württemberg, which would have been the greatest net loser if such a plan were to have been introduced, where state election was coming up in early 1988 (*Handelsblatt*, 6 August 1987, 18 January 1988, 20 January 1988). The state government's opposition was shared by the state local insurance funds' association (that is to say, by both the regional employers' and trade union organisations) (*Handelsblatt*, 6 August 1987; *Der Gelbe Dienst*, no. 25, 25 November 1987). The Baden-Württemberg local funds reckoned with the support of the Bavarian funds and the CSU, since Bavaria would have been the other main loser through the institution of an interregional financial redistribution scheme (*Handelsblatt*, 6 August 1987).[7] In Hesse, another state governed by the Christian Democrats, the employers' organisations were also opposed to any such scheme, so that on this issue the local insurance funds' association was deadlocked (*Der Gelbe Dienst*, no. 25, 25 November 1987).

The Baden-Württemberg local funds counted on the southern states being able to defeat such a proposal, were it be made, in the *Bundesrat* (*Handelsblatt*, 6 August 1987). In effect the coalition abandoned it earlier – the December 1987 agreement between the three parties provided for no more than *voluntary* interregional financial redistribution measures (BMASO, 1987, p. 8). A scheme providing for redistribution between different kinds of funds was explicitly ruled out. As the reform bill went to the committee stage in the *Bundesrat* however, some CDU-governed states broke the coalition ranks – a majority of the Labour and Social Affairs Committee voted in favour of such a scheme. This vote may be attributable to the fact that most of the Labour and Social Affairs ministers in the CDU-governed states come from the party's labour wing, which is more sympathetic to the concerns of the local insurance funds than other party factions. This was illustrated also by the committee's proposed amendments to the bill to make it more difficult for new company insurance funds to be established and for some white-collar workers to join the white-collar funds (*Die Ortskrankenkasse*, no. 11, p. 323, 1 June 1988). These and other amendments proposed by the committee were strongly attacked by the company and white-collar funds and the FDP. By the time they reached the floor of the *Bundesrat*, coalition discipline on these issues had been restored. The majority in the *Bundesrat* wanted neither a financial redistribution scheme embracing the local and other insurance funds, nor a scheme aimed at narrowing interregional differences in local fund contributions. The axis of the southern German states had won out.

The idea that manual workers be given the same freedom to choose which statutory fund they wanted to join as the white-collar workers enjoyed was evidently viewed by the funds with consternation. Their general opinion seems to have been that such a reform would result in complete chaos and do nothing to contain health insurance costs (*SDZ*, 5 September 87; *Handelsblatt*, 23–4 October 87). The white-collar workers' funds proposed that separate 'substitute' funds be created for manual workers, who could then choose whether to belong to these or to the local funds. They were not interested in recruiting manual workers, presumably because they were not such 'good risks' as white-collar workers and could be burdened by a larger proportion of unemployed or economically non-active members (Strack 1987; *FAZ*, 16 September 1987, 23 September 1987). Such a development was likely if, at the same time as manual workers were given the right to join white-collar funds, the latter were obliged to accept all manual workers wanting to join them. For the local funds, the latter measure was the *sine qua non* of any reform designed to eradicate inequalities in the legal treatment of manual and white-collar workers (Strack, 1987).

Although the various health insurance funds had radically different attitudes on most issues relating to the organisation of health insurance, on this one they formed a negative grand coalition. A reform extending manual workers the same freedom of choice of fund membership as that already possessed by white-collar workers could have brought about a radical change in the distribution of fund membership. The Christian-Liberal coalition could have implemented it only against the more or less intense opposition of the various health insurance funds, which would then have swelled the ranks of the opponents of the reform even further. The difficulties of achieving a compromise on such a reform within the coalition would thereby have been considerable. The labour wing of the CDU was pledged to oppose any measure which threatened the survival of the local insurance funds, while other factions in the CDU–CSU and the FDP, despite its social policy specialist's plea for a 'maximum of freedom of choice' for the compulsorily-insured (*FR*, 22 September 1987), would arguably have attempted to stave off any reform at the expense of the white-collar workers' funds (*Handelsblatt*, 5 July 1988; Sozialausschüsse der CDA, 1987, p. 3). The coalition made do with granting manual workers with incomes above a certain (relatively high) limit, the same right to choose between statutory and private health insurance already enjoyed by high-earning white-collar workers. Of the same 23 million persons insured by the local insurance funds, no more than 337 000, according to the funds' estimate, would have this choice (Daniels, 1988). For the time being at least, only this very small group of manual workers would enjoy the same freedom of health insurance choice as their white-collar counterparts.

CONCLUSION

Unlike the reform attempts of the Christian Democratic Labour Minister Blank in the 1960s, the Christian-Liberal coalition's health insurance reform reached the statute books. Unmoved by the campaigns of the trade unions, the SPD and some voluntary doctors' and dentists' associations, and the pleas of the north German Christian Democratic state governments and the one or other FDP state organisation for the reform bill to be postponed, the coalition stuck to its objective of getting the bill through the Federal Parliament by the end of 1988, so that the unpopular reform would not be a burden for the governing parties in the numerous state and federal elections in 1990.[8] In contrast to the 1960s, the CDU–CSU Parliamentary party did not disintegrate into irreconcilable factions of reform supporters and opponents, and the chancellor did not desert his Labour Minister in the midst of the battle.

However the triumph of Labour Minister Blüm was akin to that of the Old Man in Hemingway's novel. Like the Old Man, he succeeded in landing the big 'fish' that had got away from Blank, but the victory was largely Pyrrhic. In the lobby-infested health insurance 'sea', the 'fish' was so badly molested that by the time he got it ashore not much more than the skeleton was left. For the most part, the original proposals formulated by the coalition commission had themselves not been very adventurous (Gehrmann, 1987). The issues of limiting the number of doctors, containing hospital costs and restructuring the health insurance to moderate differences in the levels of contributions and right the unequal status of manual and white-collar workers were largely put off. The coalition did not want to carry out a reform 'against the doctors'.

Nonetheless, of the proposals that were accepted by the coalition in December 1987, many were savaged beyond recognition during the ensuing year-long political struggle over the reform. Ultimately only three structural reforms were still identifiable in the 'health reform bill': the burden of providing home care for the disabled was to be partially collectivised; the costs of various kinds of medical treatment partially reprivatised; and the prices of (an uncertain proportion of) prescription drugs (and medical aids) were no longer to be set by the 'market', (insofar as this could be said to exist in the statutory health insurance), but by the health insurance funds. In the final coalition compromise on the bill, the CDU–CSU conceded the FDP the introduction of higher or new patients' charges in return for the FDP's acquiescence in the other two measures (*FR* and *SDZ*, 14 October 1988).

Why was little bar the skeleton of the health insurance reform left at the end? This analysis suggests that the *substantive* defeat of the reform may be attributed to the same variables that condemned to failure previous attempts to carry out major reforms of the health insurance. The fact that a reform 'against the doctors' was never contemplated is explained most plausibly by the comparatively modest growth of doctors' fees, which in turn, it was argued, is related to the greater capacity of the insurance doctors' associations, compared with other suppliers' organisations, to make advance fees policy concessions to the government. Through the *Bundesrat* and, at least in the case of Bavaria, through direct representation in the federal coalition, the state governments stymied plans for at least a 'mini-reform' of the hospital sector. The Christian Social or Christian Democratic southern German state governments also coalesced with the trade union, employers' and local health insurance funds' associations in their respective states to help ensure that there would be no interregional financial redistribution scheme for the local funds. Within the federal coalition, the FDP blocked numerous proposals which would have curtailed prerogatives of medical care providers and suppliers (doctors, dentists, chemists, pharmaceutical manufacturers) or succeeded in having them substantially diluted. It retreated from plans in which it had originally acquiesced as the lobbies of the medical professions and the pharmaceuticals industry mobilised against the reform and, for electoral–political reasons the 'cooperative' strategy pursued by the then party leader, vis-à-vis the CDU and CSU, fell into increasing disfavour. In turn the FDP's own latitude, in concert with the neo-liberal forces in the CDU-CSU, to implement a more radical privatisation of the risk of illness was restricted by the labour wing of the CDU, which insisted that benefit cuts and new or higher patients' charges be offset, at least in part, by hardship clauses and the introduction of a new fund-financed programme, which was widely feared to be more costly than the Labour Ministry projected.

The eventual coalition compromise constituted in effect the lowest common denominator between these two health policy 'wings' of the coalition, neither of which could majoritise the other, and given the overall consensus in the coalition that something had to be done to contain growing health care costs, neither was prepared or willing to see the reform attempt collapse completely.

There is much evidence that by the mid-1980s the federal government had effectively forfeited its formal right to make authoritative decisions on health policy issues in favour of negotiating 'deals' with monopolistic or oligopolistic groups of health care providers and financiers (Scharpf, 1988, pp. 22–3). The Christian-Liberal coalition's decision to attempt to reform the health insurance signalled its (at least partial) disillusionment with this mode of steering the health system, and the unilateral suspension (at least by the Labour Minister and in some sectors) of consensus-oriented decision-making. For the Labour Minister, the health insurance reform became a test case for the capacity of 'democratic majorities to facilitate changes' against the opposition of powerful organised interests (Blüm, 1987 and 1988).

According to Müller, the increasing over-capacity in the 'medical industry' had changed the 'strategic situation' of health care providers and suppliers in the FRG since the 1960s, and increased the federal government's attitude to reform the health system (Müller 1985). To be sure, the insurance doctors' associations were prepared to exercise incomes policy self-restraint (but not to acquiesce in structural reforms at their cost) in return for the government's promise of legislation to curb the growing number of doctors, and the Labour Minister's plans via fixed drug prices to reduce the insurance funds' prescription expenditures. This bill would have been inconceivable had it not been for the increasing availability of generic pharmaceutical products. The outcome of the conflicts over the Christian–Liberal health insurance reform indicates however that, under the political and institutional conditions which typically obtain in the FRG, the existing medical care providers and suppliers can still make a thoroughgoing reform of the health system politically impossible.

Notes

1. Thus, the head of the health insurance division in the Labour Ministry said: 'We will not rely . . . only on patients' charges. Our position is that parties – the insurance fund members, the pensioners, the service providers, the health insurance funds and the government – must make a contribution to the reform. . . . Only if all sides make the necessary sacrifices will it be possible to solve the financial problems of the health insurance' (Jung, 1987, pp. 190–1).

2. In the frank description of a leading figure in the labour wing of the CDU, higher or new patients' charges would be acceptable to the labour faction in the CDU–CSU Parliamentary party only provided the 'political damage' that they might cause was not much higher than the monetary savings that they could be expected to yield (*FR*, 16 October 1987).

3. An insight into the reasons for the CSU's intense opposition to a reduction in the state governments' responsibilities concerning the hospital sector is offered by the memoirs of the late and long-time party chairman, Franz-Josef Strauβ, who wrote in his memoirs: 'For the citizens, the hospital sector is one of the most important problems, because it affects, or can affect, everyone. I find in conversations with local government politicians that 40 per cent or more of the points they raise have to do with local hospital problems. I make the same experiences at election rallies. Although there is great interest in the major national and international issues, in European and disarmament policy and policy towards East Germany, the first question everywhere after my speech is mostly about the hospital' (Strauβ, 1989, p. 541).

4. On the problems posed for a 'corporatist' management of the health system by the structure of suppliers' or producers' organisations, see Wiesenthal, 1981, pp. 201–2.

5. In addition to the structure of suppliers' (or financers') organisations, there are other potential obstacles to corporatist techniques of managing the health system in the FRG. A formal price-restraint agreement between the pharmaceuticals industry and the health insurance funds, for example, would require the authorisation of the Federal Cartel office or, if that was not forthcoming, that of the

Federal Economics Minister. Similarly the Federal Labour Minister can not honour the fees policy self-restraint of the insurance doctors by curbing the number of medical students because education policy is the domain of the state governments. Thus the law and the structure of government may stand in the way of the corporatist management of health care.

6.		A third, as it turned out, non-issue relating to the insurance funds had to do with their relations with the service-providers. The autonomy of the substitute funds to negotiate independently with the providers' associations, and so on, and the perceived capacity of the latter to play the different funds off against each other, had long been seen in some quarters as one factor contributing to growing health insurance costs. The Labour Ministry's first draft bill contained some measures which, if implemented, may have curtailed the autonomy of the substitute funds. When the FDP learned of these proposals, which would have been anathema to the private-practising doctors as well as to the substitute funds themselves, its social policy spokesman let the Labour Minister know that they were unacceptable (letter from Dieter-Julius Cronenberg to Norbert Blüm published in *Dienst für Gesellschaftspolitik*, no. 1, 7 January 1988). They were then absent from the bill formulated by the Ministry after the initial coalition agreement over the reform in December 1987.

7.		According to one source (*Ärztezeitung*, 7 December 1987), the CSU was the driving force behind the coalition decision to postpone any major reform of the health insurance funds.

8.		One public opinion survey found that opponents of the health insurance reform outnumbered the supporters by five to three. Barely a half of the supporters of the governing parties were in favour of the reform (*Der Spiegel*, no. 18, p. 37, 2 May 1988).

Bibliography

Ärztezeitung, various issues from 1987 and 1988.

Ausschuß für Arbeit und Sozialordnung (1988) 'Stenographisches Protokoll der öffentlichen Anhörung von Sachverständigen zu dem Gesetzentwurf der Fraktionen der CDU–CSU und FDP zur Strukturreform im Gesundheitswesen' (*Gesundheits-Reformgesetz/GRG*) (Bonn).

BMASO (1985) (Bundesministerium für Arbeit und Sozialordnung), 'Pressemitteilung' (text of speech by Labour Minister Norbert Blüm to the 17th meeting of the Concerted Action for the Health System) (Bonn, 18 November).

BMASO (1987) *Sozialpolitische Informationen*, no. 19 (Bonn, 8 September).

BMASO (1988a) '. . . gute Besserung' (Bonn).

BMASO (1988b) *Sozialpolitische Informationen*, no. 6 (Bonn, 12 April).

Blüm, N. (1987) 'Solidarität und Eigenverantwortung in ein neues Gleichgewicht bringen', *Handelsblatt*, 31 December.

Blüm, N. (1988) 'Der Zug fährt auf den Abgrund zu', *Der Spiegel*, no. 10, pp. 21–23, 7 March.

Daniels, A. (1988) 'Die armen Kassen', *Die Zeit*, no. 4, 22 January.

Der Gelbe Dienst: issue no. 25, 25 November 1987.

Der Spiegel, various issues from November 1985 onwards.

Deppe, H.V. (1987) *Krankheit ist ohne Politik nicht heilbar: Zur Kritik der Gesundheitspolitik* (Frankfurt-am-Main: Suhrkamp).

Deutscher Bundestag (1988a) 'Gesetzentwurf der Fraktionen der CDU/CSU und FDP., Entwurf eines Gesetzes zur Strukturreform im Gesundheitswesen' (*Gesundheits-Reformgesetz – GRG*), *Drucksache* 11/2237, 3 May.

Deutscher Bundestag (1988b) 'Plenarprotokoll', 11. Wahlperiode, 78. Sitzung, Freitag, den 6 May.

Deutsches Ärzteblatt, various issues from 1988.

Dienst für Gesellschaftspolitik, various issues from 1987 and 1988.

Die Ortskrankenkasse, issue no. 11, 6 January 1988.

Die Zeit, various issues from 1987 and 1988.

Döhler, M. (1987) 'Politics versus Institutions: Comparing Health Policy under Neo-Conservative Governments in Britain, the United States and West Germany' (unpublished paper, West Berlin).

FAZ (*Frankfurter Allgemeine Zeitung*), various issues from 1984 onwards.

FR (*Frankfurter Rundschau*), various issues from 1984 onwards.

Fink, U. (1987) 'Wir schlagen Pässe, hinter denen andere herlaufen', *Frankfurter Rundschau*, 22 October.

Forster,J. (1985) 'Die Krankenkassenbeiträge sollen unauffällig steigen', *Süddeutsche Zeitung*, 30 November.

Gehrmann, W. (1987) 'Jetzt kommt das Grobe, *Die Zeit*, no. 46, 6 November.

Gehrmann, W. (1988) Gewaltkur ohne Wirkung, *Die Zeit*, no. 17, 22 April.

Groser, M. (1986) 'Selbstregulierung durch Pharmaverbände', in Boettcher, P. Herder-Dorneich, E. Schenk (eds.), *Jahrbuch für Neue Politische Ökonomie*, 5. Band (Tübingen: J.C.B. Mohr (Paul Siebeck), pp. 211–24.

Handelsblatt, various issues from 1984 onwards.

Jung, K. (1987) 'Zum Erfolg Verurteilt – vor der Reform der gesetzlichen Krankenversicherung', in Bundesminister für Arbeit und Sozialordnung (ed.) . . . *Es begann in Berlin* . . . *Bilder und Dokumente aus der deutschen Sozialgeschichte* (Bonn), pp. 184–93.

KBV (Kassenärztliche Bundesvereinigung) (1987) *Tätigkeitsbericht der Kassenärztlichen Bundesvereinigung 1987* (Cologne).

Kudella, p. (1988) 'Ja zur Strukturreform', *Soziale Ordnung*, no. 4, 30 March, pp. 6–7.

Kölner Stadt-Anzeiger, various issues from 1987 and 1988.

Limbach, E. and H.J. Arentz (1987) 'Christlichsoziale Positionen zur Strukturreform im Gesundheitswesen: Fragen, Anstöße und Forderungen zur vorbereitenden Diskussion' (manuscript, Bonn).

Mittelstandsvereinigung der CDU/CSU: Kieler Beschlüsse (1987), in *Mittelstandsmagazin*, no. 7, July 1987, pp. 54–58.

Müller, A. (1985) 'Krankheitskosten: Soll man handeln oder abwarten?' *Die Welt*, 21 November.

Münnich, F. (1987) 'Arzneimittelpreise sind konstant. Sicht der pharmazeutischen Industrie', *Das Parlament*, no. 11, 14 March.

Sachverständigenrat zur Konzertierten Aktion im Gesundheitswesen (1987) *Jahresgutachten 1987 Medizinische und ökonomische Orientierung: Vor-*

schläge für die Konzertierte Aktion im Gesundheitswesen (Baden-Baden: Nomos).

Scharpf, F.W. (1988) 'Verhandlungssysteme, Verteilungskonflikte und Pathologien der politischen Steuerung' (Discussion Paper no. 1, Max-Planck-Institut für Gesellschaftsforschung, Cologne).

Schwarz, A.P. (1983) *Die Ära Adenauer: Epochenwechsel 1957–1963* (Stuttgart and Wiesbaden: Deutsche Verlagsanstalt/F.A. Brockhaus).

Schwefel, D. and R. Leidl (1988) 'Bedarfsplanung und Selbstregulierung der Beteiligten im Krankenhauswesen', in Gérard Gäfgen (ed.), *Neokorporatismus und Gesundheitswesen* (Baden-Baden: Nomos) pp. 187–207.

SDZ (*Süddeutsche Zeitung*), various issues from 1985 onwards.

Sozialausschüsse der CDA (1987) 'Strukturreform im Gesundheitswesen: Beschluß' (manuscript, Königswinter).

Soziale Ordnung, issue no. 11/12, 3 December 1987.

Strack, G. (1987) 'Auch Arbeiter sollen ihren Gesundheitsschutz frei wählen', *Frankfurter Rundschau*, 22 September.

Strauß, F.J. (1989) *Die Erinnerungen* (West Berlin: Seidler).

Webber, D. (1988) 'The Politics of German Health System Reform: Successful and Failed Attempts at Reform from 1930 to 1984' (unpublished paper presented to the Joint Sessions of the European Consortium of Political Research, Rimini, Italy, April).

Wiesenthal, H. (1981) 'Die Konzertierte Aktion im Gesundheitswesen: Ein korporatistisches Verhandlungssystem der Sozialpolitik', in Ulrich von Alemann (ed.), *Neokorporatismus* (Frankfurt–New York: Campus) pp. 180–206.

Wirtschaftswoche, various issues from 1987 and 1988.

Zöllner, D. (1988) 'Die Beeinflussung der Ausgaben durch Steuerungsinstrumente' (text of address delivered to conference of the Gesellschaft für sozialen Fortschritt, Bonn, May).

4 Privatising from Within: The National Health Service under Thatcher[*]

Wendy Ranade and Stuart C. Haywood

INTRODUCTION

A major political phenomenon of the 1980s has been the scale and range of privatisation policies which sought to return state enterprises and activities back to the market. Such policies have flourished not only in Europe, the USA and Japan but more surprisingly in many Third World countries too in spite of the previous statist preferences of their nationalist governments.[1]

The widespread nature of these policies provides rich material for comparative policy analysis. The purpose of this paper is to examine the constraints and opportunities for governments wishing to reduce the role of the state by drawing on the recent experience of the British National Health Service (NHS). Paradoxically, carving out a more limited role for the state and changing the public-private boundaries requires a government strong enough to defeat powerful vested interests and change long-established expectations of public welfare services. The background to the paper is the debate on the role and the autonomy of the state in the context of the alleged 'crisis' of welfare and policy preferences for privatisation. The examination of the NHS experience since 1979 consequently focuses on change rather than continuities.

* This paper was prepared for presentation at the XIVth World Congress of the International Political Science Association on August 28 to September 1, 1988 at the Sheraton-Washington Hotel, Washington DC, USA. It was written in July 1988. There are references in it to the Government Review of the NHS, the results of which were published in January 1989 in a White Paper 'Working for Patients'.

AN ANALYTICAL FRAMEWORK

The paper starts from recent arguments which reassert the autonomy of the state in shaping social and economic policy in ways which are not simply reflective of the demands or interests of classes, social groups or society.

The 'state capacity' approach[2] views the state as a political actor with its own goals and varying capacities in differing policy fields to effect their attainment. Understanding policy involves not only specifying the policy instruments and resources states may have for dealing with particular problems but how these inter-relate with particular kinds of political and socio-economic environments. A state's capacity to change behaviour, transform structures or oppose demands in a given policy arena may in part depend on historical legacies which condition the expectations and organisation of key societal groups whose support and cooperation is essential. A key concept is the notion of 'policy networks',[3] a structure of patterned relationships between state and non-state institutions and actors which has developed around particular policy areas and may be extraordinarily stable and difficult to change.

The 'state capacity' approach suggests a common research agenda to discipline comparative inquiries on the success or failure of neo-conservative governments in 'reprivatising' areas of social and economic life. A complete analysis would examine:

(a) The content of new right ideology and its different emphases in different contexts.

(b) The reasons for its emergence and ascendancy as an intellectual and political force in a historical context.

(c) The institutions and policy networks through which policies were framed and implemented.

(d) The strategies available to the state to effect change in different policy arenas and the policy instruments in its repertoire. This would involve analysing more clearly the different faces and meanings of 'privatisation' and their applicability in different contexts.

(e) The obstacles faced in implementation.

(f) An assessment of policy outputs in terms of the scope and significance of change and the ways in which the policy networks and the boundaries between public and private have been redrawn.

Such a comprehensive analysis is probably a counsel of perfection given our current state of knowledge, and is certainly beyond the contraints of this paper. Nevertheless we will attempt to address these questions, though inevitably partially and briefly.

THE CRISIS OF WELFARE AND THE 'NEW RIGHT' RESPONSES

The vocabulary of crisis has permeated contemporary analyses of the welfare state, though the reality, nature and causes of the crisis are subject to intense debate. What is indisputable is the reality of the *definition* of the current situation as one of crisis and the political ascendancy of neo-liberal explanations and policies to deal with it.

The signs and symptoms of the crisis are familiar. Keynesian economic management seemed unable to deal with the onset of 'stagflation' in the late 1970s and the growth of large scale unemployment. A yawning gap between anticipated social expenditures and resources was forecast due to a combination of demographic pressures, low economic growth and taxpayer resentments at the 'burden' of welfare. The achievements and role of the welfare state came under increasing critical scrutiny and the post-war 'Butskellite' political consensus on the managed mixed economy and Beveridgian social welfare began to fragment in the United Kingdom. At an academic level Mishra[4] argues that the intellectual issues raised by these events could not be adequately analysed within the 'social administration' paradigm which had dominated the study of social policy in Britain and contributed powerfully to a shared perspective between senior politicians, civil servants and academics about the role of the state in tackling social problems. Sociological approaches to welfare based on either functionalism or 'post-industrial' technological determinism were similarly deficient. Theoretically only Marxist and liberal explanations seemed able to address these issues and due to a combination of political circumstances the way was open for neo-liberal doctrines and policies, previously considered anachronistic, even eccentric, to come in from the cold and be considered as a serious political alternative.

The contents of the New Right ideological attack on the interventionist state are too well known to bear repetition in detail, but the main outlines have been concisely summarised by Clarke *et al.*,[5] on which we draw here.

The central theme of neo-liberal analysis centres on the relationship between the state and the economy, and the need to free enterprise and initiative from state interference. This interference takes a number of forms. First, state planning and regulation of the economy inhibits its efficient operation by distorting market forces. Secondly, the government taxes its citizens excessively to fund public expenditure which blunts risk taking and economic effort. Thirdly, a large public sector in the economy aids economic decline, since it does not create wealth, whereas the private sector does.

Excessive state intervention has political as well as economic effects by inducing unrealistic expectations on the part of voters and electoral trade-offs between political parties bargaining for votes and demands for government action on the part of sectional interest groups for new 'needs' they have identified. This in turn leads to the 'overload' thesis. Excessive demands are placed on governments, beyond their political or administrative capacity to meet. Repeated government 'failure' results not only in a withdrawal of support from specific administrations by the electorate but eventually disillusionment with the institutions and processes of political democracy itself.

These general arguments for 'rolling back the state' underpin a more specific critique of the state's role in welfare which revolves around two themes, moral values and economic efficiency. Comprehensive state welfare induces dependency and reduces incentives to work, individual and family responsibility, initiative and enterprise. It is held to undermine the social obligations of citizens to others by undermining charitable and voluntary provision. (Such arguments have, of course, a long history stretching back to the Poor Law Amendment Act of 1834).

On the second theme, provision of welfare by state monopolies is held to lead to economic 'waste' since they are 'insulated from the efficiency – inducing pressure of market competition. This monopoly position (means) that welfare services (are) more likely to serve the bureaucratic and professional interests of their staff . . . rather than the needs of their consumers (clients)'.[6] Therefore monopolistic state welfare limits the freedom of individuals in two ways: as taxpayers forced to pay for wasteful services, and as consumers denied any choice over the level and type of service they wish to consume.

These views were considered something of an academic curiosity throughout the 1960s and 1970s, relatively unheeded from within the political consensus but kept alive in the United Kingdom by organisations like the Institute of Economic Affairs and the Adam

Smith Institute. They briefly received a more sympathetic reception from the Conservative Government elected in 1970, which however soon returned to more conventional policies. Interest in neo-liberal policies quickened in the mid-1970s, boosted by the new leader of the Conservative Party, Margaret Thatcher, a devotee of writers like Hayek. Since the election of the first Thatcher government in 1979 'privatisation' as an ideological vision and policy strategy has reshaped major sections of the British economy and welfare.

CONCEPTS OF PRIVATISATION

Definitions of privatisation vary considerably but Stephen Young argues for a broad approach to the concept which has utility in analysing the experience of the NHS.

> In very broad terms privatisation can be taken to describe a set of policies which aim to limit the role of the public sector and increase the role of the private sector, while improving the performance of the remaining public sector.[7]

Operationally such policies contain one or more of the following elements:

1. Policies that change the existing balance between public and private sectors by reducing the size, scope and role of the public sector and attracting private resources into the resulting vacuum.
2. Policies that aim to change the existing balance in the longer term by creating opportunities for the private sector to grow, for example, by changing regulations.
3. Policies that aim to make use of private resources to help carry out tasks and solve problems facing government. This involves mobilising private sector resources on a wide front to help government implement schemes which support the thrust of its policies, for example, investment finance, the secondment of personnel, use of business and management practices, etc.
4. Policies that bring increased market pressures to bear on the use of assets staying in the public sector. This may involve forcing more internal and external competition on public organisations.

Using these four elements of privatisation Young argues that seven different *forms* of privatisation are identifiable in Conservative policy since 1979.

(a) Selling off public sector assets to the private sector, for example British Telecom, British Petroleum, sales of council housing, and so on.

(b) Relaxing state monopolies (referred to as liberalisation). Exposing individual parts of the public sector to increased competition, for example, changing regulations to allow the private sector to provide bus services, generate electricity, compete with the Post Office over some aspects of mail delivery.

(c) Contracting services out through policies which force public sector organisations to put part of their work out to tender to private firms. The aims are twofold: to create the opportunities for more private sector involvement in the long term and stimulate greater efficiency in similar services remaining in the public sector.

(d) Private provision of services. Policies that aim to increase private provision of services at present provided by the public sector. They may continue to be financed from public funds or from private funds and sponsorship.

(e) Investment projects – the process of leveraging the private sector to complete development projects in deprived areas, for example, Urban Development Grant scheme, London Docklands Development Corporation.

(f) Extending private sector practices into the public sector, which may involve the secondment of personnel from the private sector to draw on their expertise. Young argues this still falls within the sphere of privatisation since 'part of the thrust of the whole privatisation strategy has been to imbue the public sector with practices tested, developed and refined in market conditions. . .'[8]

(g) Reduced subsidies and increased charges. Some services provided in the public sector have had their subsidies reduced and charges levied so that consumers either pay the total cost or a greater proportion of the real cost of providing the service.

Young makes two further important points. Privatisation in all its forms is not new and there are *ad hoc* instances under both Labour and Conservative governments. What distinguishes the approach of the Thatcher governments is the notion of a sustained strategy based on coherent philosophy which applies privatisation principles and where it can, '. . . not just to the headline grabbing issue of selling government assets but also the detailed operations of little known quangos like the Forestry Commission'.[9]

Secondly, the policy has been implemented by changing the administrative style of government and the application of considerable political clout. The Prime Minister has personally monitored the progress of individual ministers. Promotion and demotion in Whitehall has partly depended on enthusiasm and resourcefulness in applying privatisation principles.

THE NEW RIGHT AND THE NHS: POLICY PRESCRIPTION AND POLITICAL REALITIES

The Critique

The nature of the NHS makes it an exemplar of publicly provided services which attract the criticisms of the 'new right'. It has a seemingly irresistible momentum for growth, demanded by most of its one million employees supported by public opinion which, in the past, politicians disregarded at their peril. Enoch Powell, reflecting on his experience as Minister of Health in the 1960s, observed:

> Anyone in the National Health Service below the Minister, who professed himself satisfied with what was being spent could not be unreasonably represented as a traitor to his colleagues, his profession and his patients on the basis, namely, that more money means improvement, and that complaint and dissatisfaction are essential to extracting more money. However instances of such treasonable conduct are rare indeed.[10]

The dynamics of this situation still exist and arise from two institutional features of the NHS which, as Klein points out, try to square two circles.[11]

First, the NHS accounts for 90 per cent of total health care spending and is almost totally dependant on government funding, but responsibility for delivering services is delegated to local health authorities. Consequently the locus of responsibility for the quantity and quality of services is blurred.

The second dilemma involves squaring the circle between public accountability and professional autonomy. Ministerial accountability to parliament for the use of taxpayers' money sits uneasily with the doctrine that only doctors and other clinicians can make judgements about the way resources are used at individual patient level. In the absence of fiscal incentives for clinicians to economise or consumers to limit their demands (since services are still largely free at the points of use) the pressures for increased spending have not abated, and indeed became a major political issue in 1987–8, prompting a Ministerial review of the NHS.

The NHS has also been criticised for restricting consumer choice over the level and quality of health services they wished to consume, as this extract from an article by Rhodes Boyson in 1971 makes plain:

> The National Health Service was introduced by men of compassion who wished to improve the health of the poor and to remove the worry of medical bills. The end result has been a decline in medical standards below the level of other advanced countries because people are not prepared to pay as much through taxation on other people's health as they would pay directly on their own and their families'. Long queues in surgeries, an endless waiting list for hospital beds and the emigration of many newly trained doctors are among the unexpected results. Small wonder that more and more people are looking to some form of private insurance to give them wider choice in medicine and surgery.[12]

'PRIVATISATION' AND THE NHS

The new Conservative government quickly showed its enthusiasm for a much bigger private sector in health care after its election in 1979. In any event there was a rapid growth of private medicine in 1979 and 1980 and Gerard Vaughan, Minister of Health at the time, remarked that he expected it to ultimately reach one-quarter the size of the NHS. The Government helped the process along by disbanding the Health Services Board set up by Labour to regulate private sector growth, stopped the phasing out of NHS paybeds, and in 1980 allowed consultants on full time contracts to earn up to 10 per cent of their NHS salary from private practice without any deduction from their salary. Before, they had forfeited two-elevenths. Some commentators believe this measure was the most effective and least costly fillip to private sector growth.[13]

In the early days there is evidence that more radical measures were at least discussed. Leaked 'think tank' proposals in 1982 advocated the replacement of taxation funding by some form of health insurance and the Department of Health examined a variety of continental insurance schemes. However subsequent support for the private sector, though still strong, is more guarded and Ministers, including the Prime Minister, have repeatedly affirmed their support for the underlying principles of the system. Thus Mrs Thatcher at the 1982 Conservative Party conference said:

> The principle that adequate health care should be provided for all, regardless of their ability to pay, must be the foundation of any arrangements for financing the health service.[14]

while in 1988 her Secretary of State for Social Services, John Moore, reiterated:

> Our commitment to the principle that no one should be denied necessary treatment because they are unable to afford it remains unshakeable.[15]

It seems clear that the high level of political support for the NHS which has marked its history shows no sign of weakening. The state of the NHS was a significant issue in the 1983 and 1987 elections and public opinion surveys suggest this support continues, albeit combined with tolerance of a complementary private sector.[16] Public opinion is powerfully reinforced by medical support, expressed vociferously through the Royal Colleges and the BMA.

Nevertheless there have been changes consistent with ideas from the privatisation stable. Most fall within Young's categories of contracting out (c) and incorporating private sector practices (f). While the paper concentrates on these manifestations of privatisation we summarise others for the sake of completeness.

Measures falling within the scope of Young's category (a) include requiring health authorities to review their estate and sell off under-used assets; under (b), changes to consultant contracts mentioned earlier and changes in the income limits of tax relief on group health insurance offered by employers to encourage wider take-up. Ministers have exhorted health authorities to co-operate with the private sectors in a number of circulars. The first of two examples, in 1981, overturned the previous policy of not allowing health authorities to contract with profit-making health care organisations by telling them

> When planning the provision of NHS services (including short-term needs) health authorities should take into account the current and planned facilities available in the independent sector.[17]

The second, in February 1983, sent to Chairs of Regional Health Authorities gave examples of the kind of co-operation the Department had in mind.

> Independent sector capital might be used to provide expensive equipment for, say, a district general hospital on the basis of a leasing/rental agreement (or for joint use by an NHS or independent hospital). Pay-beds could be 'managed for a fee by the independent sector'; wards could be 'sold to the independent sector which would run (them) outside the NHS but would have guaranteed access to the main hospital facilities.[18]

There are examples of initiatives which fall into Young's category (d), the extension of private provision. Changes in Supplementary Benefit regulations on board and lodging allowances have financed a large expansion of private residential and nursing homes for the elderly, mentally handicapped and mentally ill. There are also instances of greater cost-sharing with consumers (category g). Prescription charges have been increased thirteenfold since 1979 (from 20p to £2.60 per item), and more competition introduced for the supply of spectacles. Under the Health and Medicines Bill under consideration by Parliament (summer 1988) all forms of dental treatment will be subject to higher charges, and new charges introduced for sight tests and dental examinations although low income, age and disability exemptions still pertain.

Contentious as some of these policies have been, they do not mark significant discontinuities with the past. The distinctive contribution of the Conservative Government lies in the efforts to recast management structures, systems, norms and values in line with the perceived virtues of the private sector, in particular its efficiency and dynamism. The investment of effort cannot be explained by pressures from within the NHS. The Merrison Commission[19] while criticising some aspects of its structure and management arrangements did not advocate change on the scale introduced since 1979. The attention to management has its roots in the Government's attitude to the public sector and its doubts about its efficiency.

THE CHANGES: A SUMMARY

Management Arrangements

The Conservatives moved quickly to abolish an area tier of organisation to rectify 'well-founded' criticism of existing arrangements. The White Paper 'Patients First'[20] speaks of:

- too many tiers;
- too many administrators in all disciplines;
- money wasted (para 3).

District Health Authorities (DHAs) were created in 1982 and following the practice of the previous Labour Government, the proportion of the budget spent on administration was reduced. The new arrangements were intended to:

enable health authorities to be planned and managed most efficiently, and within which decisions can be taken quickly by those who are close to and responsive to the needs of patients (para 5).

However these and associated changes left the intra-NHS balance of power undisturbed, maintaining the arrangements agreed in 1972–4.

The Government has rejected the proposition that each authority should appoint a chief executive responsible for all the authority's staff. It believes that such an appointment would not be compatible with the professional independence required by the wide range of staff employed in the service (para 11).

Annual formal review of performance of the 14 Regional Health Authorities (RHAs) by Ministers and the DHSS began in 1982, subsequently extended to RHA reviews of DHA's and DHA reviews of unit managers. 'Performance indicators' first developed in 1983 have increasingly informed these reviews, concluded by a letter outlining agreed action which then provides the basis for subsequent reviews.

The reviews have reinforced the importance of Ministerial and RHA views on policies and priorities and *upwards* accountability. The latter has also been reinforced by changes in appointments of chairmen of health authorities which increasingly have the character of political appointments.

General Management

Further changes in NHS management were effected under the rubric of 'general management' recommended by the NHS Management Inquiry chaired by a businessman from the private sector.[21] Official endorsement related the changes to effectiveness: ensuring 'the expenditure devoted to the Service . . . does reach its target'. The changes, and other initiatives to improve management were 'designed to provide the efficient use of what must always be limited resources.[22]

The main effect of these changes was the appointment of a general manager at each level of management. While 'the importance of consensus in a multi-professional organisation' was not undervalued it was insufficient as a 'management style' to 'secure effective and timely action' (para 5). Also a supervisory board at national level was quickly established 'to help establish policies and priorities'. These provided the context for a newly established Management Board, responsible for 'planning, implementation of the policies . . . leadership . . . control performance . . . achiev(ing) consistency and drive . . .'.[23] The first two chairmen were appointed from the private sector.

The position of managers within the organisation has been enhanced. It is reflected in the pay of general managers which has been brought more in line with that of hospital consultants. Previously managers (administrators, nurses) had been paid less. Their higher profile in the organisation is well illustrated by phrases in the DHSS circular on implementation:

'leadership', 'bringing about a constant search for major change and cost improvement'; 'securing proper motivation of staff; ensuring that the professional functions are effectively geared into the overall objectives and responsibilities of the general manage- ment process'; and 'making sense of the process of consultation'.[24]

The change in the nature of the position of managers was further underlined by three new features. General managers were appointed on short-term contracts and a performance-related element was introduced in their remuneration in 1987. A national performance appraisal system has also been introduced. Unsurprisingly appointments of general managers extended beyond the original deadlines, well into 1986. More significantly the majority of posts went to ex-NHS administrators, usually with their previous authority. This was in spite of interim arrangements for pay and conditions which favoured external applicants and doctors.

The importance attached to these changes was underlined by considerable central involvement in implementation, with Ministers approving nominations for appointments to regional and district posts. There were well publicised cases of individuals whose nominations were unacceptable to Ministers. Shortlists were also checked to ensure balance and the acceptability of candidates. Job descriptions and management structures required approval from higher authority.

The Drive for Efficiency

The motivating force behind these and other changes was the Government's determination to improve efficiency in the public sector, as a means of controlling costs and giving the taxpayer 'value for money'. The 1985 Annual Report on the Health Service asserted:

> Getting the best out of resources in terms of maximizing the services to patients is . . . a fundamental challenge . . . for the Government.[25]

The appointment of general managers was mentioned as one of a 'series of major steps to that end' (*ibid*). Also mentioned were 'improving the accountability of health authorities'; 'encouraging the better utilization of manpower' which included the introduction of manpower targets; and a requirement of health authorities that they 'carry through substantial and sustained cost-improvement programmes' which included the controversial programme of competitive tendering for 'hotel' services, better management of the estate, and the programme of Rayner efficiency scrutinies.

We examine the implementation of one of these initiatives, competitive tendering, below to illustrate the general tenor of government expectations. However another theme in the general management saga merits a mention at this point, given its relevance to neo-liberal criticisms of state welfare. The report which ushered in general managers also put considerable emphasis on the need for more attention to the needs and wishes of consumers and underlined the prime importance of considerations of quality. The most tangible outcome has been widespread appointments of directors with responsibility for consumer relations and quality, usually from the ranks of partially displaced senior nurse managers. However the main thrust of the value-for-money initiatives has been to obtain more services for the same input of resources (which does improve access to health services) or the same for less.

COMPETITIVE TENDERING

Private supply of goods and services previously provided by NHS authorities, was not unknown before the Conservative Government's initiative on competitive tendering. For example, hospital authorities progressively withdrew from the production of pharmaceutical products in the 1960s switching to direct purchases from private manufacturers. There have been similar changes in other areas, for example, architectural, sterile supply and maintenance services without them becoming ideological issues. Also private cleaning, catering and particularly laundry firms had supplied services to some hospitals for many years, accounting for 13.7 per cent of expenditure on NHS ancillary services in 1982–3.[26] The possibility of more contracting of laundry, cleaning and catering services was first raised in 1981 and followed in 1983 by a draft circular for comment on competitive tendering. The issue was considered sufficiently important for inclusion in the Conservative Party's manifesto for the 1984 election and definitive guidance quickly followed.

DHAs were asked 'to test the effectiveness of their domestic, catering and laundry services by putting them out to tender' and 'submit . . . a timed programme for implementation'.[27] Rules have been developed to ensure 'fair' competition, with a requirement that the contract was to be let to a private contractor if his price was lower, rather than the tenders being used 'to establish a new base cost for running the in-house service'.[28] Also tender documents were not to specify the terms and conditions of employment for contractors' employees. This particular requirement led to a strong letter from the Minister in 1984, rebuking authorities which had insisted on disregarding this requirement and asked that tenders be based on Whitley Council agreements on pay and conditions of service for NHS staff.

> This is contrary to the advice given by the Department . . . and it is, as John Patten made clear in his letter this summer, unacceptable to Ministers.[29]

A review of arrangements in 1984 led to further instructions to ensure fair competition. Health authorities were asked not to introduce 'unreasonable conditions and ask for unnecessary information', such as the 'automatic demand for performance bonds, union recognition or details of grievance procedures . . . or stipulate detailed requirements for staffing and length of time needed to undertake tasks'. The RHAs were asked 'to ensure that only essential questions are included' (in pre-tender questionnaires) and the need to give tenderers 'adequate time to complete them'. There was also advice on selection of tenderers and evaluation of tenders.[30]

The avowed purpose of the exercise was to increase the efficiency of the ancillary services, not necessarily to 'contract out' the services to private suppliers. In the early stages of the process, however, four out of five contracts were awarded externally but as the process got under way the situation changed. Overall only about 15 per cent of contracts have been awarded to private suppliers. Nevertheless the programme had achieved substantial annual savings by the end of 1986, amounting to 30 per cent on cleaning contracts, less though still significant savings on catering and laundries. In March 1988 net annual savings were reported as £106 million, about 1 per cent of the hospital and community health budget. By that time virtually all domestic and laundry services and 76 per cent of catering services had been put out to tender.[31]

In terms of the Government's avowed intentions the programme must be judged a success.

> savings are growing all the time . . . health authorities now have a good deal of extra money to use on improving services to patients.[32]

The programme has succeeded in stimulating greater efficiency by concentrating (painfully) management time on a relatively neglected

and undermanaged part of the service and changing employee
practices. Talbot comments:

> Service managers have had to be educated to think like their
> external competitors and also to keep their employees very aware
> of the probable level of external competition. Under the ever
> present threat of redundancy unproductive bonus schemes have
> been scrapped and some cosy 'working practices' eradicated.[33]

Critics of course would argue that the savings have been achieved at
the cost of already low paid employees, and the substitution of full
time by part-time workers with fewer rights and benefits and by a
poorer quality of service though there is little substantial evidence for
the latter. Initially many managers, chairmen and members of health
authorities voiced fears about these possible consequences and
dislike of the whole exercise[34] but now that the savings represent an
important part of the mandatory minimum cost improvement
programme which managers have to achieve in a climate of increasing
financial stringency, reliance on the savings quells unease about
effects.

THE NHS EXPERIENCE: IMPLICATIONS FOR POLICY DEVELOPMENT

The Conservative Government's experience of changing the NHS
since 1979 provides an interesting paradox. It illustrates both the
Government's limited power to effect change and how much can be
achieved.

There is considerable evidence that the NHS did not fit neatly with
Government views on the role of state welfare and their policy
preferences. Yet the general picture is in great measure one of policy
continuity. There have been no drastic changes in the method of
funding and provision and the basic structure and dominance of the
NHS in health care remains intact. Longstanding policy priorities
(reducing geographical inequalities, rundown of long-stay hospitals)
have been continued, in some cases with increased vigour. The
founding principles underlying the NHS have been reaffirmed many
times and the NHS remains the pre-eminent supplier of health care in
the United Kingdom. Additional finance has also been forthcoming,
although not on the scale to which the NHS was accustomed before

he fiscal crises of the mid-1970s. The 'real' cost to the economy of he NHS (a measure of how much money the Government has made vailable) increased by 17 per cent between 1979–80 and 1984–5. The proportion of Gross Domestic Product consumed by health care as also risen steady. However the input costs of health care have been rising more quickly than general prices on which Government stimates are based. Robinson calculates that when programme-pecific indices are used 'new' monies rose by only 5 per cent in the ame period.[35] Health authorities were asked to free resources from llocations for current activities through redeployment and efficiency avings to make good any shortfall above this for additional demands rom a growing number of elderly people, introducing new technol-gy and meeting 'above average' pay awards.

But the general picture is one of increased public spending, a near nonopoly for public provision of health care and a renewed commitment to the principles on which the NHS is based. Anything ess would have been unsustainable.

Within this general constraint the Government has nevertheless ursued policies which have effected considerable changes in the way he service is organised and run. A form of privatisation is being ntroduced. First by defining a new model of management for NHS nanagers to emulate, derived from private sector practices and recepts. Secondly, by raising the profile and responsibilities of nanagement through the introduction of general management hroughout the service. Thirdly, by creating new mechanisms to einforce the political accountability of health authorities and the nanagerial accountability of managers upwards to Ministers, the NHS Management Board and RHAs, coupled with a willingness to xercise considerable 'political clout' in using these mechanisms. Examples already mentioned include the control of chairman ppointments (non-reappointment of critics or less than enthusiastic mplementers of Government policy, and drawing in outsiders, new o the NHS for business and finance), the accountability reviews, and nore prescriptive policy 'guidance' from the centre. By the use of hese instruments as illustrated in the example of competitive endering Ministers have succeeded in changing managerial behaviour to ensure concepts of efficiency, cost effectiveness and roductivity are accorded more weight in the organisational culture. The harder financial climate and reduced rates of revenue growth ave also been important in changing expectations and forcing hange.[36]

There are two noteworthy aspects of this strategy. The first is an implicit assumption that the definition of management is unproblematic, and as such is not properly part of the ideological debate. Significant change in the nature of an organisation can be effected by developing a particular definition of management and enhancing its position within that organisation.

The second point concerns the content of that definition. The report on general management emphasised control, consumer sensitivity, quality and efficiency. The reality reveals considerable emphasis on the latter. Consequently, cost-containment and cost-improvements increasingly engage the attention of managers in practice. The effect of this has been to produce a system more concerned with this rather narrow definition of efficiency than at any time in the history of the NHS.

Introducing this particular brand of privatisation within the general framework of a publicly provided welfare service with the institutional features of the NHS is producing new contradictions and tensions. Examples are legion. For instance with central allocations and cash limited budgets increased efficiency leading to greater throughput of patients does not lead to increased revenue, simply greater costs. DHAs cannot control referrals from general practitioners and a high quality or efficient service may attract referrals across authority boundaries greatly in excess of the number of patients the DHA is funded to treat. Yet it is unable to charge either the patient or the district they came from. Clinical decisions are still the main determinant of how resources are used but managers possess only weak formal controls over consultants, not even holding their contracts outside of teaching districts.

While the nature of these rather obvious contradictions is well understood it remains to be seen whether the elaboration and development of the Government's 'privatised' concepts of management can be reconciled with notions of a publicly provided welfare service. The former leads in the direction of individual choice, market satisfaction, competition and opportunities to use alternative suppliers: the latter is still rooted in collective choice, search for justice and equity, collective action and public protest. The limits to change through the 'privatisation of management' may have been reached in the NHS.

References

1. See for instance discussion in A. Kaletsky, 'Everywhere the state is in retreat', *Financial Times*, 2 August 1985 and D. Wilson, 'The Privatisation of Asia', *The Banker*, September 1984.
2. P. Evans, D. Rueschemeyer and T. Skocpol, *Bringing the state back in*, Cambridge University Press, 1985.
3. P.J. Katzenstein (ed.), *Between power and plenty: foreign economic policies of advanced industrial states*, Madison, London, 1978.
4. R. Mishra, *The welfare state in crisis*, Harvester Press, 1984.
5. J. Clarke, A. Cochrane and C. Smart, *Ideologies of welfare: from dreams to disillusion*, Hutchison, 1987.
6. Ibid, p. 137.
7. S. Young, 'The nature of privatisation in Britain 1979–85', *West European Politics*, 9, pp. 235–52, April 1986.
8. Ibid, p. 240.
9. Ibid, p. 246.
10. E. Powell, *Medicine and politics*, Pitman Medical, London, 1966.
11. R. Klein, 'Performance evaluation and the NHS: a case study in conceptual complexity and organisational perplexity', *Public Administration*, pp. 385–407, winter, 1982.
12. R. Boyson (ed.), *Down with the poor*, Churchill Press, 1971.
13. See for instance, G. Rayner, 'Health care as a business', *Policy and Politics*, pp. 439–59, autumn, 1986; and Joan Higgins, *The business of medicine: private health care in Britain*, Macmillan Education, 1988.
14. Quoted in J. Le Grand and R. Robinson, *Privatisation and the welfare state*, Allen and Unwin 1984.
15. Reported in NAHA News, June 1988.
16. See P. Taylor-Gooby, 'The politics of welfare: public attitudes and behaviour' in *The Future of Welfare*, R. Klein and M. O'Higgins (eds), Blackwell, 1985, and 'Extra money for the NHS should come from taxation: latest MARPLAN poll', *NAHA News*, June, 1988.
17. From DHSS Circular HC (81)1, quoted in Rayner *op. cit.*
18. Rayner, op. cit.
19. *Royal Commission on the Health Service* (The Merrison Commission), HMSO, 1979.
20. *Patients first*, DHSS:HMSO, 1979.
21. *Inquiry into NHS management* (Griffiths Report), DHSS: HMSO, 1983.
22. DHSS Circular HC (83)13, Health Services Management. Implementation of the NHS Management Inquiry Report.
23. Griffiths Report, op. cit., paras 1–3.
24. Circular HD(83)13, paras 9 a–e.
25. *The Health Service in England,* Annual Report for 1985, HMSO.
26. House of Commons, 27.2.1984, written answers.
27. DHSS Circular HC (83)13 Health Services Management, *Competitive tendering in the provision of domestic catering and laundry services.*
28. Ibid, para 8.
29. Letter – Minister of Health to Health Authority Chairmen, 1984.

30. *Competitive tendering: further advice for health authorities*, DHSS 1985.

31. House of Commons, 6.7.1988, written answers.

32. DHSS Circular HC (85)5, *Resource assumptions and planning guidelines*.

33. P. Talbot, 'Are local authorities ready for competitive tendering?' *Public Finance and Accountancy*, 5 December, 1986.

34. See for instance S.C. Haywood and W. Ranade, 'District health authorities: tribunes or prefects?', *Public Administration Bulletin* June, 1985.

35. R. Robinson, 'Restructuring the Welfare State: an analysis of public expenditure, 1970/80 to 1984/5', *Journal of Social Policy*, 1986.

36. S.C. Haywood and W. Ranade, 'Resources and innovation in health care', *Policy and Politics*, October, 1986.

5 Nordic Health Policy in the 1980s[*]

Richard B. Saltman

INTRODUCTION

The Nordic countries developed perhaps the Western world's most comprehensive welfare states in the decades following World War II. During long periods of Social Democratic political hegemony, Sweden, Denmark and Norway created wide-ranging public sector systems for the delivery of human and social services. Finland, governed by a centre-left coalition of agrarian (now centre) and Social Democratic parties, developed its own equally comprehensive mix of 'municipal socialism' with nationally mandated welfare programmes.

The major tenets of Nordic health policy similarly appeared – at least upon initial viewing – to be internally comprehensive and externally consistent. The centrality of tax-based funding, of universal access, of public ownership of hospitals, or publicly salaried hospital specialists, and of decentralised regional and–or municipal responsibility for administration have all characterised Nordic health systems since at least the 1960s. Viewed from outside the region, these commonalities still suffice to speak of a 'Nordic model' for health care.

In the 1980s however, this unruffled external appearance came to belie an increasingly unsettled policy reality. Both within and between countries, the proper emphasis for future health sector development has become contested and uncertain. Broad changes in international economic expectations, particularly in the form of pressures to reduce overall public sector consumption and to reduce high marginal tax rates, have pincered government revenues and

[*] Support for this study was provided by a research fellowship from the German Marshall Fund of the United States, the Swedish Center for Working Life in Stockholm, and the University of Massachusetts at Amherst.

111

generated substantial pressure to impose painful programmatic changes. New intensive clinical procedures have been developed which threaten the core health policy emphasis upon expanding primary and preventive services while keeping hospital inpatient expenditures on a tight rein. Lastly, and most controversially, a growing willingness among Nordic citizens to insist upon convenient and responsive as well as competent clinical care has forced tightly planned public sector providers to reconsider important aspects of service design and delivery. Among the consequences, the traditional 'allocative' or command-and-control models that have been the backbone of Nordic health planning have been increasingly discredited in favour of less rigid, more 'innovative' public sector techniques (Saltman, 1987).

While these pressures have developed to different degrees within different national contexts, contingent upon differing national industrial and trading as well as health sector decision-making and administrative patterns, the underlying commonality has become one in which policy formulation reflects a pressured present and an uncertain future environment. It is this set of perceptual changes, more than particular policy departures, which reflects the fundamental shift in Nordic health policy over the course of the 1980s. While policy formulation and implementation remain careful and pragmatic, many national officials and analysts no longer automatically presume that it need remain so. Although the discussion below will concentrate on this transition in two countries – Sweden and Finland – this shift now pervades the policy formulation process not only in other Nordic countries but throughout publicly operated health systems in Northern Europe (Saltman and von Otter, 1990).

THE HEALTH POLICY CONTEXT

Viewed retrospectively, most Nordic health officials and commentators had a generally optimistic and self-confident view of public sector capabilities through the 1970s and early 1980s. The central clinical theme of increasing emphasis upon primary and preventive health services represented a policy which would require considerable ingenuity to translate into institutional reality. The dominant organisational theme of decentralising administrative (and subsequently policy) decision-making to regional (county in Sweden; province and–or central hospital districts in Finland) reflected growing confidence in the ability of representatively constituted (except Finnish province) regional government to maintain clinical standards while adapting service delivery to local conditions. The overall objective appeared to be the full articulation of an increasingly comprehensive, financially and administratively independent, regionally based, publicly operated health system.

This health policy process was most extensively pursued within the Swedish and Finnish health systems. The thrust both toward primary care and toward decentralised administration was initiated in Sweden with the 1948 publication of the Hojar Report (Serner, 1980). In the same year that Aneurin Bevan launched a centralised, hospital-oriented national health service in the United Kingdom, the head of the Swedish National Board of Health issued a landmark if controversial report that set a rather different policy tone in Sweden. Indeed it can be argued that much of the subsequent evolution of Swedish health policy involved the gradual adoption of Hojar's broad vision (Saltman, 1988a). Central aspects of this public sector, regionally based consolidation of health care decision-making include the 1955 introduction of county responsibility to develop primary health centres; the 1970 'Seven Crown Reform' that obligated hospital specialists to become fully salaried county employees; and the 1973 Primary Care Act which adopted a primary and preventive emphasis to future resource utilisation. This process toward public sector consolidation was capped by the 1983 Health Act, which effectively empowered the 26 health provider governments (23 counties and three municipalities: Göteborg, Malmö, and the island of Gotland) to act as independent regional health systems. In combination with the subsequent 1985 'Dagmar Reform', which transformed the prior fee-for-service national ambulatory insurance programme into a system of capitated annual payments channeled exclusively through the 26 regional providers, the 1983 Act represented the culmination of a publicly planned, regionally operated, primary-care-based health strategy (Saltman and von Otter, 1990).

In Finland, a similar if differently configured policy transition also was underway. In a parallel approach to that which was adopted in 1949 to develop the acute hospital sector, the 1972 Primary Health Act established a network of 100 free-standing and 100 federated (two or-more facilities) municipally operated 'health centres' which assumed central responsibility for developing primary care services. This explicitly public sector strategy was buttressed by a strong national planning role in the form of tight controls over new personnel and capital, and a sliding national subsidy, which on average provided 50 per cent of health centre operating costs (Saltman, 1988b). One unique component of the Finnish programme was to attach new and–or existing skilled nursing facilities to these health centres as 'primary care hospitals', an approach which increased both the budgetary and political presence of the public primary care sector (Pekurinen *et al.*, 1987).

Three subsequent changes were introduced which were intended to consolidate the Finnish primary care strategy. In 1979 partial responsibility for allocating new resources in the national planning process was decentralised to Ministry of Health appointees within the twelve provincial governments. In 1984 the national planning and subsidy mechanism was extended to the social service sector, thus officially integrating within one planning process what typically are separately organised sectors within publicly operated health systems (Saltman, 1987). Lastly, in 1985 the Personal Doctor Program began a series of demonstration projects which, by introducing patient lists for health centre physicians reinforced by a modified system of performance-based salaries, sought to strengthen the position of the publicly operated system vis-à-vis the private and occupational health components of primary care delivery in Finland (Vohlonen *et al.*, 1989).

Viewed conjointly, both Finnish and Swedish health policy pursued a consistent and relatively similar set of objectives through the mid-1980s. The central emphasis was to build up the primary care sector of the delivery system, to emphasise preventive as against curative models of care, and to reinforce the role of the publicly operated, regionally and–or locally administered primary care delivery system.

Although the specifics are different, the broad emphasis upon locally organised primary care also formed the core of health policy development during this period in Norway and, to a lesser degree, Denmark. The Norwegian approach, like that of the Danish, placed greater emphasis upon the independent general practitioner, although 1983 legislation shifted the contracting (and financing) public sector body from regional (county) to municipal level (Siam, 1986). The Danish model is similar in concept to the British system, although general practitioners are supervised by elected regional (county) rather than centrally appointed (District-level General Practice Committee) officials. While neither system stressed preventive team-based primary care to the extent visible – in policy and practice – in Sweden and Finland, the Norwegian emphasis upon a strong municipal managerial role did give that system a more locally controlled, publicly influenced character than the Danish approach.

THE POLITICAL CONTEXT

The broad Nordic policy thrust toward a locally controlled, publicly operated, primary-care-based health system had been established during the extended period of Social Democratic (Sweden, Denmark, Norway) or centre-left coalition (Finland) political domination. The central tenets of this health strategy reflected concerns with distributional equity and social justice that formed the core of Social Democratic ideology generally (Castles, 1987). In the Swedish and Finnish as well as a part of the Norwegian approach, the emphasis upon decentralised administration (but not necessarily policy formulation) fit less comfortably with the official Social Democratic position, since it entailed at least the possibility of a divergent process-driven rather than a centrally imposed content-driven understanding of how a democratic society should be organised (Saltman and von Otter, 1989).

A further factor in the political mix was the adoption by the World Health Organisation during this period of an explicitly primary-care-based strategy, reinforced in the European Region by a series of documents which appeared to be broadly modeled on the Swedish and-or Finnish health centre model (WHO, 1981; WHO, 1984). This European 'Health For All' strategy was officially adopted by the member states by a vote of the Regional Committee, in which Nordic governments not only committed themselves to this strategy but were seen as its progenitors. While commitments made in international bodies are not legally binding on national policy, the highly visible Nordic profile during the policy formulation and, subsequently, implementation phase undoubtedly generated additional pressure on the Swedish and Finnish governments to adhere to a primary-care-oriented policy format at home.

In the midst of this longstanding Nordic health policy process, the political substratum upon which it was at least officially based – Social Democratic hegemony – began to crumble. As small states with a high reliance upon exports to maintain domestic production, the Nordic region was severely affected by the economic dislocations of the world economy during the late 1970s and early 1980s

(Bosworth and Rivlin, 1987). As traditional Social Democratic distributionist formulas appeared increasingly unsuited to the emerging problems of a stagnant economy, key elements within carefully nurtured national voting coalitions began to split off and vote more independently. In Sweden in 1978 a non-socialist coalition took national power for the first time since the 1930s. In Denmark in 1982 a centre-right coalition government was formed, overturning what had been a largely unbroken generation of Social Democratic national leadership (Einhorn, 1987). In Norway, despite several intermittant periods of non-socialist rule, the election of a conservative-led government in 1981 similarly signaled the end of the Labour Party's post-World-War-II political dominance (Einhorn, 1987). Lastly, although the special Finnish relationship with the Soviet Union had been presumed to preclude participation by rightist parties, the success of Finnish foreign policy during the latter half of the Kekkonen era (after the 1962 'night frost' incident) and the subsequent presidency of former Social Democratic Prime Minister Mauno Koivisto, as evidenced in Finland's increasingly independent foreign policy and trading patterns (Jutikkala and Pirinen, 1984), culminated in the formation of a left–right national government in 1987. Despite the return to national power of the Social Democrats in Sweden in 1983 and in Norway in 1986, the perception of a new political heterogeneity in the Nordic region, and the end of the Social Democratic era, is now acknowledged even by Social Democratic theorists (Esping-Andersen, 1985).

With regard to health policy specifically however, it remains important to recognise the key role played by regional and–or municipal governments (Bogason, 1987). Partly as a legacy of national history (particularly Finland), partly as a consequence of prior Social Democratic efforts to decentralise administrative responsibilities (particularly Sweden), the influence of national governments upon key health issues is leavened (if not in some instances neutralised) by the relatively powerful role of regional and–or municipal government. In Finland, despite the importance of 'municipal socialism', the national government has perhaps the greatest influence in the Nordic region due to the combined influence of the national planning process for new resources and the scope of the subsidy programme for existing operations (Saltman, 1988b). In Denmark, although elected county councils (and two health provider municipalities – Copenhagen and Fredericksberg) are officially autonomous and have the power to tax, the historically powerful role of the national Parliament combined with the only recent (1970) establishment of the county council system, creates an environment in which the national government has legislative as well as considerable financial authority over the long-term behaviour of regional government (Amstrådsforeningen I Danmark, 1986). The role of the Swedish national government, particularly as a consequence of the progressive decentralisation to the counties of state responsibilities in health care, was largely limited to financial matters by the end of the 1970s. As noted above, the national government's zone of discretion was further delimited by the reforms of 1983 and 1985, which in principle freed the counties to develop new policies as well as to administer services in the pursuit of broadly conceived national objectives.

Given the centrality of regional level government both in the administration and, depending upon the system, in the formulation of policy, the importance of an increasing political heterogeneity in the composition of national governments is somewhat contingent upon the existence of political heterogeneity at the regional level as well. That is, conservative political parties in national government require willing (or coercible) allies at the regional and–or municipal level to effectively implement new policy departures. Viewed tactically, non-socialist national governments thus require a mixture of prior dissatisfaction and–or conservative regional allies in order to successfully alter policy direction.

POLICY DEVELOPMENTS IN THE 1980s

The 1980s has been a period of ferment in Nordic health policy. The settled presumptions of the previous decade – in particular, emphasis upon primary care and structural decentralisation – have come under renewed scrutiny and, increasingly, criticism. One component in this policy reassessment has been the rise of potential and–or electorally successful conservative parties at the national level, injecting neo-classical economic concerns about increased productivity and reduced public sector consumption into social policy debates. National conservative parties in Sweden, Denmark, and Finland also harbour preferences for a larger private sector role in the provision (although not necessarily the finance) of health services.

However Social Democratic parties have also begun to question many of the prior policy orthodoxies in the health sector. Both at the national level (in Sweden and Finland) and at the regional and–or municipal levels throughout the Nordic region, socialist as well as non-socialist parties have begun to discuss alternative delivery mechanisms and, increasingly, alternative policy strategies as well. Rather than reflecting concerted ideological pressure from conservative parties then, in Sweden, Finland and Denmark alike the thrust toward new policy and delivery solutions in the latter half of the 1980s has been driven by broadly visible, broadly recognised but pragmatic structural considerations.

National Developments

The first pragmatic change reflected increasing recognition that exclusive policy emphasis upon primary care services was no longer tenable. While the hospital sector was not starved of new resources, the rate of growth in posts and funds had been substantially lower than hospital specialists had desired. This had been particularly true in Sweden and Finland, where the political consensus in support of developing primary care, as well as the organisational arrangements for channeling institutional resource flows, were strongest. In a widely publicised incident in Sweden in Spring 1988, the chief of the Radiology Department at Karolinska Hospital in Stockholm announced that capacity shortages were delaying vital chemo-therapy treatments for cancer patients (Dagens Nyheter, March 1988).

A second non-political factor had been the relatively rapid shift in clinical indications and–or acceptance of certain elective surgical procedures, especially for intra-ocular lens transplantation, full hip-replacement and coronary bypass procedures. In combination with relatively rigid public budgeting structures, along with central emphasis upon developing primary care facilities, this shift in clinical indications resulted by the mid-1980s in substantial (often one to two years) waiting lists for these and other therapeutic procedures. While there has been some debate about the consistency and appropriateness of clinical criteria used in developing these waiting lists (for a Swedish example, see Socialstyrelsen 1988), their similar length and character across publicly operated health systems not only in the Nordic region but, most controversially, in the United Kingdom as well (Yates, 1987) suggests that the fundamental problem is both real and structural in nature.

This growth of elective surgical queues combined with a third, essentially sociological factor created a volatile situation in Sweden,

Finland and Denmark alike by the end of 1987. Very simply, this was the increasing insistence of Nordic citizens that they be treated less like the object and more like the subject of their publicly operated delivery systems. The celebrated 1983 case in Denmark of Mrs. Sorensen, who personally confronted the Danish Interior Minister in order to extract permission to undergo a then-experimental liver transplant in The Netherlands (which was in her case successful), symbolises the new tone of individual activism. By 1988 both Swedish and Finnish health authorities found themselves subjected to media campaigns about elective surgical queues, with the Finnish press going so far as to suggest that the public authorities, in the case of postponed coronary bypass surgery, were complicit with murder (*Helsingen Sanomat*, 21 February 1988). Beginning in 1986 but with greater urgency in 1987 and 1988, health sector officials in Denmark, Sweden and Finland began sending substantial numbers of bypass patients abroad; Copenhagen County to Wisconsin and London, Stockholm County to London (as well as to two private Swedish hospitals in Stockholm and Göteborg), and Finland to Pamplona, Spain and to Talinn in Soviet Estonia.

As a result of these three structural forces: capacity shortages in the hospital sector; a shift in clinical indications for newly developed surgical procedures; and growing citizen activism in response to the rationing of elective procedures, it became clear that the prior primary-care-based strategy would have to be modified. In Sweden, in the words of one Ministry of Health and Social Affairs official, 'The wind has shifted completely'. As explained by a senior national planning official, the new policy would be a joint emphasis upon low intensity services to the elderly, particularly in the social services, alongside a renewed investment in intensive hospital-based activities (Wennstrom, personal communication, 1988). In Finland in April 1987 the traditionally docile municipalities refused to accept the proposed 1988 national health and social services plan from the National Board of Health. Insisting that the municipalities could no longer afford to expand their primary care and social service sectors as the national plan required, the municipalities demanded and won the right to shift personnel posts among categories in the plan. This in effect 'melted' the tightly controlled national framework that had been utilised specifically to expand the primary care sector (Saltman, 1988b). In Denmark, although the maiden speech of the national government's first Minister of Health promised fealty to WHO's Health For All policy, the very formation of the new Danish Ministry as separate from the Ministry of Social Affairs, which then remained responsible for municipally provided social services, violated the central objective of the WHO strategy. It also broke ranks with the Swedish and Finnish model of combining social and medical care into one integrated administrative unit.

While softening their prior, primary-care-based policy, the Swedish, Finnish and Danish national governments have simultaneously sought ways to consolidate and–or expand their own policy-making power as sitting governments. Effort has concentrated on rearranging a variety of prior organisational patterns so as to enhance the national government's voice in the policy formulation process. The formation of the new Danish Ministry serves as the most visible indication, creating a new national vehicle through which to temper and potentially counterbalance the operating autonomy of the 14 Danish county councils.

Perhaps the most interesting indication of commonality in the perceived national dilemma has been the serious discussions in Finland, Sweden and Denmark alike during 1987 and 1988 about subsuming their respective National Boards of Health – traditionally independent professional planning and advisory bodies – directly into their Ministries as downgraded 'development centres' and–or auxiliary planning departments. Although the national governments were headed by political parties of divergent ideologies; Social Democratic in Sweden, a conservative-led coalition in Denmark, and a left–right coalition in Finland, in all three instances the National Boards (which date back to 1663 in Sweden, 1812 in Finland, and 1909 in Denmark) were perceived as physician-dominated and unresponsive to the new political concerns of the national government. The fact that by 1989 the Danish government had decided to press ahead with its reorganisation plans, the Finnish government had decided to merge the previously separate National Board of Social Welfare with the National Board of Health, while the Swedish government reversed course and reinvigorated the National Board as an instrument to monitor the quality of county-produced services, indicates less about the impact of political ideology than about alternative strategies through which to strengthen the national government's health policy hand.

Beyond revitalising the National Board of Health, the Swedish government has set in motion a variety of initiatives in an effort to reverse the policy vacuum created at the national level by the 1983 Health Act. A new national centre for technology assessment has been established within the Ministry, despite considerable feeling that such a centre should logically be placed within the National Board of Health and Welfare. This new centre has a mission to help educate hospital specialists about the costs and benefits of new diagnostic and therapeutic procedures. A joint national-federation of county council committees has been reconfigured, chaired by the Prime Minister, with the unofficial task, in the private comment of a Ministry of Health official, to 'negotiate treaties' between the two Social-Democratic-led bodies. As one national official expressed the prevailing sentiment in early 1988, 'Sweden is a single country, not a federation of 26 governments. We should have one national health policy'.

The Finnish national government, although also having attempted to absorb its independent National Board of Health, has faced a rather different set of national-regional policy tensions. Finland has had a substantially higher level of national authority over health policy, as expressed by such mechanisms as the national plan and the 50 per cent national operating subsidy, and by the legal requirement that the annual allocations made through these instruments must be adopted by both Cabinet and Parliament. Conversely however, despite its wide formal authority, the role of the national government in Finland is in certain policy areas viewed to be less legitimate than that of municipal government; a constraint which reflects residual resentment of the national government's pre-1917 role as a proxy for foreign powers (Jutikkala and Pirinen, 1984).

This political context, coupled with the still segmented character of regional health sector administration in Finland, has created an environment in which the current national government has sought more to consolidate and exercise its substantial policy authority than to pursue new avenues of control. In particular, two specific nationally-led proposals have been put forward, each intended to streamline and clarify administrative authority within the delivery system, and in the process simplify the national government's ability to monitor and direct policy formulation and execution. One reform, at the regional level, will consolidate the several existing hospital districts (central hospital, district hospital, and mental hospital) into a single Central Health District. A second, inside the health centres at the primary care level, will introduce patient lists and performance-related salaries for general practitioners (Vohlonen *et al.*, 1989). A central objective of this Personal Doctor Program, currently in a second round of demonstration projects, is to improve the quality of both clinical care and patient satisfaction so as to reduce further growth in private ambulatory and occupational health services (Vohlonen *et al.*, 1989). Both reforms, seen from a Swedish or Danish perspective, continue to pursue a type of decentralisation strategy, albeit in a nationally mandated manner. Moreover, and equally distinct from its Nordic neighbours, the Finnish National Board and Ministry intend increasing the existing publicly operated component of the delivery system, especially at the primary care level.

Regional Developments

Having explored the shift in policy focus at the national level, it remains to consider the degree of development and congruence at the several different health sector operating levels. While the picture varies somewhat between the three countries, the overall perspective is one of uncertainty and experimentation with a variety of alternative delivery arrangements. Beyond intraorganisational approaches like the Finnish personal doctor program, there also have been across-sector attempts to better integrate and coordinate existing public sector services, as well as carefully bounded efforts to redefine the traditional borders between public and private sector providers.

Intraorganisational developments have included a new willingness by publicly operated regional and–or municipal provider agencies to introduce differential payscales based on performance incentives, particularly for physicians. Along with the Finnish personal doctor program, in Denmark's Copenhagen county, general practitioners were recently (1987) moved off full salary back to a base-salary-plus-volume-adjustment, similar to the model in the other Danish counties (Teilmann, personal communication, 1988). In Sweden a new national contract between the Federation of County Councils and the Swedish physicians' union will allow county councils to introduce individually negotiated performance-related pay for hospital chiefs-of-service beginning in 1989. These and other differential salary arrangements, while accepted by private sector labour unions in Nordic counties, are both new and controversial in the public sector, especially in Sweden with its longterm policy of wage solidarity. They also create a variety of complications for integrating pay schedules for nurses and other health care team members (Vohlonen *et al.*, 1989).

Cross-sector developments, while still within the public sector, reflect external pressures to increase service efficiency, but also efforts to improve continuity of care and overall service quality. The ongoing Swedish experiment with 'Free Municipalities', reinvigorated by the newly installed (national) Minister of Public Administration in late 1988, has sought to improve linkage between the clinical services delivered at the county level (especially primary care services) and the municipally provided social services. While attempts to move responsibility for primary care to county municipal control have thus far not been successful (Saltman and von Otter, 1990), expected 1990 legislation to give municipalities central coordinating responsibility for all care received by the elderly represents a new effort to bridge the regional-municipality gap. In Denmark, pursuing much the same objective although in less dramatic fashion, the new Ministry of Health has funded a North Jutland pilot project in which the municipal social services, once notified by a hospital, must accept a 'finished' patient within five days or begin paying a daily fine directly to the hospital (Christensen, personal communication, 1988). In Finland, in a departure from traditional allocative planning principles, the next stage of the personal doctor program may include mechanisms to transfer unutilized hospital funds to the primary care centres if general practitioners reduce their referral rates (Vohlonen, personal communication, 1989).

The question of contracting out clinical services to private providers, particularly with regard to ambulatory physician visits, reflects the extent to which regional administrative authorities can control existing revenue flows. In Finland private sector physician visits are reimbursed by national insurance funds at 60 per cent of charges on a fee-for-service basis, while the municipally operated health centres receive annual prospective budgets (supplemented by a similarly prospective national subsidy). Thus in the Finnish instance the municipal public sector lacks a direct financial level over private providers, while it is required by law to utilise most of its own prospectively-allocated revenues within the public sector. In the Danish case, the two-track public insurance system, in which patients who prefer to self-refer directly to hospital specialists pay an additional fee beyond the publicly reimbursed figure, effectively enfolds major elements of a private ambulatory sector into the publicly operated system. This model's reliance upon independent general practitioners with individual practices serves to moot the issue of increased private primary care provision in Denmark.

Consequently the main Nordic arena for public sector contracting out for privately produced ambulatory services is in Sweden, where the administrative autonomy of the county councils, in combination with complete control over the ambulatory revenue flow, has generated a suitable environment for experimentation. Although the number of counties and the percentage of patient visits and–or revenues involved remains very small, there are currently a number of different contracting models under exploration. The main alternatives appear to be leasing existing or new health centres to private entrepreneurs (Stockholm and Hallands counties) and funding private sector walk-in ambulatory clinics (Stockholm, Göteborg and Malmö) (Saltman and von Otter, 1990). Although a spring 1988 survey suggests that non-socialist-led counties are more likely than socialist-led to explore contracting possibilities (von Otter *et al.*, 1989), socialist-led counties have pursued privatisation strategies as well.

The question of increased private provision of hospital inpatient services also revolves in considerable part around revenue-related issues. A major factor in all three countries is the availability of a private revenue stream, typically provided by private insurance companies, and (given high marginal tax rates) the existence of national tax policies that facilitate personal and–or corporate deductions for the purchase of private cover. In Denmark, where the cost of private insurance is not tax deductible, there are neither private hospitals nor private specialist companies staffed by moonlighting publicly salaried physicians. Two recent efforts to establish for-profit specialist clinics, one in Jutland and a second in Copenhagen, failed to attract sufficient numbers of subscribers to commence operations (Christensen, personal communication, 1988). In Denmark consequently, the issue of private provision at hospital level has focused on public sector county council decisions to utilise tax-generated revenues to send patients abroad – to Holland, England or the United States – for specific acute procedures like coronary bypass or liver transplantation. The structural character of the pressures which continue to require 'exporting' certain patients can be seen in the fact that the Social-Democratic-led Copenhagen county has been the largest purchaser of these (foreign) private hospital services.

In Sweden by comparison, there is a small private insurance sector with approximately 15 000 subscribers, predominantly senior executives in large companies or key officers of smaller service-oriented businesses (Saltman and von Otter, 1990). While these private policies are intended mostly to provide 'business class' ambulatory care, they often cover certain elective inpatient procedures as well. The absence of a national tax deduction for individual purchase of private health insurance may help explain why almost all private cover is purchased by businesses. Moreover the January 1988 removal of tax deductibility for businesses can be expected to slow down the recent pattern of growth in corporately purchased policies.

Reflecting the limited amount of private insurance in force, privately provided inpatient services in Sweden are overwhelmingly purchased, as in Denmark, with public sector funds by the county councils. In Sweden elective procedures have been purchased from the two privately operated hospitals (typically staffed by off-duty specialists from the nearby university hospitals) but also, in several counties, from private surgical groups composed of publicly salaried physicians working at night or during the weekends, often in their publicly funded operating theatres. Additionally, as previously noted regarding coronary bypass procedures, patients have been sent abroad, most commonly to private hospitals in London which solicit Nordic business with aggressively-priced package arrangements. As in the primary-care sector, 1988 data indicated that socialist as well as non-socialist-led counties were utilising private sector contracts to reduce waiting lists (von Otter *et al.*, 1989). Indeed a national initiative by the Swedish Ministry, which began in autumn 1987 and established financial incentives for Swedish counties to have their waiting list patients treated within only publicly operated institutions, was beaten back the next year by the equally Social Democratic Federation of County Councils as an infringement upon the legal responsibility of county councils to set medical priorities.

The Finnish picture with regard to the private provision of hospital inpatient services is, in a structural sense, the oldest and most institutionalised arrangement of these three Nordic countries. Finland has four privately owned hospitals, all in Helsinki, with the largest (Mehilainen) staffed primarily by off-duty specialists from Helsinki University Hospital. Finnish law allows both individual as well as corporate deductions for private medical expenses and–or private insurance cover. A considerable number of Finns carry supplemental private insurance, and in Helsinki private cover is often expected as an employee benefit. Hence privately supplied elective procedures are available through private Finnish institutions, without requiring prior public sector physician referral nor public sector funds for individuals with appropriate private cover and–or sufficient personal resources. The number of beds and procedures however represents only a small fraction of the services provided by Finland's publicly operated institutions, which also (as in Sweden) provide extensive and expensive back-up facilities in emergencies.

In 1987 and 1988 this private hospital sector in Finland was supplemented from two directions. Seizing upon popular discontent with extensive waiting lists, new three to five bed clinics have been established in Oulu, Tampere, and Turku, staffed (as elsewhere) by off-duty publicly salaried specialists. Additionally, as noted, coronary bypass patients are being sent abroad. One type of private initiative which has not yet been allowed in Finland, at the joint insistence of the Ministry of Health and the National Federation of Municipalities (the legal owners of Finnish publicly operated hospitals), has been to permit salaried specialists to continue to work nights and–or weekends in their institutions as private entrepreneurs.

This review of private activities in clinical provision in Sweden, Denmark and Finland suggests the tentative and careful character of current initiatives. Perhaps the most striking aspect of privatisation in the Nordic region is the overwhelming extent to which private production is dependent upon public sector revenues, in most cases channeled through public sector provider agencies, and to a lesser degree the off-duty time of publicly salaried physicians. This pattern of provision, coupled with the existing prohibitions against tax deductions for private sector expenditures in Sweden and Denmark, suggests that privatisation may remain simply a useful tool; in the words of one Swedish official, 'to prod the public elephant'. Indeed another Swedish official went so far as to suggest that, once the private sector had helped eliminate Sweden's current waiting lists, private inpatient services would no longer be required by the publicly operated system. While this view of privatisation ignores its financially inertial and socially corrosive characteristics, these statements nonetheless affect the overall confidence in existing publicly operated health systems felt by Social Democratic officials in both Sweden and Finland.

CONCLUSIONS

The absence of ideological correlation between support for specific privatisation activities on the one hand, and a conservative or neo-liberal political orientation on the other, deserves to be emphasised. Sweden, with its national government and regional government federation headed by Social Democrats, has perhaps the greatest activity in the area of contracting out clinical services to privately operated providers. Finland, with a joint Social Democratic–Conservative national administration (and no elected provincial-level institutional counter-balance) has substantially less experimentation although it has the largest private sector of these three countries. Yet Denmark, with a conservative-headed national government, has almost no privatisation activities beyond the export of certain elective surgical patients. While this lack of correlation reflects only national level administration, and does not incorporate the widely varying political forces at the regional and–or municipal operating levels of their health system, the pattern is nonetheless informative and important. In the Nordic region, with the most heavily public sector health services in Western Europe, the response to the current period of organisational uncertainty, financial pressure, and popular restiveness has been pragmatic rather than political, focused on service quality and responsiveness rather than political ideology. There is of course no certainty that the policy and structural preconditions which have produced this outcome will remain in place indefinitely. For the forseeable future however it would appear that the key policy questions in the Nordic region will remain those of (a)   accommodating renewed attention to hospitals and acute procedures with the less intensive requirements of providing custodial care to the growing numbers of elderly and (b) balancing the desire of national governments to increase their influence over the policy formulation process with the insistence of regional and–or municipal providers that their operating authority not be compromised. In short, the central policy question will continue to be how these publicly operated, tax-based systems will reconstruct themselves for a second generation of service; what the new public sector models will look like, rather than whether they will survive as publicly operated, publicly accountable health systems.

References

Amstrådforeningen, I.D. (1986) *Regional Self-Government* (Copenhagen).
Bogason, P. (1987) 'Capacity for Welfare: Local Government in Scandinavia and the United States', *Scandinavian Studies*, no. 59, pp. 184–202.
Bosworth, B.P. and A.M. Rivlin (1987) (eds), *The Swedish Economy* (Brookings Institution).

Castles, F.G. (1987) *The Social Democratic Image of Society: A Study of the Achievements and Origins of Scandinavian Social Democracy in Comparative Perspective* (London: Routledge and Kegan Paul).

Dagens, Nyheter (1988) 'Vårdgarentier für sjuka' 30 March.

Einhorn, E.S. (1987) 'Economic Policy and Social Needs: The Recent Scandinavian Experience', *Scandinavian Studies*, no. 59, pp. 203–20.

Esping-Andersen, G. (1985) *Politics Against Markets* (Princeton University Press).

Helsingen Sanomat 27 February 1988.

Jutikkala, E. and K. Pirinen (1984) *A History of Finland*, Fourth revised edition (Espoo: Weilin and Goos).

Pekurinen, M. I. Vohlonen, and V. Hakkinen (1987) 'Re-allocation of Resources in Favour of Primary Health Care: The Case of Finland', *World Health Statistics Quarterly*, no. 40, pp.313–25.

Saltman, R.B. (1987) 'Management Control in a Publicly Planned Health System: A Case Study from Finland', *Health Policy*, no. 8, pp. 284–98.

Saltman, R.B. (1988a) 'Health Care in Sweden', in R.B. Saltman (ed.) *The International Handbook of Health Care Systems* (Westport, CT and London: Greenwood Press).

Saltman, R.B. (1988b) 'National Planning for Locally Controlled Health Systems: The Finnish Experience', *Journal of Health Politics, Policy and Law*, no. 13, pp. 27–51.

Saltman, R.B. and C. von Otter (1989) 'Voice, Choice and the Question of Civil Democracy in the Swedish Welfare State,' *Economic and Industrial Democracy*, no. 10, pp. 195–209.

Saltman, R.B. and C. von Otter (1990) *Planned Markets and Public Competition: A Framework for Strategic Reform in Health Systems* (forthcoming).

Serner, U. (1980) 'Swedish Health Legislation: Milestones in Reorganisation Since 1945,' in A.J. Heidenheimer and N.J. Elvander (eds), *The Making of the Swedish Health Care System* (New York: St. Martin's Press).

Siam, H. (1986) *Choices for Health* (Oslo: Universitetsforlaget).

Socialstyrelsen (1988) Köer I. Sjukvården: Sammanfattande Redovisning Och Uppföljning Effectiverna Av Statsbidraget (Stockholm: Socialstyrelsen).

Vohlonen, I., M. Pekurinen, and R.B. Saltman (1989) 'Reorganising Primary Medical Care in Finland: The Personal Doctor Program,' *Health Policy* (forthcoming).

von Otter, C., R.B. Saltman, and L. Joelsson (1989) 'Välmöjligheter, Konkurrens, Entreprenader M.M., Inom Landstingens Sjukvård – Enkätrëultat', Working Paper (Swedish Center for Working Life).

World Health Organisation, (1981) *Regional Strategy for Health for All (Copenhagen): WHO.*

World Health Organisation (1984) (Regional Targets in Support of the Regional Strategy for Health for All (Copenhagen: WHO).

Yates, J. (1987) *Why are We Waiting?* (Oxford: Oxford Medical).

6 Heart Disease in Israel: Curative or Preventive Policy?

Yael Yishai

THE PROBLEM

Ischaemic heart disease is the number one killer in the modern world; it is the 'plague' of the 20th century (Stamler, 1985), a source of much concern to the public and health authorities alike. In Israel the figures are striking: in 1986 the ratio of deaths due to heart disease among 100 000 Jews was 243 (one-third of the total – 752) (Budget Proposal, 1989, p. 74). The standardisation rates per 100 000 also present a gloomy picture: in Israel they stand at 188.69 (in 1986), compared with the European average of 154.11 (Health System, 1988, p. 31). Although a considerable decline in the death rate was identified (particularly in the 1970s) (Epstein, 1979) the problem looms large, calling for medical and political action.[1]

Policy-makers face two alternatives in dealing with the high death toll exacted by heart disease: the preventive option and the curative option. Numerous studies conducted in the last thirty years have substantially increased our knowledge of the possible causes of heart diseases and of the means for their prevention. Several intervention studies, including some community-based trials, have confirmed the feasibility of preventing ischaemic heart disease (Modan, 1989; Rywik and Kupske, 1985). It is hard to believe that only some two decades ago the identification of high risk factors conducive to this ailment took place. These include high blood cholesterol, lack of physical activity and, primarily, cigarette smoking. The 'high risk factors' are significantly influenced by a number of personal and population characteristics acting separately or in combination. Health authorities assert that the identified factors are largely determined by sociocultural conditions and are therefore modifiable. Appropriate eating habits, low alcohol intake, regular exercise and primarily refraining from smoking are likely to reduce the chances of being afflicted with a heart disease. Raising public awareness of the dangers of unhealthy eating habits and smoking is thus a prime national objective.

The WHO urged health authorities to initiate countrywide programmes aimed at promoting healthy life-styles supported by an appropriate social policy. However, while preventive measures were expected to reduce the occurrence of the disease, complementary programmes were required to prevent deaths as well as the increase and recurrence of acute myo-cardial infarction and strokes (Targets, 1986). Sophisticated medical technology consuming immense financial resources was geared to this purpose.

The expediency of employing both preventive and curative measures is self-evident, but the scarcity of resources necessitates choosing between alternatives, that is determining priorities regarding the preventive and the curative options. Rhetorically, human welfare necessitates investment in whatever may advance and maintain individual health, but the exigencies of reality require that choices be made. The question of 'who gets what when and how' is highly pertinent to coping with the threatening killer. Should available resources, limited as they may be, be invested in the acquisition of highly expensive equipment? Or should an extensive preventive campaign be launched aimed at curbing the problem before it arises? Answers to these questions are not based on an ideal type model, but on observations regarding the actual pattern of policy-making in Israel. What are the values that determine the priorities of decision-makers? What are the forces and constraints that shape them? What are the outcomes of policy decisions, and how and by whom are they formulated? These are the questions addressed in this chapter.

Choosing between the curative or the preventive options is not only a technical matter of allocating scarce resources. It also touches upon fundamental questions of state and society. The issue of heart disease is highly 'politicised' because it involves authoritative decision-making and determination of national priorities by ruling elites. At the same time, as a major health problem, it is also of high concern to the individual and therefore belongs to the sphere of society. Theoretically those promulgating the preventive option believe it is the state duty to influence society, to exercise its authority and to interfere with individual behaviour. Those in favour of the curative option assume that society predominates, that resort to health risk factors is an individual choice. The state can provide means for curing disease; it is the people's responsibility to watch their own health.

The underlying assumption is that the choice between the preventive and the curative options is determined by:

(a) The benefits available to policy-makers derived from the policy alternatives.
(b) The constraints impeding the articulation of either of the alternatives.
(c) The characteristics of the policy universe.
(d) The characteristics of the policy process.

More specifically, a policy is likely to be chosen:

- When ideological and political benefits outweigh those of the alternative.
- When constraints, in terms of political pressures, are weaker compared to the alternative.
- When the structure of decision-making tends to be centralised and institutionalised.
- When 'entrepreneurs' seize the opportunity to advance an issue through an 'open window'.

Israel deviates from this pattern. It is a highly politicised society since governments have invariably promoted a 'big' state. The left-wing coalitions that ruled the country for nearly thirty years (1948–77) established a government apparatus which is the largest in the democratic world in terms of resources and involvement. The ascendance of the right-wing Likud to power did not alter the scope of state control. The government remains big, highly centralised and preoccupied with functions which usually belong to the social domain (Sharkansky, 1987). Security imperatives, economic exigencies and political structures have so far impeded any change. Policy-making regarding heart disease thus takes place within an environment in which politics looms large and where society is conspicuously within the reach of government. Under these circumstances 'politics' is expected to predominate. It in fact did, but not in the expected form since in Israel the curative option has had a clear priority over the preventive one.

This chapter will delineate the Israeli case against the common assumptions. It will proceed by discussing some dimensions of the outputs and the impact of the chosen alternative in terms of public policy.

THE EXPECTED BENEFITS: VALUES AND INTERESTS

The underlying value which guides decision-making is the need to diminish the rate of deaths caused by heart disease. In this respect however, cardiovascular illness is not substantially different from other causes of mortality. The deep concern with heart disease is a reflection of the salience attached to human life. This may be a universal feature, especially in Western liberal societies where individual life and liberty are cherished and inscribed in legal norms. In Israel these norms have been reinforced due to specific sociocultural circumstances. Jewish tradition regards the individual as an incarnation of the Holy entity. A proverb frequently cited asserts that 'He who saveth one person saveth the whole world'. In fact saving life overrides all other religious commandments, including the sacredness of the Sabbath. A Jew is permitted to desecrate the holy day if saving a human soul is involved. This attitude reflects the social aspect of health care underpinning individual rights. But there are also state oriented values.

The country's precarious security condition has necessitated the elevation of health to the top of the national agenda. The numerical inferiority of Israel via-à-vis its enemies generated pressures for comprehensive provision of health services. Israel simply could not afford an ill society. The health of its population has become an important component of national power. The state's commitment regarding the health of its citizens has had economic and political implications. Israel was established as a welfare social-democratic society based on the principles of mutual aid. The government was mandated to be responsible for the health and well-being of its citizens. A wide network of public health systems has thus been established based on public funding and centralised (political) control. Private medical care has constituted a marginal portion of health care. The state has been unswervingly committed to looking after its citizens' health, either by its own means or through public associations.

Both prevention and cure of heart disease is thus a prime national need in the Israeli case. However, within this broad category of pro-life orientations, values seem to have provided higher incentives for curative policies, which could be manipulated as a means for fulfilling other ideological objectives. The curative option provides a good example of such a 'value transplant' from one policy domain to the other, namely from health policy to population dispersion.

The transfer of human and material resources from the centre to the periphery has been one of the state's promulgated (though much less applied) social policies. Israel's coastline is densely populated, with approximately 70 per cent of the population inhabiting the metropolitan areas and smaller cities. Its peripheral zones have been vulnerable from a defence perspective and have suffered continuous economic shortage (Borukhov and Werczberger, 1981). Population dispersion was aimed at increasing the country's facilities to integrate newcomers; it was intended to spur the state's economic development and to provide a security belt for the hinterland. As a democratic society Israel could not compel its citizens to 'disperse' and reside in the periphery. It could however offer social-economic incentives in order to attract individuals to these remotef often under-developed areas. For example, one of the paramount disadvantages of living in the periphery was the absence of advanced medical services which were available only in the big health centres located in metropolitan areas. The distribution of curative techniques to peripheral hospitals was thus congruent with the often quoted national goal of population dispersion.

The introduction of curative techniques has also provided a means for emphasising the Israeli authorities' commitment to egalitarian health services. Many political battles have been fought for this principle, which more often than not has consumed a heavy toll of scarce resources. It has been inconceivable to apply rational calculations to decisions affecting access to health services. Therefore the right of every Israeli to enjoy the benefits of modern medical treatment has been almost unrestricted. Conventional criteria (such as age) have not been applied in the Israeli health system.

Adherence to ideological tenets could also be rewarding in terms of political interests. The politicians' desire to reap immediate fruits and enjoy the crop of their labour while still in office is a truism. Yet in the case under consideration this factor has been highly conspicuous. Preventive policy rewards only in the long run. It is most likely to encounter opposition and its outcomes are unlikely to be seen during the politician's incumbency. Curative measures on the other hand show almost immediate results. They confer power upon decision-makers and enable them to turn their authority into electoral assets.

Curative techniques are easily translated into the language of statistics and provide tangible proof of the administration's effectiveness and competence. These values are most likely to induce the adoption of curative measures, regardless of their long-term contribution to diminishing the death rate caused by heart disease.

CONSTRAINTS ON DECISION-MAKERS

The determination of each option under consideration, the preventive or the curative, is grounded in a different set of constraints and economic imperatives. The curative technique is based on a wide variety of treatments including artificial hearts, heart transplants and simpler forms of heart surgery, all of which consume immense human and material resources which are highly expensive. This chapter focuses only on one of the medical techniques available to alleviate a heart condition: catheterisation. This particular type of treatment was chosen because of its recent introduction and its rapid expansion. Tracing the diffusion of catheterisation facilities provides an opportunity to analyse the process of decision-making regarding priorities in a health care system.

The cost of installing catheterisation machinery approximates 450 000 dollars. Operating these instruments puts a heavy load on health budgeting. Although the percentage of the GNP spent on health in Israel is not lower than that of many other European countries (see Table 6.1), the analysis of trends reveals growing budgetary constraints.

Health expenditure per capita in 1980 was $459, in 1986 it amounted to $477; that is an average annual growth of only 0.6 per cent. This increase lagged behind the rise in income and standard of living (Health System, 1988, pp. 51–2). Not only has growth of resources devoted to health care been extremely limited, but there are additional factors which contribute to financial stringency. First, the proportion of the population aged 65 or older has dramatically increased from 7.4 in 1974 to 8.9 in 1985.[2] Secondly, the demand for sophisticated medical treatment has been constantly growing; but the government's share in financing health services has continuously declined. During the years 1979–83 the state financed 58–61 per cent (respectively) of health expenditure. In 1987–8 its share was only 50 per cent.[3] The diminishing government investment in the provision of health services has not had much impact on their demand. One of the

Table 6.1 National expenditure on health as a percentage of GDP in selected European countries (1983)

Country	Percentage
Sweden	9.6
France	8.8
FRG	8.2
Austria	7.3
Israel	**7.0**
Norway	6.9
Denmark	6.6
Belgium	6.5
UK	6.2
Greece	4.7

Source Budget Proposal 1989, based on OECD Measuring Health Care 1960–1983, Expenses, Cost and Performance, OECD, Paris

direct results was a growth in local initiative, with hospitals launching programmes in response to narrow parochial pressures. These, according to health authorities, 'were not based on an objective, integrative view of the needs of the population and the needs of the health system at large' (Health System, 1988, p. 61). As will be indicated below, these initiatives have had a direct bearing on advancing the curative option.

Constraints on the curative option have thus been limited to the reality of financial resources. In theory no-one opposes the unlimited acquisition of catheterisation equipment as long as qualitative essential medical conditions are fulfilled. The general opinion is that the wider the dispersion of curative measures, the higher the public access to treatment and the higher the chances of maximising medical effects. The picture is different with regard to preventive measures, implying restrictions on smoking and on the intake of certain kinds of food. The issue has triggered both outright and more tacit opposition of economic enterprises.

Preventive policy has included three major strategies: legislation (including regulation) restricting (or banning) the use of high-risk factors; educational campaigns aimed at persuading the public to refrain from resorting to high risk factors; and the introduction of comprehensive preventive measures such as regular checking of high blood pressure or high cholesterol level. The last strategy has never been implemented because of the high price involved. In fact it has not even been subject to rational evaluation based on long-term cost-benefit analysis, the main reason being the shortage of short-term resources. Legislation and educational campaigns have encountered opposition mainly by the tobacco industry, the Advertisers' Association and the food industry.

The tobacco industry

Israel is a smoking society. According to a recent survey (conducted during June–July 1988) 36 per cent of the Jewish population in Israel (20 years of age and older) stated that they smoke cigarettes (Ben Sira, 1988). This was an increase on the previous year's rate and a continuation of the fluctuations (presented in Table 6.2) seen in the rate since studies began in 1970. Admittedly, when judged by international standards, Israel is only seventeenth among 26 countries of the European region in its rate of per capita consumption of cigarettes (Smoke Free Europe, 1988). But the rate is growing.

The high incidence of smoking is allegedly influenced by the tensions caused by the precarious security situation in the country, and by the cost of cigarettes.

Table 6.2 Percentage of cigarette smokers by date of survey

Date of Survey	Percentage of cigarette smokers
June–July 1970	42
March–April 1971	37
October–November 1972	35
November 1973	38
March 1974	40
March 1975	36
March–April 1976	39
January 1979	36
January 1981	37
February–March 1983	36
July–August 1987	32
June–July 1988	36

Source Ben Sira 1987:61; 1988:3

Evidently the price of a packet of cigarettes (fixed by state authorities) is cheaper in Israel than in most other European countries. In 1987 the cost of one packet amounted to only $0.64; the third cheapest (after Greece and Spain) among 11 European Common Market countries. The main reason for the low cost of cigarettes is the amount of tax in the total price, which in Israel was only 62 per cent (Table 6.3). This rate placed Israel in the second lowest position among European countries, with only Spain imposing a lower rate of taxes (49 per cent). It is worth noting that in Denmark, taxing of cigarettes is as high as 87 per cent of their price.[4]

Table 6.3 Tax on cigarettes in European Common Market countries (1987)

Country	Price ($)	Tax (%)
Denmark	3.60	87
Ireland	2.77	74
U.K.	2.45	74
Germany	2.19	72
Italy	1.21	72
Portugal	0.72	72
Holland	1.65	71
Belgium	1.54	79
Greece	0.48	63
Israel	**0.64**	**62**
Spain	0.55	49

Source Adapted from the *Jerusalem Post*, 17 March 1989.

A further major lowering of taxes on imported cigarettes occurred in February 1988 with the changing of the tax ratio from approximately 60 per cent tax and 40 per cent actual price to 40 per cent tax and 60 per cent actual price. As a result, imported cigarettes have become cheaper in Israel than in their countries of origin and the Israeli market has been flooded with them.

The administrative decree which lowered taxes on imported cigarettes was issued following a strike in the only Israeli cigarette company, Dubek. The strike was unique in the sense that it was not a regular labour dispute between workers and employers. Rather the two joined forces together in order to influence authorities to allow the cigarette enterprise to increase the price of its products. The stoppage of work in the factory, which immediately created an acute shortage of cigarettes, prompted the government to hit back. The Ministry of Commerce and Industry, together with the Ministry of Finance, lowered prices for imported cigarettes in order to break the cigarette monopoly in one of the goods most favoured by the Israeli public. The fear that the rise in the price of cigarettes would have a detrimental effect on the Consumers' Price Index was the major reason behind this unusual step. There were also personal considerations involved, as top officials in both ministries aligned against the controversial manager of the cigarette industry.

It has been estimated that the damage caused by cigarette smoking to the Israeli economy is as high as $500 million; this equals five times the income derived from taxes on cigarettes.[5] Nevertheless the state has been ready to sacrifice income from levies in return for economic stability. It has granted priority to short-term monetary considerations over long-term consequences for public health.

The tobacco industry has also been a major obstacle to legislation regarding restrictions on smoking. This branch of the economy includes not only the powerful monopoly of Dubek and its workers, but also a myriad of other interested bodies such as tobacco-growers (not very powerful because the growth of tobacco is concentrated mainly in the Arab sector) and, primarily, the Chamber of Commerce, whose members enjoy the benefits of selling the cigarettes. The constraints created by these associations are sustained by a favourable environment. Israel is a stress-ridden society, with compulsory military service for three years (in the 18–21 age group; two years for women) and continuous annual reserve service for all men up to the age of 55. The precarious security situation is conceivably one of the reasons for the relatively high smoking rate of the Israeli population. In fact the army is a hot-bed of smokers, many of whom are introduced to the practice during their military service. In the framework of the October (1973) War effort, cigarettes were given free to soldiers on the front by the voluntary Committee for Soldiers and by the cigarette company. Cigarettes were presented as a good friend for soldiers and for the homefront as well as a way to cope with tension. In fact Dubek was declared a vital industry and key production employees were freed from military duty to ensure cigarette supplies to the army. Representatives of the company were quoted as stating that the small flame of the cigarette contributes greatly to lowering the soldiers' stress. Trucks bearing the name of the company were appropriated by the military and served as mobile advertisements for cigarettes throughout the war.

Notice has to be taken of the smokers themselves. There are no reliable data on the incidence of smokers among decision-makers but some of the state's top leaders (for example, Yitzhak Rabin, the Defence Minister) are known to be heavy smokers. Smoking is permitted in government meetings (Premier Begin was the only one who banned the practice). The delay in anti-smoking legislation was attributed partly to the strong lobby of smokers among Knesset members.

Finally, the Ministry of Finance may have contributed to the constraints (there is no evidence to this regard), due to the economic impact of the taxes. Although, as noted earlier, taxes are relatively low, the total income derived from excise duty on alcohol and tobacco amounted (in 1987) to $71 000 (Israel Statistical Abstract 1988, p. 561).

The Advertisers' Union

Cigarette advertisements take the lion's share of the press advertising budget (amounting to 4.3 million shekels in 1988).[6] In the first quarter of 1989, there was a considerable rise in the income from cigarette advertising. Out of 1.9 million shekels, 1.5 million were spent by foreign companies.[7] In 1988 approximately $160 000 was spent on advertising imported cigarettes in Israel. This amount was greater than the Health Ministry's budget available for smoking prevention. The dependence of the written media on the cigarette companies for such a huge revenue has impeded the access of the anti-smoking groups to this important source of influence on public opinion and public behaviour. Cases have been cited (by an activist in the anti-smoking group) where a journalist who dared to write against smoking lost his job. The press is thus perceived by the anti-smoking groups as a foe rather than a friend.

Since television advertising is very expensive, the lack of press support is considered to be a major barrier to the anti-smoking campaign.[8] Furthermore, reportedly the Advertisers' Union officially opposes any banning on cigarette advertisements. The association maintained that 'advertisement in all its forms is inseparable from marketing. As long as there is no limit on cigarette production and sale, there is no logic in curbing advertising'.[9]

The Food Industry

Unofficial data indicate that some half of the sample of Tel-Aviv residents suffer from a 'very high' or 'high' rates of cholesterol in their blood.[10] Furthermore, according to a study conducted in 1987, approximately half of Israel's adult population is overweight (although only a small proportion will admit it). Some of the respondents (14 per cent) even think that fat-rich foods have the most important nutritional components (Ben Sira, 1987). These findings indicate that food consumption may contribute to the frequency of heart disease and should therefore be subject to regulative policy.

The sale of cholesterol-rich foods (such as hard cheeses and beef) is controlled by statutory agricultural marketing councils (the Milk Council and the Beef Council respectively) which operate under state auspices. Initially the Councils were aimed at promoting cooperation between the government and the numerous farmers' associations. In practice however the Councils have largely become instruments for implementing a two-pronged official policy. Whilst the Ministry of Agriculture's goal was to secure the highest prices for food products and to maintain the high rate of subsidies to farm products, the Treasury aimed at reducing the prices in order to lower the cost-of-living index and simultaneously minimise the state's heavy subsidies to agriculture.

The two objectives were made compatible by cutting subsidies on the one hand and encouraging the farmers to increase marketing on the other. One of the means for achieving this purpose was granting the Councils access to public service broadcasts. Television advertisements claimed to serve legitimate public causes on the ostensibly noncommercial network. However the agricultural Councils represented strictly commercial advertising in the guise of serving the public. In fact they did a disservice to the public and may even have posed a danger to it. In an attempt to cover up the commercial aspect of their TV advertising, the Dairy Council took great pains to assure the public that ice-cream and hard cheeses contain 'calcium drawn directly from nature'. Likewise the Beef Council claimed that 'soft calf meat' is invigorating and healthy. Not one single word was mentioned with regard to the fat that turns into cholesterol. Authorities who were supposed to veto the 'public service' broadcasts approved them, in what was termed by the press 'a dereliction of public duty'.[11] Clearly the state's economic stake in the marketing of farm products has inhibited effective measures against health risks related to coronary diseases.

THE STRUCTURE OF THE POLICY UNIVERSE

Mapping the process of decision-making reveals a set of actors focusing on major issues relating to heart policy. At the centre of the policy universe is the Ministry of Health, vested with the formal authority of making decisions regarding health policy. In addition two types of policy networks can be identified for each of the policy options: a *diffused* network with many actors pulling the strings in different directions; and a *coordinated* network, where power is hierarchically ordered. The preventive policy universe is more congruent with the first pattern. It includes, in addition to the governmental agencies and legislative organs involved in the process of formulating policy, public interest groups and professional associations. The curative policy universe is more compatible with the second pattern. The issue is elaborated mainly by bureaucratic agencies or their extensions.

The Ministry of Health

The Ministry of Health is, on paper, one of the more important welfare departments in the Israeli cabinet. Not only is it politically responsible for the provision of health services to the Israeli population, but it operates the major network of hospitals in the country. The Ministry is thus both a provider and a coordinator of health facilities. It is vested with wide authority to plan, allocate and determine priorities in all spheres pertaining to physical and–or mental health (Budget Proposal, 1989). In reality, for two major reasons the powers of the Ministry are extremely limited. First, traditionally the Ministry of Health was granted to a minor coalition party whose influence on general policy was negligible. Second, the marginality of the Ministry has resulted from the fact that health policy in Israel has been determined to a large extent by a non-governmental institution, that is the General Sick Fund (Kupat Holim). The Sick Fund, insuring some 75 per cent of the population has been, by all indicators, far more powerful than the Ministry officially responsible for the provision of health services.

Data comparing human and material resources demonstrate Kupat Holim's prominence. The budget of Kupat Holim (in 1986) was almost twice as high as that of the Ministry; 1.2 billion shekels and 777 million shekels respectively. The number of physicians employed by the Sick Fund was 5200 compared to 2393 employed by the state. On the Ministry's payroll were some 20 000 employees; Kupat Holim employed 28 000 workers. The Sick Fund's investment in fixed assets has also been far higher than that of the state: 39.3 per cent of the total compared with 23.6 per cent of the total respectively (Yishai 1989b). The most striking figure pertains to ambulatory care, which has virtually been controlled by Kupat Holim, owning 83.2 per cent of the country's clinics.

Under these circumstances it is not surprising that the Ministry has often been helpless in determining priorities. Kupat Holim has turned into the tail that wags the dog. In addition the Ministry of Health is largely subject to decisions made by the Treasury, one of the most powerful organs in the Israeli system of government. The monopolisation of wage negotiations and budgetary allocations by the Finance Ministry has also curbed the power of health authorities.

The Preventive Arena

The Health Ministry

A small sub-division within the Ministry of Health is responsible for 'Public Health' with a token budget of some 1000 shekels or $500 (in 1989) (Budget Regulations, 1989, p. 48), and activities which focus mainly on anti-smoking campaigns. This department does not play any role in the process of policy-making. Lip-service is paid to the target of Promoting Health, but not much is being done about it. Nevertheless, as will be indicated below, some output in the form of anti-smoking legislation has emerged. Responsibility for policies designed to introduce preventive practices has been shared with the Ministry of Education, Ministry of Justice and with the Knesset and its committees.

Public Interest Groups

Three major interest groups focus their prime attention on heart-related issues: the Cancer Association, the Israeli Heart Society, and the Anti-Smoking group. In addition there are several small groups, such as the Society for the Prevention of High Blood Pressure, whose activity and resources are extremely modest. The groups have some characteristics in common; they are elite organisations, whose major work is done by rank and file volunteers, prompted by altruistic motivations. The associations, whose finances are secured mainly from private contributions, play an advocacy role (Kramer, 1976, 1981), thus fulfilling a major function in a domain where the government has failed to act. The groups operating in the health sector not only supplement state activity but in effect, substitute for it (Yishai, 1989a). However, as Table 6.4 shows, the groups vary with regard to resources and scope of activity.

Table 6.4 The organisational attributes of interest group actors

	Cancer	Heart	Anti-Smoking
Year of founding	1952	1985	1971
No. of hired workers	80	7	–
Annual budget (1988) IS mil.	10	1	0.1
No. of branches	60	6	3
Forum of decision-making	professional committees	formal executive	informal executive

Source Interviews with groups' leaders

The Cancer Association is the most resourceful of the three. It was formed in the early 1950s by oncologists aiming at channeling national funds to the prevention and cure of cancer. The Cancer Association has been successful in enlisting wide public support. At present it is a well-staffed organisation, with some 80 workers on its pay-roll (including those who work on a part-time basis) and thousands of volunteers. Its annual budget for 1988 was 10 million shekels (nearly $6 million), which is very high by Israeli standards. The Association is highly institutionalised with a firm bureaucratic basis. It has a centrally controlled organisational setup including sixty branches. Among its leaders are well-known public figures, such as Suzy Eban the former Foreign Minister's wife. The Cancer Association's activity covers six major domains of rehabilitation and prevention of the disease, including public education targeted mainly against smoking.

While lobbying activity is not one of the Association's declared strategies, it has nevertheless been active in promoting the anti-smoking legislation. The Cancer Association was an active actor in putting the issue of smoking on the parliamentary agenda. Its constant pressures triggered authorities to enact an anti-smoking bill. The Association has also strongly protested the proposal to lower the price of cigarettes in Israel. In fact it has called upon the government to consider increasing the tax burden on smokers and use the extra tax revenue to maintain and improve health services in the country.[12]

The Heart Society is smaller than its counterpart both in terms of organisational attributes and in its scope of activity. It was established (on a national basis) in the mid-1980s by an ex-high-ranking IDF (Israeli Defence Forces) officer who was personally afflicted by the disease. The Association's organisational framework is more modest than that of its counterpart; its annual budget amounted (in 1988) to less than one million shekels. Human resources are also on a smaller scale, with only seven hired employees and a few hundred volunteers. The leadership of the Heart Society includes high-ranking cardiologists, as well as noted people in other walks of life. The Heart Association is highly centralised, with the central headquarters located in Kfar Saba (a small town near Tel Aviv) virtually controlling the activities of the other branches. While the major party (75 per cent) of the group's funding is derived from the branches, their share in the expenditure is only half. Centralisation is regarded as an organisational asset despite the defection of a major branch.[13] As one activist put it, 'branches shun responsibility, they would prefer the centre to handle the association's affairs'.

At its inception the Society targeted its strategies more on curative than on preventive goals. Its major functions included the provision of resuscitation courses to interested citizens, and increasing public awareness of this means as a life-saving instrument. Anti-smoking activity was not on the Society's agenda since it was already addressed by the Cancer Association. Blood pressure was also taken care of by Kupat Holim. The unique contribution of the Heart Society to the prevention of heart disease has therefore been confined to the issue of cholesterol. A scientific committee established by the Association (including cardiologists, internists and nutrition experts) proposed a campaign strategy for diminishing the intake of cholesterol. Consequently an international conference was convened as a means to capture public attention. The Heart Association also carries out blood tests in public domains in order to detect high cholesterol rates and to prompt medical treatment. This initiative however is criticised by health authorities who are highly suspicious of the utility attached to 'street screening' of medical problems.

The Society for the Prevention of Smoking was formed in the early 1970s. Its prime goals have been to prevent youngsters from smoking and protect non-smokers from damage inflicted upon them by tobacco users. The group, whose organisational structure is extremely tenuous (without paid staff and only two branches), targets its activities both at the wide public and at political authorities. Funded by a Los Angeles tycoon, the Anti-Smoking group produces media advertisements, and lobbies the Knesset and government to enact anti-smoking legislation. The Society works in close cooperation with the Public Health Services of the Ministry of Health to increase the budget for public campaigns against smoking. Headed by a lawyer, it also employs litigation strategies, appealing occasionally to the

Supreme Court of Justice to ban cigarette advertisements. The activity of the Anti-Smoking group overlaps with that of the Cancer Association; however the former claims that 'you cannot expect only (the Cancer Association) to focus on the issue of smoking. The problem is so severe that further public activity is necessary'. The two organisations have had some success in their struggle against tobacco. In 1987 the official IDF weekly (*Bamachane*) banned cigarette ads as a result of a petition to the Supreme Court issued by the Cancer Association and the Anti-Smoking group. In the course of 1988 the two associations submitted two additional petitions to the court. The first petition was against the Minister of Health for not fulfilling her duty to issue Public Health regulations on forbidding smoking in the work place. The second one was submitted against the Ministry of Commerce and Industry on its readiness to subsidise (in accordance with the investment law) a cigarette factory that was to be built in a development zone. These petitions, limited as they were, aimed at creating pressure on government to formulate an overall policy on smoking prevention.

The Israeli Medical Association (IMA)

The IMA, founded in 1912, is a powerful interest group. It is the only organisation representing the 12 000 Israeli doctors, 95 per cent of whom are salary-earners employed by public health institutions. The IMA is not only the sole spokesman of the country's physicians on wage negotiations, it is also active on the professional medical scene. The Scientific Council of the medical association was legally granted the responsibility to award specialisation titles in numerous medical branches. It conducts examinations, and in effect regulates the profession. Since 1987 the IMA (in cooperation with Israel's four medical schools) has also been responsible for the administration of a nostrification process which requires doctors who are not graduates of Israeli universities to pass qualifying examinations. From its inception, the IMA has regarded itself not only as a trade union defending the professional and economic rights of its membership, but also (perhaps mainly so) as a 'public' organisation whose interest lies in the welfare of society. In reality however, genuine issues of public welfare are not often present on the IMA's agenda. The Association is usually concerned with the economic plight of physicians and the deteriorating conditions of their employment. It acts more as a trade union safeguarding the interests of its members than as a professional association promoting collective benefits. Its activity in maintaining the scientific level of the medical community is regarded as a major contribution of the profession to public welfare.

One notable exception to this rule was the IMA's attempt in the early 1980s to launch a campaign aimed at inducing anti-smoking legislation. In June 1982 the IMA sent letters to ministers and influential members of the Knesset urging them to advance legislation regarding the restriction of smoking in public places, which was already pending and discussed by a Knesset committee. Worth noting is the fact that the IMA did not initiate legislation but acted in order to accelerate the process. It also urged the Health Ministry to issue orders banning smoking in hospitals. The surprising activity of the IMA regarding a public issue was reportedly prompted by the advice of a public relations agency as part of a campaign to improve its image. The idea was not original. British physicians were already widely engaged in an anti-smoking campaign (Royal College, 1977). The American Heart Association was also involved in the promotion of preventive policies.

In the early 1980s the IMA manifested considerable weakness in persuading authorities to grant wage increases to doctors. Its image was marred by recurring strikes and work stoppages. The IMA had to mobilise resources for the big struggle to improve salaries. Only half a year later (in March 1983) a three-month strike was staged, the longest in the rich tradition of medical work disturbances in the country. The promotion of the anti-smoking campaign, adequately publicised by the press, could thus be employed as a strategy in the physicians' abortive attempts to defend their economic interests. However it soon became evident that the anti-smoking activity would not increase the doctors' income. The campaign was short-lived and not very effective.

The General Sick Fund of the Histadrut (Kupat Holim)

Kupat Holim, which as already noted is a major actor on the health field, is not very active in preventing heart disease. Despite the enormous costs entailed in the provision of curative services to its some 2 million members, the Sick Fund suffices with limited educational activities. Kupat Holim dispenses some information material, including posters for voluntary compliance with no-smoking in ambulatory clinics (not yet included in law). The Health Education department also provides training and guidance for smoking prevention upon request and initiates activities, particularly in the framework of the Fund's Health Report, the results of which have not yet been studied or evaluated.

The Curative Arena

Health Ministry

Despite its inherent weaknesses, the Health Ministry can exercise authority with regard to the issue under concern by controlling the process of licensing. The Law of Public Health authorised the Ministry to control the diffusion of specified medical equipment – linear accelerators, computer tomographers (CT), magnetic resonance imaging (MRI), lithotrypters and instruments for heart catheterisation – whose acquisition required state approval. Formal certification of need was applied in the early 1980s only to the public health service. Since 1988 however, it has been extended to all medical institutions, including those operated by private resources. Although the dwindling health resources do not allow for state funding to acquire the sophisticated medical technology, the issue is regarded as having far-reaching public implications in terms of manpower (derived from public health services) and general level of health care. Each individual hospital obtaining the certificate of need is thus expected to acquire the equipment out of its own funds, generally solicited with the aid of Friends' Associations from contributions abroad. However, once purchased the Health Ministry is expected to be financially responsible for the installation and the daily operation of the machinery. The approval is hence mandatory not only because it is a legal requirement, but also because in its absence the hospital will not be funded for using the expensive equipment.

Within the Ministry, the Top Hospitalisation Committee (THC) has been identified as a major actor in the process of decision-making regarding the formulation of the curative policy. The THC includes eight members representing the various sectors of the health services. The Committee is chaired by the Health Minister (or the General Manager), the Hadassah hospital manager, the IDF's chief surgeon, the head of the Ministry's budgetary department, the Kupat Holim's general manager, his or her deputy and the head of the Sick Fund's treasury. The composition of the THC is aimed at ensuring a 'national outlook' not based on narrow interests of any one health sector. In other words it is designed to provide a balance between the two major actors, Kupat Holim and the state, and to grant a voice to other important organs, such as Hadassah. The THC, whose function is to determine policy based on comprehensive considerations, is often aided by experts whose judgement is based on proficiency and professional competence. As will be indicated below, this has been the case regarding the treatment of heart disease.

The huge sums of money needed for the acquisition of medical instruments puts a heavy burden on the shoulders of those responsible for dispensing them. While the final decision remains within the Ministry, it is adopted by a body which also includes people outside the state bureaucracy. As noted by a senior official: 'we do our best to avoid adopting decisions arbitrarily, on the basis of two, three or five lay members of the Ministry's executive. Hence we are often aided by experts' counseling committees' (Mashiah, 1989, p. 55). On the basis of this principle, the Ministry of Health formed (in 1986) a committee (headed by Professor Shlomo Laniado, a noted cardiologist) whose mandate was to recommend certificate of needs regarding the distribution of catheterisation equipment. The seven-member Committee included noted cardiologists from major hospitals throughout the country. After the conclusions of the Laniado Committee had been submitted, another forum was created, headed by Professor Agmon, also a senior cardiologist. This committee however was not staffed only by professionals, but also included high officials, experts in budgets and administration. The Agmon Committee was designed to recommend, on the basis of national medical data regarding heart surgery, ways and means to implement the recommendations of its predecessor, the Laniado Committee, and further the facilities for modern heart treatment in the Israeli health system.

The curative alternative has thus enjoyed a clear advantage over the preventive option. Although numerous actors advocating prevention have attempted to persuade decision-makers to act in favour of their cause, their activity has not been coordinated. Each organisation has pursued its own course, targeting its efforts at different objectives. Diffusion is also evident in the administrative domain. Not one state agency has been singled out as responsible for designing an overall preventive policy. Alternatively the policy universe of the curative alternative has been characterised by internal coordination, with the actors hierarchically linked in a cohesive network of decision-making and information.

THE BEHAVIOURAL ASPECTS OF THE POLICY UNIVERSE

The two policy options regarding heart disease, namely the preventive and the curative, have not been rationally weighed in terms of costs, constraints and predicted outcomes. Yet the formulation of the curative option has been successful in terms of policy agenda because entrepreneurs who have a high stake in promoting the issue have been present.

Policy entrepreneurs are people willing to invest resources in return for future policies they favour (Kingdon, 1984, p. 214). They are motivated by combinations of several things: their concern about the problem; their pursuit of self-serving benefits; and–or their promotion of policy values. The function the entrepreneurs perform in the policy process is invaluable. Their activity, in all stages of the process, is central to forging policies. As noted by Kingdon (1984, p. 215), they bring several key resources into the process: their claims to a hearing; their political connections and negotiating skills; and their sheer persistence. These factors become politically significant when a 'policy-window' opens, that is when the opportunity for advocates to push their solutions to their problems occurs. The test of successful entrepreneurship is in taking advantage of this opportunity. This has been the case regarding those promoting the curative option.

Preventive Policy

In the past, preventive policy was a one-man initiative prompted mainly by scientific interest. It was also an emulation of out-state activities. The prevention of coronary diseases in Israel was first put on the public agenda by Professor Henry Neufeld, a noted cardiologist whose interest in the issue was both humanitarian and medical. In the mid-1960s Dr. Neufeld initiated large-scale research comparing populations with a low frequency of heart disease to that of a high risk constituency (of government officials). The results of the study (published in Medalie *et al.*, 1973), increased interest in the scientific aspects of prevention, and encouraged him to raise the issue on the public agenda for deliberation and possibly concomitant implementation. The entrepreneurship of Professor Neufeld did not fall on barren ears. It did invigorate public activity. It prompted the Cardiologist Association within the IMA to jump on the wagon and play a considerable role in the medical association's anti-smoking campaign. However the initiative was not forceful enough to command additional resources. The entrepreneurs were preoccupied with their professional interests and were conspicuously amateurs in politics.

Only on 6 July 1988 was a committee established by health authorities, mandated to recommend strategies to promote the prevention of heart disease. The Committee (headed by Professor Kaplinski)[14] has not yet (at the time of writing) issued its final report and recommendations. Its interim conclusions reveal little novelty. The report emphasised the need to refrain from smoking, to eat 'wisely' and to engage in some form of physical activity. Reportedly the committee would urge the government to further legislation banning the advertising of cigarettes and to launch educational campaigns encouraging the youth to adopt a healthier life style. These recommendations would probably be congruent with the manual of 'healthy living'. As such they are likely to remain policy guidelines rather than policy outlines ready for application and implementation. Worth noting is the fact that the Committee has not included any epidemiologists and has not seriously considered data available on the influence of high-risk factors. It thus has neither set priorities nor calculated the cost-benefit balance entailed in each of the alternatives. The lack of scientific data, the lack of public visibility and the priorities of the Committee's members has prevented successful entrepreneurship. The preventive option has remained dormant and has not been seriously considered. No policy windows have been opened and no entrance was ever made.

The interest groups involved have also failed to induce action. Policy analysts distinguish between various stages of influence (Yishai, 1984), extending from mere 'access' to decision-makers to a comprehensive solution of the problem which gives rise to organised action. Access is a necessary condition: it enables those having a grievance to present their case and to be heard. The absence of access commits the issue to the domain of 'non-decision' where the mobilisation of bias precludes elite attention and impedes further action (Bachrach and Baratz, 1962). Access however is only the first step along the road to influence. It is an essential condition for raising the issue on the formal agenda (Cobb, Ross and Ross, 1976), but unless contenders are granted the right of participation, preferably 'integrated participation' (Olsen, 1981), access may easily dissolve into inaction. The second step is thus the acknowledgement that those having a stake in the issue may take part in forging solutions. Public interest groups seem to have reached only the first stage of influence. They have been granted free access; never, when they have so requested, have they been refused a meeting with high officials or even with the Health Minister. But access has not led to further phases of influence. The groups are not represented in any policy formulating body. Their claim to a hearing has remained intermittent and equivocal. No window has been available to them for entrance.

The Curative Option

The chief entrepreneurs in the curative domain have been the medical professionals, the executives of hospitals and the heads of cardiological departments. Decision-making has been vested only in the Ministry of Health, but authority has been widely shared, enabling the entrepreneurs to play an active role in the process. The circumstances facilitating the opening of the 'window' have been clearly visible.

The first catheterisation instrument in Israel was installed in 1981 in the Sheba hospital, the largest state hospital in the country. The operation of this medical technique revolutionised the treatment and cure of heart disease. The news rapidly spread across the country and public demands to enjoy the benefits of the new equipment escalated. The shortage of catheterisation facilities became unacceptable in a country advocating egalitarian medical service. But supply was far shorter than demand. The number of people waiting for preventive catheterisation has been constantly on the rise, with the queue extending for several months. The State Comptroller (1988, p. 199) reported that 1800 patients were waiting (in 1987) in line for catheterisation. The gap between demand and supply was not bridged despite the fact that catheterisation treatments doubled from the previous year. Public pressures to receive the best available medical treatment mounted.

The inability of the health care system to yield to these pressures put a heavy burden on scheduled medical services. Patients requiring elective catheterisation often returned to the cardiological centres in need of emergency treatment, which is not only more expensive, but also disruptive of the planned medical workload. The result was further clogging of the heart departments and longer queues for elective treatment.

The introduction of the balloon technique (angioplasty) to heart treatment accentuated the need for catheterisation and added a dramatic flavour to its operation. Since its invention (by Dr. Andreas

Gruentzig) in 1977, angioplasty (PTCA) has gained wide acceptance as a form of nonsurgical treatment for many patients with coronary artery disease. Long-term results have been encouraging and the treatment has rapidly spread. The line of cardiological centres throughout the country requesting permission to acquire catheterisation technology grew simultaneously with the line of patients waiting to enjoy its benefits.

The rush of hospitals to acquire the equipment has not been prompted by pure humanitarian interests to cure the sick; neither were funding considerations the major trigger for joining the catheterisation club. On the contrary, since hospital budgeting is based mainly on hospital days, the expensive operation of the catheterisation technique is more a financial liability than an asset. What is mainly at stake is the hospital's prestige (especially that of its cardiology department). Hospitals without catheterisation facilities are considered second rate and are doomed to deteriorate. They do not attract prominent cardiologists, nor specialising practitioners. Pressures have been most effective when applied on colleagues manning positions of consultation and–or authority in the Ministry of Health. When wrapped up with considerations of 'public health', pressures have been more often than not irresistible.

The establishment of the Laniado Committee was the first step in the road to influence. The Committee was a vivid example of successful entrepreneurship; it based its conclusions on the medical facilities of the hospitals requesting catheterisation equipment. It took into consideration the available professional manpower and expertise for performing the treatment. Also relevant became the number of patients receiving this kind of treatment in other public hospitals in the area. The Laniado Committee was not concerned with the economic aspects of introducing the expensive equipment and limited its recommendations only to medical facilities. For its members, experts in cardiology, certification of catheterisation equipment was not dependent on the rules of the zero-sum game. Scarcity of resources was irrelevant to its decisions. In its conclusions the Committee noted that 'the needs of public health services in the area of cardiology have dramatically changed in the last five years'. Consequently the issue of catheterisation turned into 'a prime national health issue' (Laniado Committee, 1987). The deliberations and the final report clearly reflected the entrepreneurs' needs and demands. The Laniado Committee recommended the addition of six hospitals to the ten already administering such treatment, regarding catheterisation as a technique essential to any modern hospital. In fact it recommended the approval of all requests, regardless of their financial cost.

The Agmon Committee further exhibited the entrepreneurs' influence. It fully endorsed the conclusions of the Laniado Committee, although it recommended that regional arrangements should be imposed in order to provide short-term solutions to the mounting demands manifested in the growing queue for catheterisation. In fact it added another hospital to the list, bringing the number of new catheterisation centres up to seven. It emphasised the hospitals' responsibility for soliciting the funds required for purchasing the equipment, although it did not deny the commitment of public authorities to finance its operation (Agmon Committee, 1987).

The recommendations of the two committees were discussed by the Top Hospitalisation Committee, whose final authorisation paved the way for the approval of catheterisation equipment. The predominance of the curative option was thus officially established. The voice granted to the entrepreneurs throughout the policy process was unmistakable. Their access was made possible not only because of their competence, but also because it matched the interests of top decision-makers. The THC was authorised to forge decisions and allocate resources on the basis of national needs. But it has not escaped sectoral interests. In fact it has been chaired not by a senior official but by the Minister, whose influence on decision-making has been considerable. As noted by one of its members, the manager of the Hadassah hospital: 'The voice of the Minister is always the voice that determines decisions in the Hospitalisation Committee'.[15] Admittedly this assertion was qualified by other members of the committee. The head of hospitalisation services in the Health Ministry said that 'there were instances, in this forum, as well as in others, where people *dared* (emphasis mine) to speak out against the Minister's opinion. There were even cases when the Minister conceded to majority opinion'. He also noted however that there were instances in which 'people were not free to express their views in full'.[16]

The Hospitalisation Committee is thus a political organ whose resolutions reflect and are affected by partisan considerations. The entrepreneurs are not necessarily experts in politics. But their recommendations have coincided with the politicians' interests. As noted above, curative techniques could be turned into tradable assets in the competitive political market. The coincidence of professional demands presented by the entrepreneurs' and politicians' needs alike has opened a wide window through which the curative option could easily emerge.

OUTPUTS AND IMPACT OF POLICY PREFERENCES

Despite the constraints on both preventive and curative options, policy outputs are identifiable. The major output on the preventive scene is the legislation restricting smoking. On 26 July 1983 the Knesset passed a law prohibiting smoking in public places, including closed halls used for entertainment or other forms of public gathering, such as hospitals, elevators and public transportation.[17] In 1988 the law was further extended (by administrative order) to supermarkets, restaurants,[18] kindergartens and sports clubs.

A study of smoking habits conducted about half a year after the regulations were issued indicated that an overwhelming majority of the public were aware of the banning of smoking in public transportation (80 per cent); a sizeable majority knew about the restrictions in cinemas and hospitals (51 per cent and 46 per cent respectively). However only a negligible minority knew about the restrictions pertaining to other public domains (Ben Sira, 1988, pp. 32–3). In fact the enforcement of the law in these areas is extremely lax. There are no restrictions on smoking at the workplace or prohibitions on the sales of cigarettes to minors, which is common in other Western societies (Roemer, 1987, pp. 34–6).

The 1983 legislation also restricted the advertising of tobacco products on radio and television broadcasts or public inland transport.[19] However it has not banned press advertising other than that intended for children and young people. Although those advertising or marketing tobacco products were required to print a warning stating that 'The Ministry of Health has Declared that Smoking is Harmful to Health', advertisements whose scope was described above have remained uninterrupted. A proposal to extend the bill to ban all types of advertising is currently being discussed by the Knesset. Nevertheless it appears that the chances of such a bill being approved are dim. The impact of the anti-smoking legislation remains unclear. As noted earlier, there has not been a discernible effect on the size of the smoking population, which has remained fairly stable.

Various other outputs can be identified, including programmes and activities in the education system. For example, a joint committee of the Ministry of Education and the Ministry of Health was established which has undertaken as its first project the preparation of a syllabus on healthy life-style. Efforts have been made to promote health education in schools, to distribute printed and audio-visual material to all schools and to prepare background material for communication and curriculum units for elementary school children. As of the academic year 1987–8, the subject of smoking prevention was made obligatory for all schools. Israel thus joined nine other European countries (out of 26) where anti-smoking education in schools is mandatory (Roemer, 1987, p. 43). Educational activities have extended to the mass media with paid anti-smoking commercials, prepared by official authorities in cooperation with the voluntary associations, creating an anti-smoking atmosphere. Worth noting is the fact that TV ads have been financed by the anti-smoking groups and not by the Ministry of Health. Since these activities are geared to produce long-term effects it is much too early to estimate their impact.

Outputs of the curative policy are more readily discernible. The decisions adopted by the Top Hospitalisation Committee have substantially increased the potential of administering catheterisation treatment to Israeli patients. Unofficial data reveal that the queue for catheterisation has shrunk from as long as a year to only a month or two in most places.[20] Since the newly certified hospitals started to operate this technique only in 1988 it is too early to estimate the advantages of this equipment or the efficiency of its use. But the impact remains ambiguous.

The most prominent conclusion is that, after the United States, Israel (and The Netherlands) rank prime among selected countries regarding the availability of sophisticated heart treatment. Table 6.5 reveals that in 1986, 1103 patients received PCTA (angioplasty) for treatment of coronary artery disease, that is 0.3 per capita. This rate is not only far higher than in, say, Brazil (0.01 per capita), but also compared to industrialised countries such as France (0.07 per capita). Even in Canada the rate of angioplasty per capita is 0.2, far lower than the Israeli standard. In Britain, whose population is much larger than Israel's (approximately 57 million compared to 4.5 million respectively), the number of angioplasties carried out in 1988 was 6000.[21]

Table 6.5 Coronary angioplasties in selected countries – 1986

Country	Population Number of Procedures	Procedures p.c.
United States	159 643	0.6
Israel	**1 103**	**0.3**
The Netherlands	3 508	0.3
Canada	5 535	0.2
FRG	8 000	0.1
France	6 880	0.07
Belgium	1 706	0.05
Japan	6 233	0.05
Argentina	581	0.01
Brazil	1 681	0.01

Source Special Report Circulation, ISFC–WHO Task Force 78, (3 September 1988) p. 781.

The high dissemination of catheterisation facilities clearly seems to improve the possibilities of individual citizens receiving adequate health care for one of the most devastating diseases in the modern world.

When outputs are judged in terms of ideological concerns the picture is more ambiguous. One of the major values guiding the provision of health services, the equal right of every citizen to equal access to medical treatment, has been partly materialised in the case of coronary disease. Peripheral hospitals were in the past seriously disadvantaged in their facilities to provide the latest treatment for the patients in their region. In comparison with the quantity of heart treatment equipment in the big cities, they were seriously handicapped. The various committees dealing with the issue did some justice to the countrys' periphery. Three (out of eight) peripheral hospitals (in Safed, Hedera and Afula) joined the prestigious club of catheterisation centres. Others have not joined the club.

However correcting one fault may have been responsible for the creation of another. Examination of the catheterisation map indicates that economic consideration did not rank prime in the process of allocating permission to acquire the facilities. In the Tel Aviv area (extending from Holon to Petach Tikva), where the ratio of catheterisation per capita was already the highest in the country before certification (see Table 6.6), a third hospital was allowed to introduce the technique, despite the fact that occupancy in the heart department at one of the hospitals was as low as 56.1 per cent.

Table 6.6 Catheterisation treatment, by hospitals, regions and population, 1986

Region	Hospital	Population (thousands)	No. of cath.	Share per hospital pop.	Share per region pop.
North	Safed	104			
	Poria	71			
	Naharia	190			
	Afula	258			
Total		650			0
Haifa	Rambam	319	412	1.2	
	Rothschild	140			
	Carmel	104	1 187	11.4	
Total		563			2.8
Coast line	Hillel Yaffe	204			
	Meir	288	243	0.8	
Total		492			0.4
Center	Hasharon	161			
	Assaf Harofe	230			
	Kaplan	233			
Total		624			0
Tel Aviv	Ichilov	250	825	3.3	
	Wofson	283			
	Sheba	313	1 451	4.6	
	Beilinson	232	1 143	4.9	3.1
Total		1 078			
Jerusalem	Hadassah		1 503		
	Shaarei Zedek	531	190	4.2	
	Bikur Holim		550		
Total		531			2.5
South	Barzilai	130			
	Soroka	277	177	0.6	
	Yoseftal	22			
Total		429			0.4

Source Files of the Ministry of Health.

The picture in Haifa was even more striking. Haifa has three major hospitals which offer medical services to over half a million people. One of these hospitals (Carmel) is famous for its heart surgery; the ratio of catheterisation per head of population in the region is as high as 11.4. Yet certification of a neighbouring hospital (Rambam) took place although the heart department occupancy at this particular hospital was only 68.9 per cent, and the catheterisation ratio was (in 1986) as low as 1.2 per capita. Notwithstanding these facts a third hospital in Haifa, situated but a short distance from the two others, was also certified to purchase the equipment. The stated reason echoed the voice of the entrepreneurs: 'The professional aptitudes of the staff in the cardiology department is such that they enable the establishment and development of a catheterisation centre' (Laniado Committee, 1987).

Furthermore, notwithstanding the norms of equality, geography is not a trustworthy indicator for dispensing medical technology. Only one peripheral hospital (Yoseftal in Eilat) is remotely situated. Other medical centres are located at a relatively short distance (less than one hundred kilometers) from the big cities – Jerusalem, Haifa and Tel Aviv (see Table 6.7). It is highly dubious whether the installation of catheterisation facilities is absolutely necessary in terms of national resources. Data moreover indicate that the further the hospital is from the centre, (that is, Meir in Kfar Saba, and Soroka in Beer Sheba), the smaller is its output in terms of catheterisation per capita (hospital's population).

The addition of more peripheral hospitals to the list may have its benefits – the attraction of new senior physicians and the higher

Table 6.7 Distance (in kilometers) of peripheral hospitals from urban centres

Peripheral hospitals	Tel-Aviv	Haifa	Jerusalem
Safed	72		
Poria (Tiberias)		69	
Naharia	35		
Haemek (Afula)		44	
Hillel Yaffe (Hedera)		51	
Meir (Kfar Saba)	25		
Hasharon (Petach Tiqua)	15		
Assaf Harofe (Tzrifin)	15		
Kaplan (Rehovot)	23		
Barzilai (Ashkelon)	54		
Soroka (Beer Sheba)			81
Yoseftal (Eilat)			309

Source Karta's Israel Road and Touring Guide, 8th ed. (Jerusalem: Karta, 1985).

prestige conferred upon those already practising medicine in the area – but whether or not the residents of the area reap the fruits of the sophisticated medical technology remains an open question. The expertise and competence needed for the successful utilisation of sophisticated technology is not likely to be present in peripheral hospitals, with a smaller number of patients and much less experience.

So far there are insufficient tools to determine whether the extravagant dispersion of catheterisation equipment in Israeli hospitals has indeed had a prominent impact on public health. The performing of so many catheterisations has considerably increased the burden on cardiac surgery departments because many patients who undergo this examination are found to need open heart surgery. The difficulty in assessing the impact of the expansion of catheterisation facilities is grounded not only in the absence of adequate data but also (perhaps primarily) because of the lack of calculated alternatives.

CONCLUSIONS

The foregoing discussion has probed the circumstances under which priorities are determined regarding the preventive and curative alternatives in the treatment of heart disease. The study indicates that the curative option overrides the preventive one. Policy-makers have (a) taken more administrative action regarding the curative aspect of heart disease and (b) been willing to invest more resources in this alternative. To prevention they have paid lip service; to curative measures they have allocated immense funds. Four major reasons seem to be responsible for this hierarchy of preferences.

(1) Although health authorities have been staunchly committed to the promotion of health through the use of all available strategies, the curative alternative has been more promising in terms of short-term *political benefits*. At stake has been the distribution of tangible goods which could yield immediate political fruits. The allocation of curative resources has also been congruent with a broader set of values, such as commitment to an egalitarian health system and to population dispersion. The promotion of the curative policy has thus provided an opportunity to secure both power and symbolic rewards; that is to adhere to undisputed national goals while at the same time advancing one's vested interests.

(2) *Constraints* have also been less powerful with regard to the curative policy. This is surprising in view of the fact that the equipment needed for curing heart disease is extravagantly expensive. The cost of the installation and operation of one single catheterisation centre could provide adequate financial resources for a full-scale preventive campaign, the results of which, regarding expenditure on health care, could have been substantial. Yet the curative alternative faced no opposition. Not one single body (except for the State Judicial Committee whose recommendations have not yet been issued) challenged health authorities with regard to their expenditure on catheterisation equipment. At the same time the scene abounded with oppositional activity aimed at curbing any preventive policy. Tobacco users, producers and influential advertisers vetoed any progress toward strict measures of prevention. Dairy manufacturers and meat producers, whose links with political parties and their affiliated institutions have turned them into a powerful lobby, strengthened the constraints put on the preventive option.

(3) The *structure* of the *policy universe* (described in Figure 6.1) adds another dimension to the understanding of the determined priorities. A variation of the preventive and the curative alternatives is clearly visible. In the curative category there are numerous actors. Apparently the Ministry of Health has been reluctant to carry the responsibility of making important decisions and has shared its authority with committees of experts. However the bodies that were established to advise and counsel have formed a *policy network* in the sense that they are all defined by a common *policy focus* (Pross, 1986). The internal integration between the actors has enabled a forging of policy, whose essence could further the curative technique.

This has not been the case with regard to the preventive category. Here too a variety of actors can be identified as having some part in the policy process. However all actors either captured part of the problem or, alternatively, were preoccupied with a broader set of issues. Kupat Holim did not pay a heed. The Cancer Association and the Anti-Smoking group advocated restrictions only on the use of tobacco; the Heart Society focused mainly on cholesterol. The IMA simply manipulated the promotion of health for its own use. Its scope of interests was far broader than prevention of heart disease. Lack of coordination between the actors, whose rivalry fragmented action, hindered the promulgation of effective preventive policy.

(4) Finally, choosing between and, especially, within alternatives has also been a product of the *process* of policy-making. Entrepre-

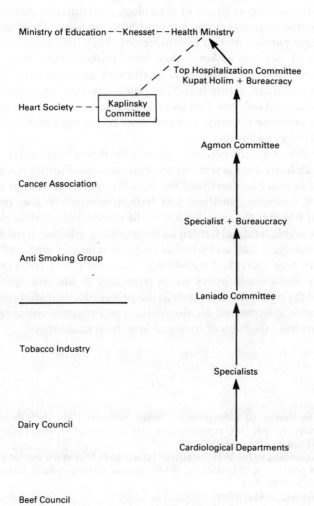

Preventive Policy   Curative Policy

Ministry of Education – –Knesset – –Health Ministry

Top Hospitalization Committee
Kupat Holim + Bureaucracy

Heart Society – – – Kaplinsky Committee

Agmon Committee

Cancer Association

Specialist + Bureaucracy

Anti Smoking Group

Laniado Committee

Tobacco Industry

Specialists

Dairy Council

Cardiological Departments

Beef Council

Figure 6.1   The policy universe

neurs have not been visible on the preventive arena. To be sure there are myriad actors anxious to advance preventive measures, but none have qualified as 'an entrepreneur' in the political sense. They have lacked the skill, devotion and the resources that make effective entrepreneurship. Entrepreneurs have excelled on the curative scene. The members of the professional community act in numerous capacities: they are internists specialising in heart disease, senior physicians serving as heads of cardiology departments, members of professional committees and administrative agencies. Their multiple roles have enabled mutual reinforcement. They have penetrated the process of decision-making; they have pushed their case at the propitious moment. They have performed an impressive role of coupling solutions to problems. The political receptivity of the health system has certainly been an asset in advancing the curative option, but the presence of competent and devoted entrepreneurs has been critical to its conclusion.

Whether or not the curative option is the most effective strategy to cope with heart disease remains an open question. Further research is needed in order to determine the benefits of catheterisation on the basis of economic, medical and human criteria. It also remains dubious whether the introduction of the new technique does not put an unbearable financial burden on its operators, whether it influences epidemiological data and whether or not it relieves human suffering and advances individual well-being. The case under concern does indicate that even in policy issues pertaining to life and death, the rules of the political game (such as the power of anticipated rewards, constraints, coordinated decision-making and effective entrepreneurship) override the rules of 'rational' long-term calculations.

Notes

1. The number of admissions to Cardiac Intensive Care Units decreased from 31.1 per 1000 population in 1985 to 2.9 in 1987. *Israel Statistical Abstract*, 1988; p. 673.
2. According to the WHO statistics Israel ranks fifth in the rate of growth of proportion of its elderly. WHO *Annual Demographic Yearbook*, 1975, 1986, N.Y.
3. *Haaretz*, 1 May 1989.
4. *Jerusalem Post*, 17 March 1989.
5. *Haaretz*, 2 May 1989.
6. The budget for imported cigarettes advertisements was 1 million shekels; Dubek had the larger share. *Haaretz*, 5 May 1989.
7. *Haaretz*, 5 May 1989.
8. Noteworthy is the fact that on 2 May 1989 an anti-smoking advertisement appeared on a full page in the daily press, which gladly accepted the huge sums required for this kind and size of publicity.

9. *Haaretz*, 5 May 1989.
10. *Haaretz*, 12 May 1989.
11. *Jerusalem Post*, 24 February 1989.
12. Information is based on interviews with the Cancer Association's staff and the Annual Reports 1984–8.
13. The Haifa branch withdrew from the association on account of over-centralisation, charging the centre with neglecting the periphery.
14. The committee included nine members: three representative of the Ministry of Health; five senior physicians; representatives of government and public hospitals; and one representative of Kupat Holim.
15. S. Mashiah, State Judicial Committee for the Examination of the Functioning and Effectiveness of the Israeli Health System. Meeting no. 86, 28 March 1989 p. 74.
16. S. Mashiah, *ibid.* pp. 76–7.
17. *Sefer Hachukim* (The Book of Laws) 1983, no. 1074, p. 148.
18. The law applies only to restaurants which seat 20 or more diners in which case there must be a no-smoking area clearly posted.
19. *Sefer Hachukim, op. cit.,* no. 1090.
20. *Jerusalem Post*, 16 June 1989.
21. *Observer*, 21 May 1989.

References

Agmon Committee (1987) *Recommendations*.

Bachrach, P. and M. Baratz, (1962) 'Two faces of power', *American Political Science Review*, no. 50, pp. 947–52.

Ben Sira, Z. (1987) *Health Promoting Behaviour: Trends and Constraints* (Jerusalem: The Israel Institute of Applied Social Research, October Pub. No. (z) ZBS/1013/H.

Ben Sira, Z. (1988) *Smoking: Habits, Attitudes and Knowledge in Public Places* (Jerusalem: The Israel Institute of Applied Social Research) July Pub. No. (s) ZBS/1035/H.

Borukhov, E. and E. Werczberger (1981) 'Factors Affecting the Development of New Towns in Israel', *Environment and Planning*, no. 13, pp. 421–34.

Budget Proposal (presented to the 12th Knesset) January 1989.

Budget Regulations (Jerusalem: Health Ministry) April 1989.

Cobb, J.K., K.-J. Ross and M.H. Ross (1976) 'Agenda Building as a Comparative Political Process', *American Political Science Review* no. 70, pp. 126–38.

Epstein, L. (1979) 'Ischaemic Heart Disease in Israel: Change Over 30 Years', *Israel Journal of Medical Sciences*, no. 15, p. 993.

Ganor, A., *Haaretz*, 23 April 1986.

Health Ministry (1988) *Healthy System in Israel* (Data & Trends) November.

Israel Statistical Abstract (1988) (Jerusalem: Central Bureau of Statistics).

Kingdon, J.W. (1984) *Agendas, Alternatives, and Public Policies*, (Boston: Little, Brown).

Kramer, R.M. (1976) *The Voluntary Service Agency in Israel* (Berkeley:

64   *Heart Disease in Israel*

University of California Press).
Kramer, R.M. (1981) *Voluntary Agencies in the Welfare State* (Berkeley:
    University of California Press).
Laniado Committee (1987) *Recommendations*, 8 February.
Mashiah, S. (1989), *State Judicial Committee for the Examination of the
Functioning and Effectiveness of the Israeli Health System*, March 28.
Medalie, J.H., H.A. Kahan, H.N. Newfeld *et al.* (1973) 'Myocardial
    Infarction over a Five-Year Period: Prevalence, Incidence and Mortality
    Experience', *Journal of Chronic Disease*, no. 26, p. 63.
Modan, B. (1989) 'The Misery of the Decline in Mortality of Ischaemic
    Heart Disease', *Harefua*, p. 117 (in Hebrew).
Olsen, J.P. (1981) 'Integrated Organisational Participation in Government',
    in P.C. Nystrom and W.H. Starbuck (eds) *Handbook of Organisational
    Design* (Oxford University Press).
Pross, A.P. (1986) *Group Politics and Public Policy*, (Toronto: Oxford
    University Press).
Roemer, R. (1987) *Legislative Strategies for a Smoke-Free Europe*
    (Copenhagen: WHO Regional Office for Europe).
Royal College of Physicians (1977) *Smoking or Health: Report*, (London:
    Putman Medical).
Rywik, S. and W. Kupske (1985) 'Coronary Heart Disease Mortality Trends
    and Related Factors in Poland', *Cardiology*, no. 72, p. 81.
Sharkansky, I. (1987) *The Political Economy of Israel* (New Brunswick:
    Transaction).
Smoke Free Europe: A 5 Year Action Plan (1988) (Copenhagen: WHO
    Regional Office for Europe).
Stamler, J. (1985) 'The Marked Decline in Coronary Heart Disease
    Mortality Rates in the United States, 1968–1981: Summary of Findings
    and Possible Explanations', *Cardiology*, no. 72, p. 11.
Starr, P. and E. Immergut, 'Health Care and the Boundaries of Politics', in
    C.S. Maier (ed.) (1987) *Changing Boundaries of the Political* (Cambridge
    University Press).
State Comptroller (1988) *Annual Report*, No. 38.
Targets for Health for All (1986) (Copenhagen: WHO Regional Office for
    Europe).
Yishai, Y. (1984) 'Responses to Ethnic Demands: The Case of Israel', *Ethnic
    and Racial Studies*, no. 7, pp. 283–306.
Yishai, Y. (1989a) 'State and Welfare Groups: Competition or
    Cooperation?', paper presented at the Conference on Voluntarism, Non
    Government Organisations and Public Policy (Jerusalem, May 22–4).
Yishai, Y. (1989b) *The Israeli Medical Association: The Power of Expertise*
    (Jerusalem Institute for the Study of Israel, forthcoming).

7 Two Kinds of Conservatism in US Health Policy: The Reagan Record[*]

William P. Brandon

As a presidential candidate in 1976 Jimmy Carter promised to bring America universal, comprehensive national health insurance (NHI) if he became president. By the end of the decade intellectuals and policy analysts began reaching the educated public with 'procompetition' or 'market-reform' challenges to the emphasis on regulation that health policy and its analysis had developed in the early 1970s. The critiques of government regulation, and increasingly specific proposals for an alternative, were pure rhetoric in the nonpejorative sense that they were intended to be persuasive. The alternative policies suggested by these insurgents became the official policies of the Reagan administration when it came to power in January 1981.

The objective of this chapter is to summarise the rhetoric and then to assess its reflection in reality. The second part of this task involves answering two questions. Was this policy rhetoric the actual policy of the Reagan administration – or was it *mere* rhetoric? And were reasonable representations of the policy goals realised in actual federal health policies during the Reagan years?

Attention to this anti-regulation, market-reformist conservative economic agenda in health partially obscures a quite different sort of conservatism, which is sometimes called the 'social' or 'moral agenda' of the Reagan administration. Understanding the history of the Reagan administration and its health policy requires sorting out these quite different kinds of conservatism.

* The author wishes to thank Richard Adinaro, Christa Altenstetter, Hanns Kuttner and Eric Ramshaw for their comments on an earlier draft of this chapter, and Ilaina Sernick for research assistance. They of course bear no responsibility for its remaining faults.

Two Conservatisms

The modern Republican Party and the Reagan administration have contained two fundamentally different forms of conservatism. One is the traditional economic conservatism which emphasises individual economic and social freedom from government intervention. This kind of conservatism sometimes shades into political views that oppose government activism in regard to social and civil rights issues. The other conservative tradition is 'moral-agenda' conservatism. While eschewing what it pejoratively calls 'liberal' activism, moral-agenda conservatism does not shrink from using government power in support of what are believed to be traditional American moral and social values.

Other chapters in this volume call the first kind of conservatism 'neo-liberal'. In the peculiar semantics of American political discourse, 'liberal' now labels supporters of interventionist social welfare government as well as those who defend expanded opportunities for individual civil and social freedom. To avoid confusion, this essay will use the term economic conservatism.

The political tradition of economic conservatism is related to nineteenth-century liberalism, with its ideal of the 'night-watchman' state that attends to the functions of national defense, domestic public safety, monetary policy, the enforcement of legal contracts, and perhaps some infrastructure investments that exceed the capacity of private business. This litany of approved government activities can be classified under two general headings: enforcing the rules of the free market and responsibility for 'public goods' in the technical vocabulary of modern social science. Its leading modern intellectual exponent in America is Milton Friedman; Barry Goldwater is perhaps the most noted advocate in the political realm.

This conservatism is more than the glorification of unfettered capitalism. It typically involves a commitment to equality of opportunity, which logically commits its proponents to oppose racial and other sorts of invidious discrimination. Even as a politico-economic doctrine traditional American economic conservatism is not entirely straightforward in opposing government action. A populist wing, which is concerned about maintaining the necessary conditions for competition, supports intervention to break up monopolies and other restrictive trade policies. A more passive version accepts the outcome of competitive markets over time;

economic conservatives of this stripe tend to reflect the views of successful large business.

Its opposition to state intervention and its emphasis on individual freedom makes traditional economic conservatism very compatible with political libertarianism. In this more extreme view society, or at least government, should not interfere with an individual's right to do whatever he or she pleases, so long as the action does not harm others. Libertarianism became a formal political ideology in America in the 1970s. The Harvard philosopher Robert Nozick published its credo in *Anarchy, State, and Utopia* (1974), which systematically defends the 'minimal state'. A libertarian party began running candidates for the presidency during the same decade.

Moral-agenda conservatives object strongly to any libertarian implications of traditional economic conservatism. They promised to use their influence in the newly-elected Reagan administration to prohibit abortions, resist further attempts to regulate the sale and possession of firearms, attack obscenity and pornography (which in America is generally defined as explicit sexual material rather than portrayals of violence), conserve traditional 'family' values including disapproval of homosexuality and premarital sex, and prohibit recreational use of drugs (except tobacco and perhaps alcohol). The military and the sanctity of national symbols like the flag and the pledge of allegiance are valued symbols.

The rising influence of the moral-agenda conservatives in the 1970s ended the political domination of New Deal or welfare-state ideas, that is, 'liberalism' in the American vocabulary. It also obliterated libertarian expressions within the Republican party. Its rise parallels and helps to explain the US failure to progress along the path to NHI.

The history of the last decade and a half makes it easy to forget that many moral-agenda conservatives were nonpolitical in the 1960s. Those who were politically active tended to focus narrowly on particular issues such as guns or pornography rather than on building broad coalitions. The Goldwater debacle in 1964 seemed to leave all strains of conservatism in disarray. Religious conservatives had not traditionally been organised as a political group. Many US fundamentalist denominations and sects trace their historical and theological roots to Anabaptists and other dissenting sects for whom the strong division between church and state used to be an article of faith. So long as the church suffered no interference from the state, churches traditionally refrained from organised political expression.

By 1980 such views seemed quaint in light of the apparent strength of Jerry Falwell's Moral Majority and the appeal of a host of other fundamentalist televangelists. (By 1988 the Moral Majority had been disbanded and televangelism seemed to be in retreat as a result of media attention to the sexual and financial peccadillos of several of its most visible practitioners.)

The causes of renewed strength in moral-agenda conservatism are undoubtedly manifold. The Johnson domestic policies threatened established local political and social hierarchies. The Goldwater presidential candidacy, which mobilised many true believers, began the process of forging a broad-based conservative coalition. In state after state the Equal Rights Amendment (ERA), an effort by progressive feminists to enshrine guarantees of equality for women in the US Constitution, galvanised grassroots opposition which saw ERA as a liberal experiment in social engineering that threatened traditional male–female roles. A delayed reaction to the loss of the Vietnam War and a deepening sense of military decline in the face of devious enemies who were gaining strength, also contributed to the conservative resurgence. Voters influenced by these disparate sources of moral-agenda conservatism made common cause with disgruntled economic conservatives. Ronald Reagan, who had toured America making speeches to conservative groups before he became governor of California, emerged as a hero of this coalition.

Now means became available to communicate and motivate people who had not previously participated actively in politics. Thus the mastery of mass computerised mailing techniques in the 1970s by such right-wing advocates as Richard Viguerie played a key role in the conservative resurgence. Yet for all this increased activity on the right, there is no evidence that moral-agenda conservatives ever became a majority of voters.

Modern conservative thought is more complex than the two ideal types that adequately serve the limited purposes of this essay. For example, I have not dealt with those sophisticated intellectuals such as Irving Kristol, Daniel Bell and Norman Podhoretz who became known as 'neo-conservatives' during the 1970s. Although most American conservatives like to invoke Edmund Burke, it should also be pointed out that both strains of political conservatism in America are too ideological for a true Burkean or Tory conservative.

Both economic and moral-agenda conservatism were represented in health policy debates during the Reagan years. Before examining those debates however, it is necessary to understand the ideas on health care that became popular among policy analysts in the second half of the 1970s. Those ideas formed the basis for much of the rhetoric of the Reagan administration.

IDEAS AND VALUES

The political tradition of economic conservatism manifested itself in the area of health policy as the 'market-reform' or 'procompetition' approach. Proponents of this view constituted a significant policy network. It is not so important to trace the history of moral-agenda conservatism, which was less central in the day-to-day formulation of most health policies in the Reagan administration. To a large extent the pre-Reagan history of moral-agenda conservatism in health policy is found in concern over birth control, sex education and abortion.[1] Although moral-agenda conservatism played a role in determining Reagan administration health care policy, it was not sufficiently developed to provide an intellectual framework for policy-making. Perhaps only in the case of the 'Baby Doe' rules prohibiting the withdrawal of treatment, hydration and nutrition from severely impaired newborns did moral-agenda conservatism initiate and sustain policy.

In general, the moral agenda set limits to what could be proposed by economic conservatives. It was far more than just another constraint like the limited budget or federalism. The values of moral-agenda conservatism functioned as 'trumps' that intervened to overrule business-as-usual. A metaphor that is sometimes used to describe how 'rights' function is particularly appropriate because the moral agenda tends to be expressed in the language of rights.

The Context of Deregulation

It is important to understand that the market-reform position in health care was part of a wider reaction against 'liberals' and Keynesians, who are identified both with an activist fiscal policy and government intervention in private markets. Since Roosevelt's New Deal in the 1930s, conservative economists and businessmen have criticised government regulation for protecting inefficient producers. Although economic conservatives such as Murray Weidenbaum, Reagan's first Chairman of the Council of Economic Advisors

(CEA), have always been prominent in the attack on regulation and the monopolies that it supposedly encourages, the position is not exclusively a conservative one (Weidenbaum, 1988, pp. 232–5; Weidenbaum, 1975). Such consumer advocates as Mark Green and Ralph Nader (1973) make a strong case that the benefits of decreased economic regulation accrue in large measure to consumers who receive enhanced quality and–or lower prices.

Inefficiencies due to regulation offended the common sense of individuals of all political persuasions. For example, regulation of rates and territories commonly barred lorries from carrying loads on return trips. As Chairman of the Civil Aeronautics Board (CAB), Carter administration economist Alfred Kahn gained much favourable publicity for deregulating the economic aspects – fares, routes, and market entry – of airlines. In 1978 a law eliminating the CAB was passed. Airline rates fell dramatically, new airlines entered the market and access to flights, at least in more populous areas, increased.

The largest single entity to experience deregulation resulted from the antitrust suit filed by the Justice Department against American Telephone and Telegraph Company (AT&T), the giant telecommunications utility. After a number of years of litigation, AT&T and the Justice Department reached an agreement regarding the principles of 'divestiture', which involved the creation of seven regional telephone companies that would, *inter alia*, operate regulated monopolistic, local telephone networks. The agreement permitted AT&T to sell long distance telephone services in an unregulated competitive market and to compete in information transmission and processing – computer operations that had previously been closed to it.

Why Health Care is Unique

To economists and other deregulators health care seemed like a particularly fruitful area for the application of antiregulatory principles. By the mid-1970s there were a number of highly visible – but probably ineffective – regulatory agencies. Yet health care differed from other areas of deregulation, because for decades it had been generally believed that the prerequisites for a competitive market did not exist in the interaction between a patient seeking care from a health care provider. The patient was generally held to lack sufficient information to make informed consumer decisions. The physician, according to the traditional view, guided the patient in his or her health care purchases.[2] Yet in fee-for-service practice (the norm when the insurgent views of market-reformers became prominent) this 'purchasing agent's' income is tied to patients' decisions about receiving care.

The role of 'third party reimbursement' from private insurers (for employed workers) and from government exacerbates the problem of achieving market discipline in health care. Because of the power of organised medicine, insurers did not attempt to influence patients to consider cost in making health care decisions. Large-scale payment by the national government for health services only began in 1965 with the passage of Medicare (for the elderly and later the disabled) and Medicaid (for some of the poor); both Acts contained provisions that disavowed and formally disallowed any attempts to change the way medicine is practiced in the US.

In the era before the federal government became widely involved in paying for health care, formal and informal structures gave state and local medical societies great authority to discipline local physicians. Local physicians also exercised considerable control over the policies and management of local hospitals, which depended upon them for patients. Organised medicine insisted that doctors be paid on a 'fee-for-service' basis, partly to maintain professional autonomy. Its traditional dominance positioned the profession to benefit from weak regulation in Medicare and Medicaid.

The Growth of Regulation

Within five years of the inauguration of Medicare, Congress began to pass regulatory measures to contain the rate of increase in costs. By the mid-1970s, it appeared that the federal government's commitment to fund health care for a substantial number of its citizens would eventuate in a full panoply of regulation. Congress passed utilisation controls in 1972 and capital investment regulation, that was advertised as having 'teeth', in 1974. The realities of the American political system required that both efforts create decentralised institutions that would accomplish national objectives through local and–or state agendas. Adding to the confusion was the fact that the legislation generally required the founding of new nonprofit corporations or what Alan Pifer (1984) has called 'quasi nongovernmental organisations' to accomplish these ends. Significant criticisms of these efforts by market reformers include Havinghurst (1973, 1977). Equally telling objections emerged from a little noticed report commissioned by a former evaluator in the liberal US Office of Economic Opportunity. It showed that the system of grants-in-aid to states was very ineffective in persuading states to implement federal policy unless the issue was already on the state's policy agenda (Miller and Byrne, Inc., 1977).

During the deliberations regarding regulation of capital investment, the idea of hospital rate regulation was raised but rejected as too extreme. In the latter part of the 1970s individual states were permitted to have waivers that allowed them to include Medicare and Medicaid reimbursement in state experiments in setting the rates for all the payers who were responsible for reimbursing hospitals for patient care.

Economists and health services researchers began to evaluate all of these regulatory efforts almost as soon as the new institutions that were charged with implementing the federal legislation opened their doors. Sometimes researchers used data generated under prior state regulatory programmes and generalised about the likely failures of federal regulation. The research typically involved massive regression equations that were persuasive, but conceptually incapable of proving the inadequacy of capital investment regulation (through a process called 'certificate of need') and utilisation review (Brandon and Lee, 1984, pp. 106–8). The somewhat surprising result of several studies was that although capital investment regulation and utilisation controls do not hold down costs, rate regulation can restrain cost increases.

The issue between regulation and market reform is fundamentally a conceptual rather than an empirical question. The regulator will naturally respond to the failure of regulation by proposing to up the ante: regulation must have failed because its powers were too weak or the focus was incorrect. Such a response is logical unless one adopts an alternative paradigm that can ask whether the whole regulatory effort is misconceived.

Developing Market Alternatives to Regulation

Opponents of the growth of regulation in the 1970s developed alternative approaches to health policy. Paul Ellwood engineered the first apparent success of the market reformers when he invented the name 'health maintenance organisations' (HMOs) for prepaid group practices (PGPs) and convinced the Nixon administration that HMOs could solve the health policy problems that it faced (Ellwood, *et al.*, 1971). PGPs, which had struggled against efforts by organised medicine to put them out of business for forty years, were considered progressive and even politically left wing before their transformation into HMOs and subsequent apotheosis as the official health policy of the Nixon administration. An HMO combines the financing and delivery of health care in one organisation, thereby permitting the organisation and its physicians to benefit from any savings generated by efficiencies in providing care to patients. (Most efforts of the market reformers aim to reduce the rate of increase in health costs by altering the fee-for-service and cost-reimbursement incentives to provide larger quantities and more costly health services.) Passage of the Health Maintenance Act of 1973 committed the federal government to foster HMOs in local health care delivery areas. Most HMO proponents however were very unhappy with the initial Health Maintenance Act.

In a world of passive insurers who passed costs back to premium payers, the HMO was the only working example of an institution that would control costs and provide care of sufficient quality to please consumers. HMO supporters needed persuasive research to show than an efficient provider with appropriate incentives could give care efficiently, omit the unnecessary care that fee-for-service payment encourages and yet avoid negative effects on patients' health status. In particular research was necessary to prove that the apparent savings of PGPs were not due to favourable selection of healthy subscribers or to the provision of inadequate amounts of service or care of inferior quality. Another important question, which was never adequately addressed in empirical studies, was whether competition with HMOs would put inefficient traditional providers out of business or force them to change the way that they practised medicine.

By the end of the 1970s advocates of an alternative to regulation realised that a comprehensive strategy must feature much more than HMOs, which were growing more slowly than had been predicted.[3] Some focused on the professional dominance exercised by organised medicine and dentistry. Thus Clark Havighurst, an antitrust lawyer, published devastating critiques of the role of medicine in limiting competition (Havighurst, 1977, 1978, 1982). In various versions of his health plan, Alain Enthoven, an economist at Stanford who advised the Carter Administration on fulfilling its promise to enact NHI, has continuously recognised that the anticompetitive cast of medicine in the US is a major stumbling block in restructuring the health care system (Enthoven, 1978, 1988; Enthoven and Kronick, 1989). Paul Ellwood (1978), himself a physician, wanted to bring competition to physician groups.

In the 1970s there was a great deal of confusion about how insurance companies could actually control health care costs. In part, it was not clear how patient cost-sharing affected utilisation, costs, and health status. Two major empirical studies were launched to answer these questions. One study was the Rand health insurance experiment (HIE), a randomised controlled trial, in which the field work in six sites lasted from 1974 to 1982. The cost amounted to more than 70 million dollars. The other was the National Medical Care Expenditure Survey (NMCES), the only recent survey linking financial and health information from multiple sources. Its great contribution was to link insurance coverage and costs with utilisation and health status data. These two studies seemed to indicate that health care costs could be restrained if patients had to make a significant contribution at the time of receiving care. The initial HIE findings, suggesting that cost-sharing is not associated with significant decrements in health status, received wide dissemination in such prestigious journals as the *New England Journal of Medicine* (Brook, 1983; Keeler, 1987). NMCES provided the best empirical data on the comprehensiveness and depth of insurance coverage of people in differing income classes and employment statuses.

NMCES also added to a growing body of research in economics on the tax avoidance that could be gained by purchasing health insurance through one's work group. Up to four different taxes are avoided if potential employee income is used by employers for fringe benefits (Brandon, 1982). 'Tax expenditures', as these tax subsidies are formally called, are blamed for leading the American middle class to overinsure and subsequently overuse medical care. The Reagan administration put forward many proposals to abolish or modify these middle class subsidies, but they proved to be singularly unpopular on Capitol Hill.

By focusing on legislative and administrative actions, analysts and commentators often overlook the importance of judicial action in determining the context for health policy. The US courts, which both interpret statutory law and exercise the power of judicial review to ensure that state and federal law and executive acts are constitutional, provided the ultimate challenge to professional dominance of the health care system. The key case in establishing the liability of professional societies to antitrust suits for restraining competition was *Goldfarb v. Virginia State Bar* (1975), which allowed lawyers to advertise. Its extension to physicians, dentists and other professional groups effectively precluded them from using professional sanctions in disagreements over the organisation and delivery of health care. By the advent of the Reagan administration, the leadership of organised medicine was well aware of its new vulnerability to legal action. The importance of the new legal constraints on the profession can be demonstrated by comparisons over time. The possibility of a boycott gave the American Medical Association (AMA) a powerful voice in deciding the regulations implementing Medicare and Medicaid in the mid-1960s. By 1989 the AMA appeared little stronger than a supplicant pushing for some arrangements over others, as the federal government passed legislation that directly affects physicians' fees.

In summary, the complex intellectual background to the procompetition rhetoric and policies of the Reagan administration involved attacks on government regulation, attacks on practices by organised medicine that restrained trade, development of alternative delivery systems like HMOs, and the exercise of discipline in the market place by large purchasers of care using their buying power. The growth in intellectual and popular support for these insurgent views was largely due to the patent failure of the regulatory hodgepodge to deal with increasing total costs for personal health care and the federal government's rising health costs. The new ideas and values must be understood in light of the economic conditions of the 1970s, which played a large part in bringing the Reagan revolution to power.

SOCIO-ECONOMIC IMPERATIVES

A vibrant economy existed during most of the Kennedy and Johnson administrations. Early in his administration, Kennedy, who was alleged to be the first president who understood Keynesian economics, yielded on other goals to achieve a tax cut. Conventional wisdom claimed that the economic growth which resulted from this cut forestalled an expected recession and led to greater private activity, nearly full employment and enhanced federal revenues. At least Reagan became convinced of this account. It led him to accept the agenda of his supply-side advisors who wished to prime the pumps of private consumption and production with large tax cuts and simultaneously achieve massive spending reductions in a government starved of tax revenue.

Economic prosperity allowed President Johnson to fulfill the Kennedy promises to use government money and power to create a better life for the millions who were not full participants in the affluent, typically suburban middle class lifestyle of the 1950s and 60s. It was in the Johnson era that the Office of Economic Opportunity (OEO), headed by President Kennedy's brother-in-law Sargent Shriver, began funding neighbourhood health centres to provide comprehensive health services in the poorest areas of America's cities and rural areas (Sardell, 1988). Medicare and Medicaid, which were enacted in 1965, were products of the same generous impulse and flush treasuries. Both politicians and public health officials focused on access, availability and quality of care rather than on the costs involved.

By 1975 the federal share had grown to 27.1 per cent of total personal health expenditures from 10.2 per cent in 1965, and all health care spending had risen to 8.6 per cent of GNP from 6.1 per cent (Gibson, 1979, pp. 22, 32, and 1980, pp. 2, 16). Pre-Medicare (1959–66) annual increases in medical prices averaged 3.2 per cent compared with 7.9 per cent average annual increases (1966–71) before Nixon inaugurated price controls in 1971. On average the consumer price index (excluding its medical care component) rose 2.0 per cent and 5.8 per cent annually in the same periods. After price controls were lifted in 1974, the pattern for the remainder of the decade was double-digit inflation in medical costs. For example, the December 1974 to December 1975 increase in medical care costs was 10.3 per cent (Council on Wage and Price Stability, Executive Office of the President, 1976).

Faced with increases of this magnitude, the rising costs of care rather than increased access and quality rapidly became the major concern of policy makers. The career of mandated price controls under the supposedly conservative President Nixon convinced virtually everyone of the bankruptcy of price and wage controls. Some leaders, such as Senator Edward M. Kennedy (D-MA), the slain John Kennedy's brother, believed that access, quality and cost-containment could be attained together through NHI and significant amounts of regulation. In his 1976 presidential campaign Jimmy Carter committed himself to NHI. In the event, the struggle against runaway inflation, the oil crisis, an inability to reach a compromise with Kennedy and the latter's powerful trade union supporters, frustrated this latest push for NHI. Although NHI usually seems incompatible with market-reform views, some of the most influential advocates of competitive policy approaches continue to believe that it is possible to achieve universal access in a system structured by market mechanisms (Enthoven, 1978; Enthoven and Kronick, 1989).

Instead of NHI, Carter attempted to legislate a cap on hospital revenues, but was defeated when the hospitals persuaded Congress that they would voluntarily reduce their rate of cost increases. The defeat of Carter's hospital revenue cap occurred as the federal government, along with many northeastern states, became desperate to slow the rate of rising hospital costs, which constituted the largest component of health expenditures and the largest single category of federal health expenditures. Carter's ineffectual effort focused on overall national health care costs and would therefore have addressed the costs experienced by private insurers. This point becomes important in light of the Reagan administration's decision to concentrate on federal expenditures for hospital care without concern that costs would be shifted to other payers in the system.

The health policy debates in the late 1970s must be understood in light of overall perplexity and concern that something had seriously gone wrong with the 'American Dream'. Dissatisfaction with this state of affairs encouraged the electorate to vote for change in 1980. In contrast to the sixties, when economists confidently claimed to 'fine-tune' the economy to maintain just the correct balance between unemployment and inflation, the seventies produced a series of traumas that cast doubt both on Keynesian fiscal policy and the gospel of monetary theory preached by Milton Friedman. For the only period since the landmark Social Security legislation established the national pension system in 1935, the cost of living rose faster than the average workers's wage. Because Social Security retirement pensions had been indexed in 1972 to consumer prices (CPI) rather than to wages, the unusual economic conditions began to create great strains on the solvency of the largest single social welfare programme in America.[4] This combination of stagnation in growth and inflation in prices came to be called 'stagflation'. In some sectors of the economy – such as university professors – the actual purchasing power of average salaries declined over the decade.

These objective conditions generated the perception of a static or even shrinking economic pie. Thus the situation contrasted greatly with the optimistic feelings typical of the 1960s, when growth fueled increasing affluence and generated a more generous feeling about sharing with the less affluent. A tax revolt, which was first focused on the property taxes that finance local and state services, began in California and spread across the country after Reagan left the governorship. Feelings about high taxes in a no-growth economy led to resentment about high federal taxes. The Republicans began to capitalise on the anti-tax sentiment with attacks on liberal 'tax and spend' Democrats, whose bad habits the Republicans blamed for the economic impasse. The 'Reagan revolution', which was presented to the American people as standing for smaller government and balanced budgets, capitalised on this perception of economic chaos and failed government programmes.

Market reformers blamed the Democratic majority in Congress for over-regulation and rising health care costs. On his road to power, Reagan popularised the economic philosophy of the market-reformers by promising both to 'get government off our backs', that is, to deregulate health care, and to reduce the rate of increase in government funds going to health care. Thus the Reagan administration believed it was elected in 1980 with a mandate to end the panoply of 'great society' programmes.

POLICY NETWORKS

The ideas that informed the Reagan administration's procompetition policy were largely nurtured in think tanks and academia before the 1980 election. The American Enterprise Institute, a conservative think tank, sponsored a number of notable conferences under the leadership of Robert Helms, PhD, who headed its health activities. During the Carter administration a group at the Federal Trade Commission (FTC) became convinced of the validity of the new ideas and began to propagate them through vehicles like the influential conference 'Competititon in the Health Care Sector: Past Present and Future' (Greenberg, 1978). Clark Havighurst, the distinguished antitrust lawyer from Duke University Law School, spent 1978–9 as a resident consultant at the FTC's Bureau of Competition. It was in this pre-Reagan period that the FTC began challenging the domination of organised medicine in the courts.

When the Reagan administration came to power, some of the leaders in the market reform movement became government officials. For example, Robert J. Rubin, MD, became the Assistant Secretary of Planning and Evaluation (ASPE) and Robert Helms became Deputy Assistant Secretary for Health. (Later Helms replaced Rubin when the latter moved to the private sector.) Glenn Hackbarth, a young lawyer who had worked with both Helms and Havighurst, came to ASPE to draft the administration's comprehensive procompetition bill. (After several years he left to work for a hospital chain and later returned to government service as the second-in-command at the Health Care Financing Administration (HCFA), which administers Medicare and Medicaid.) The first Reagan Secretary of Health and Human Services (HHS), former Senator Richard Schweiker (R-PA), had sponsored one of the five procompetition bills in the 96th Congress. As a Senate insider however, Schweiker had acquiesced to the spending and regulatory programmes of the Democrats. The new budget director, David Stockman, was firmly in the procompetition camp. As a young Congressman he had coauthored the Gephardt-Stockman bill in the 96th and 97th Congresses, which would have legislated virtually the entire market reform agenda.

The influence of these advocates coincided with the overall administration commitment to reduce government involvement in domestic affairs – the pledge to 'get government off our backs' – and the need to cut federal expenditures because of high inflation and what were then considered to be unacceptably high deficits. (Those deficits look paltry in light of the gigantic deficits of the Reagan years.) Thus 'procompetition' became the official policy of the federal government and a bill to implement it was promised soon.

Moral-agenda conservatives mainly received their rewards in areas other than health care. For example, William Bennett became chair of the strategically placed National Endowment for the Humanities, where he could prefer the projects of conservative thinkers, like those at the Claremont complex, and discourage at least some of the funding for established liberal institutions, such as the Hastings Center Society for Ethics, Society and the Life Sciences. Although nominees for high level jobs needed to take the correct stand on issues such as abortion, the moral-agenda conservatives were not in general placed in HHS.

The most notable exception to this generalisation was C. Everett Koop, a retired professor of pediatric surgery at the University of Pennsylvania Medical School, who had been active in anti-abortion circles. Koop, who was a friend of Nancy Reagan's family in Philadelphia, had no obvious credentials in public health. Because at 65 he was over-aged for the Public Health Service, which is a uniformed or paramilitary service of the US government, Congress needed to give special authorisation for him to become PHS commander. The American Public Health Association (APHA), the liberal nonprofit professional association that serves as the watchdog of public health, took the opportunity to try to defeat the Koop appointment, but was unsuccessful. By the time that he retired in the first months of the Bush administration, Surgeon-General Koop had become such a hero of public health that he was awarded APHA's highest medal. Throughout his tenure Koop supported many mainstream public health activities (such as antismoking campaigns), but his surprising transformation came mainly in the second Reagan administration when he recognised the need for effective public health measures against AIDS, even at the risk of offending moral-agenda conservatives.

STRATEGIES, POLICIES AND CONSTRAINTS: THE REAGAN RECORD IN HEALTH POLICY

The New Federalism

The first objectives of the Reagan administration were to shed much of the federal responsibility for implementing policy and to reduce the budget. Budget reduction was part of a broader plan to reduce inflation, which by American standards had risen to unprecedented heights in the previous administration. The remarkable Stockman budget of 1981 proposed to shift much of the responsibility for health policy and other social services to the states. Although it did call for substantial cuts, Stockman recognised that fundamental administrative changes were necessary before the 'Reagan revolution' could achieve major reductions in federal domestic expenditures.

Understanding the Reagan administration strategy requires some knowledge of the peculiar American intergovernmental relationship that has developed to overcome the drawbacks of a federal structure. For the first century and a half of US independence, most health and safety issues were the responsibility of state governments, the local governments that they established and the private sector. In the first half of this century the recognition of a growing need for national policies, such as assistance for crippled children or other disadvantaged populations, led to the development of the first significant health-related grants-in-aid. Cash grants gave states or other organisations federal money to pursue activities or provide services that were specified in the law authorising the expenditure or in federal regulations promulgated by agencies in the executive branch. This voluntary mechanism reflected the constraints of the reigning constitutional interpretation, which made states responsible for health and safety while it allowed the US to develop modern national social services appropriate for an industrial nation.[5] (For example, it enabled tax dollars to flow from wealthy states to poor ones.) Although private institutions (medical schools for instance) had received substantial funding for activities such as research during the Truman and Eisenhower administrations (1945–60), the states were clearly in charge of supplying public social services. The federal government provided states with funds to carry out particular – or 'categorical' – programmes under federal guidelines that attempted to ensure minimal uniformity and standards across the country. Grants became the means for accomplishing an astounding range of national goals, from programmes paying for health care for eligible low-income patients to health statistics programmes collecting and collating data on births, deaths and disease. By the 1970s the federal government even used the threat of *withdrawing* these established grant-in-aid programmes to force states to enact such regulation as controls on capital investment under the Health Planning and Resources Development Act of 1974.

Criticism of the system of grants-in-aid came from both sides of the partnership. States complained that federal regulations required too much red tape and permitted insufficient flexibility for the money to be used where it was most needed. The federal government objected to the variability with which states implemented 'national' programmes. Outside observers often objected to inequities in which relatively wealthy states took full advantage of federal programmes, while citizens in poorer states found it difficult to qualify for benefits or received lower levels of benefits. For example, in 1967 two of the richest states – New York and California – spent 'almost half' of the federal contribution to the new Medicaid programme (Stevens, 1971, p. 479).

In the 1960s the federal government expanded the use of grants to fund – and often to establish – local private nonprofit organisations to pursue government objectives independently of local and state leaders, and sometimes in opposition to them. By the mid-1970s grant programmes to the private sector reached about a quarter of the number aiding state and local government. Neighbourhood health centres, which provided health care for low income patients and often constituted centres of political activity, were prominent examples of this phenomenon. The expansion of grants to accomplish federal aims has been so extensive in the last 30 years that one researcher uses the term 'third-party government' to designate the role that non-profits and local and state government play in carrying out federal policies. Grantees have considerable 'discretion over the spending of public funds and the exercise of public authority' (Salamon, 1987, p. 110). Yet nonprofit recipients of federal categorical grants-in-aid joined the states in complaining about restrictions imposed by the federal bureaucracy.

The 'Reagan revolution', as its proponents like to style their movement, intended to transform this complex, only partially understood web of federal, state and nonprofit activities. (In particular the role of nonprofits in the delivery of government services in the US was largely unnoticed until Reagan began cutting federal funds for nonprofits.) In virtually all areas of domestic policy Stockman's first budget proposed to combine the categorical programmes that had been subjected to so much criticism, into 'block grants' and to reduce federal expenditures through grants by 25 per cent. Administrative requirements imposed by the federal government would be cut sharply. Republicans claimed that the savings due to enhanced flexibility and lower administrative costs would make up for the reduction.

In a remarkable feat of legislative legerdemain, Stockman used recently enacted Congressional budget procedures to circumvent resistance by Congressmen and Senators entrenched in issue-specific committees. Stockman prevailed in most areas of the budget, even if his own account suggests that the victories required compromises that spelled ultimate defeat (Stockman, 1986). However he failed with health policy. In health, opposition was led by Henry Waxman (D-CA), the recently elected chair of the Health and Environment Subcommittee of the House Energy and Commerce Committee. Waxman accepted reductions in programmes for poor people but frustrated the broader aims of the administration by increasing the number of block grants and hedging them in with regulations. In some funding areas states had the option of accepting the new block grants with all their restrictions or maintaining the old categorical grants. The states almost uniformly chose the old grants-in-aid.

The fight that Waxman waged for health programmes was virtually the only Democratic success won in that first year of the Reagan administration. Greater responsibility for non-health social program-mes, such as those provided by the aging network, were shuffled off to the states, which made it easier to reduce expenditures to them in succeeding years. Aside from health, cuts in federal spending for social services were devastating. This result is especially ironic in light of the fact that the Reagan administration (like the succeeding Bush administration with its slogan of 'a thousand points of light') gave great rhetorical support to private philanthropy as the sector that would take over much of the burden that the federal government wished to drop. 'Voluntarism', Reagan said in 1981, 'is an essential part of our plan to give the government back to the people' (Bremner, 1988, p. 206).

The significance of Waxman's victory on the health front, Stockman's success in other areas of social services, and the inability of anyone to bring the increase in health costs down to the level of the general rise in consumer prices, is clarified by Salamon's painstaking efforts to evaluate the impacts of the early years of the Reagan administration on nonprofit providers:

> Although the inflation-adjusted value of total federal support to nonprofit providers remained relatively constant between fiscal years 1980 and 1985, the share of that total absorbed by health care providers increased from under 60 per cent to over 70 per cent, and the share left for all other types of nonprofits shrank from 40 per cent to under 30 per cent. (Salamon, 1987, p. 103.)

It should be added that state governments did not typically seek to take up the financial slack left by decreased federal transfer payments.[6]

The national regulatory structures quickly lost significance. The change to a deregulatory climate was very rapid at the federal level from 1979–81. Havighurst (1982, pp. 8–9) even suggested that deregulators might need to use federal power to encourage states to adopt procompetition policies. The Reagan administration and its Congressional allies only succeeded in gutting the health planning legislation after a long legislative struggle, but any effectiveness had been sapped long before final defunding in 1986. Although utilisation and quality review through the organisations of local physicians established under the Medicare Amendments of 1972 were repealed, the Tax Equity and Fiscal Responsibility Act of 1982 (TEFRA) directed the Secretary of HHS to begin contracting directly with peer review organisations. TEFRA, which initiated the movement towards a prospective system of reimbursing hospitals, reflected the Congressional conviction that at least some safeguards would have to be in place if incentives to undertreat patients were instituted.

Procompetition Legislation and PPS

HHS began work on a comprehensive procompetition bill at the beginning of the first administration. OMB, which exercised a great deal of power over policy as well as expenditures throughout the Reagan years, was very influential in formulating the centrepiece of administration policy. In 1983 Congress, in which the Republicans had just lost their Senate majority due to reverses in the midterm elections, received the 'Health Incentives Reform Plan'. It called for revision in hospital reimbursement, a plan to encourage Medicare beneficiaries to enroll in managed care programmes through a 'voucher' system, more patient copayments for brief hospitalisations (which would be counterbalanced by more generous coverage for expensive long-stays) and a cap on tax-free employer-provided health insurance. Congress adopted administration changes in hospital reimbursement, but rejected the other proposals in that Congress and successive ones. Whereas it had previously agreed to facilitate HMO and Competitive Medical Plan (CMP) enrollment of Medicare beneficiaries, Congress refused to permit private insurers to enroll Medicare beneficiaries in managed care programmes.

The aspect of the Reagan package that was accepted – the Prospective Payment System (PPS) – is undoubtedly the most important legacy in health care of the entire Reagan era. Understanding the reality of the Reagan administration's achievements requires an explanation of PPS, an appreciation of its political significance, and finally a brief look at its effectiveness as health policy.

PPS capitalised on a common criticism that retrospective reimbursement of allowable hospital costs creates an incentive to incur new expenses so long as they are reimbursable. Prospective payment systems promise a set rate of reimbursement for a given future period, typically one year. (Usually there is a *ceteris paribus* clause that allows significant changes in volume or intensity of care to change reimbursement.) If hospitals are able to provide the same general level of care for less money, they may retain any surplus. If actual costs exceed the revenues produced by the prospectively set rates (that is, the product of the rate and the number of cases), hospitals must absorb the difference. Thus prospective payment removes payment somewhat from actual costs by assuring hospitals of certain revenue for a given patient volume and intensity of care. Technical or administrative changes that produce savings under such a system will result in enhanced surpluses. Prospective payment creates the first incentive for hospitals to generate savings since hospitals quit charging patients and insurance companies whatever they wished or thought purchasers would pay. The importance ascribed to this change in incentives caused the Reagan initiative to be named 'the prospective payment system' or PPS.

The Health Care Financing Administration (HCFA) chose to base its prospective rate-setting system on a recently-developed form of the 'case' approach. In case reimbursement methods, payment to the hospital is based on the condition or disease of the patient receiving treatment rather than the length of hospitalisation (per diem) or the number of patients (capitation) or the actual services (itemised billing). HCFA selected the particular method called Diagnosis-Related Groups (DRGs), which had been developed at Yale University in the 1970s and implemented in a pilot project in New Jersey in the early 1980s.[7] The 467 categories in the DRG system were designed to group diagnoses into clusters according to similarity in the use of resources and clinical homogeneity. Rates were set to cover the typical or average case within a given DRG; extreme deviance in the resources expended on some particular patient qualifies as an 'outlier', which results in adjusted payment. Because Medicare essentially covers retirees and the disabled, the acute medical conditions of the elderly are the principal focus of the federal DRG system, which is not used to reimburse for care in long-term care, psychiatric, or children's hospitals.

In its desperation over rising hospital costs, Congress enacted and the President signed the Social Security Amendments of 1983, containing the PPS provisions, in the unheard of time of four months. The new federal legislation generated concern from many quarters. Hospitals were fearful that they would not be able to treat patients for as little as the average in their region (or for the national average that would be phased in with allowances for regional differences in labour costs). Many physicians feared that the quality of care would decline as hospitals took advantage of the opportunity to discharge patients early, thereby avoiding all the expenses associated with longer convalescent periods in hospitals. Patients have generally not understood PPS; too often they feel that their care is dictated by financial decisons made at HCFA. (Hospitals or physicians apparently sometimes lead patients to think that they are being discharged 'early' because federally-permitted 'DRG days' have expired.) Other payers expected hospitals to try to make up for Medicare's tight fists by charging nongovernment payers more.

Hospitals had good reason to be concerned. In the 1980s many hospitals experienced increased numbers of patients without any third party coverage. Yet Medicare differs from its New Jersey prototype in its unwillingness to pay hospitals for 'uncompensated care', the costs of providing care to patients without government coverage, private insurance or the personal ability or willingness to pay. Moreover by the end of the Reagan years HCFA and Congress kept the annual rates of increase in the funding of DRGs below the rate of health care cost increases. This 'ratcheting down' of DRG rate increases was justified on the grounds that funding had been generous in the first years, thereby enabling the average hospital to make substantial profits.

The adoption of PPS was a clear manifestation of the increasing preoccupation of the Reagan administration with budget deficits. Unlike Carter's proposed cap on hospital revenue, PPS does not address the overall issue of rising hospital cost, which affects employers, private insurance companies, other levels of government and individuals. PPS reflects a decision by the national government to use the buying power – monopsony – that comes from its position as the largest single purchaser of care to cut a better deal for itself.[8] Thus some commentators (for example, Glaser 1987, pp. 57–63) merely regard the federal government as a 'prudent purchaser' who invites other large purchasers to follow its lead. Yet others, who argue that Medicare reimbursement rules affect the entire health care system, see PPS rate-setting as federal regulation.

PPS has led to earlier discharge of patients from hospitals. Discharging patients early has exacerbated shortages of nursing homes and stimulated the growth of home health agencies. Anecdotes about the undue discharge of patients – the 'quicker and sicker' issue – are widespread but convincing studies of serious negative effects on patients are lacking.

Measured against Candidate Reagan's objection to government interference and his emphasis on localism, PPS looks like a great betrayal. The implementation of national Medicare hospital reimbursement rates marks an end to the great local diversity in what the federal government paid for health care across the country. The only faintly procompetitive aspect of the scheme is its prospective nature, which permits efficient hospitals to keep any surplus that they earn. The stingy increases in DRG rates demonstrate that PPS functions like the regulatory systems that squeezed hospitals in the Northeastern states in the 1970s. A hospital's financial fate is likely to depend on increasing the volume of patients with more lucrative DRGs, on serving patients with nongovernment payers to whom it can shift costs, and on attracting only a small number of patients without any third party payer.

Despite the rhetoric of 'competition' then, the upshot of the Reagan administration's most important health policy initiative has been a massive increase in federal intervention that has tied the financial fate of hospitals across the country to decisions reached by HCFA and Congress. Yet administration officials have generally been pleased by PPS, for the effort has attained its goal of reducing the rate of increase in federal hospital expenditures. Researchers have also failed to find much evidence of cost-shifting to nongovernment payers.

In health care the administration deserted its 'revolution' in favour of the traditional value of fiscal responsibility. Reducing the rate of federal increases in Medicare hospital costs and initiating deeper cuts in non-health social programmes were the practical acts of a government that had decided that it could not hand the problem of health care policy back to the states. Yet even in health, and other social services, politicians were not totally willing to gut programmes in order to balance the Reagan revenue losses. At the macro-level, in contrast, the Siren supply-side song of tax-cuts and perpetual growth, along with a massive strengthening in US military capability, triumphed over serious efforts to control expenditures, as Stockman's *Triumph of Politics* (1986) explains.

Moral-Agenda Issues

While fiscal conservatives and market reformers struggled with health policy on a day-to-day basis, the moral-agenda conservatives exerted force on a limited number of issues involving prolife policies. In addition to abortion, treatment of impaired infants and family planning in the US, foreign aid and international human rights policy received attention from the moral-agenda conservatives. They also greatly affected the outcome of Reagan administration policies on AIDS.

The official administration policy maintained that an amendment to the U.S. Constitution was needed to overturn the Supreme Court decision in *Roe v. Wade* (1973), which effectively guaranteed a woman the right to abortion during the early stages of pregnancy. That position conveniently relieved the administration of the need to fight in Congress for its policy, because the process of amending the constitution involves Congress and the states rather than the executive. Although it is possible for an administration to organise effective legislative support for constitutional change, the Reagan administration never placed a constitutional amendment high enough on its legislative agenda to threaten other achievable priorities. In the long run the administration's most effective tactic was to select candidates for appointment to the Supreme Court who hold views that can be expected to lead them to overturn *Roe v. Wade*.

Both Reagan administrations were however active in supporting the majority in Congress that refused to spend any US dollars for abortions, except in cases when the mother's life is in danger. The principal battleground came in the annual Medicaid appropriations, where states are generally left to decide what medical procedures will be provided for poor women and children who make up its largest group of beneficiaries. Fairly early in the administration, the courts helped to sort out the right of states to use their own money to continue funding abortions for welfare recipients, despite federal efforts to stop publicly-funded abortions except to save the mother's life.

In the first year of the Bush presidency however, Congress broke that anti-abortion pattern by passing a bill allowing states to use Medicaid dollars to help pay for abortions for eligible poor women who were pregnant as a result of incest or rape. President Bush angered prochoice advocates by vetoing the bill. The modest change in Congress' views became possible because the Supreme Court had generated a political resurgence in the prochoice movement. *Webster v. Reproductive Health Services* (1989) increased the scope for state regulation of the abortion rights granted in *Roe*. The Court, with a majority of justices now appointed by Reagan, appeared to be moving towards a reconsideration of *Roe*. Renewed activity within the prochoice majority in the electorate was generally regarded as an important factor in Democratic gubernatorial victories in New Jersey and Virginia in November 1989. After the election Republican National Chairman Lee Atwater began to deemphasise the right-to-life commitment of the Republican Party.

The Reagan administration did act consistently on non-Medicaid issues that involved abortion. It used federal support of family planning services to prohibit recipients of federal funding from informing pregnant women about the abortion option. In 1981 the administration backed a minor bill to authorise small sums to strengthen 'traditional' values by promoting 'teenage chastity' as a solution to the 'problem of adolescent promiscuity'. (In the conference that resolves disagreements between the Senate and House, language referring to chastity was dropped, but counsellors were forbidden to mention abortion unless teenagers or their parents specifically asked for such information.) In international affairs the administration also refused to participate in funding family planning programmes that involved abortion. Even in the case of a country so significant for the US as China, officials made plain their displeasure over the use of abortion as part of its strict one-child family policy.

Right-to-life proponents, who were generally dissatisfied with the administration's lack of energy and imagination in opposing abortion, began to emphasise the related issue of withholding treatment, hydration and nutrition from severely impaired infants. On this issue the administration responded aggressively. It plunged into an area where decision-making had always involved parents in consultation with their physicians under the largely nominal regulatory oversight of state law. President Reagan's personal interest in the issue was reported to be the source of the administration's unaccustomed diligence in making and implementing policies (Brown 1986). During the course of the controversy HHS issued three sets of regulations; one of these 'Baby Doe' regulations included provisions for a telephone 'hotline' which would allow citizens to alert federal investigators about potential violations. Each regulatory effort was struck down by the courts. The administration's remarkable assertion of federal authority was based on a creative attempt to expand the federal civil rights law (Section 504 of the Rehabilitation Act of 1973) that protects the rights of handicapped individuals. Ultimately Congress passed the Child Abuse and Neglect Amendments of 1984 (PL98–457), which defused the issue by basing the protection of infants on well-established child abuse and neglect laws that are implemented by the states. The amendments greatly reduce the draconian federal penalties for noncompliance that HHS had tried to establish in its regulations. Although the attempt to assert direct federal power over specific medical decisions did sensitise the nation to the issue, and may have had the moral effect desired by the right-to-life movement, its effort to involve the federal government in settling difficult bioethical questions was rebuffed.

One event in the first Reagan administration does seem inconsistent with administration rhetoric about the value of life. In 1981 the administration voted against a World Health Organisation agreement on an international code of ethics that would have stopped the Nestlé Corporation from vigorously marketing its infant formula in countries that accepted the voluntary code. Health authorities are convinced that breast-feeding, when possible, is a health-promoting practice. In Third World countries poverty and impure water often lead mothers to give their babies inadequate and contaminated milk substitutes when they choose formula over breast-feeding. Health experts estimated at the time that the death toll might amount to as many as one million lives a year. The US, which argued against interfering with commerce and free speech, was alone among 119 nations in opposing the code. The decision received considerable attention because two senior civil servants at the Agency for International Development resigned in outrage over the government's moral choices.

Right-to-life concerns also affected some scientific research. In general the administration permitted human genetics research to proceed, although budget problems have reduced overall growth in federal support for non-military research. In the particular area of research using aborted foetuses or embryos not required for implantation, however, the administration raised serious questions. Even though no research involving foetuses had ever received federal funds, in May 1988 federally-funded research using foetuses from elective abortions was formally suspended until a Human Tissue Foetal Transplant Research Panel considered relevant ethical and clinical issues. The advisory panel suggested that research should proceed under appropriate guidelines, but Louis Sullivan, HHS Secretary under Bush, decided to continue the ban. Since privately-funded research can use foetuses, the absence of clear regulatory guidelines increases the possibility of inappropriate or unethical use of foetal tissue.

AIDS

Patterns of symptoms that later became known as AIDS began to be recognised early in 1981. The first scientific publication to acknowledge the problem was the brief report in the *Morbidity and Mortality*

Weekly Report (Gottlieb *et al.*, 1981), which is published by HHS' Centers for Disease Control. Its cause was not established until the summer of 1983, when Dr. Luc Montagnier and associates published an article announcing the isolation of a new retrovirus, and April 1984, when Dr. Robert Gallo and HHS Secretary Margaret Heckler claimed the US discovery of the virus.

Thus the AIDS epidemic was coextensive with Reagan's presidency; it was the chief public health drama during his eight years. The federal response to AIDS measured the degree to which the Reagan administration's ideological commitment to leave health policy to the states and the private sector would be altered when faced with a genuine crisis. It also provided a test of the administration's willingness to reverse its anti-spending policies if part of the population were subject to some great natural or social risk.

For moral-agenda conservatives AIDS had several dimensions. In its earliest American manifestation, AIDS was perceived largely to be a 'gay plague'. Many moral-agenda conservatives are uncomfortable about homosexuality, which is considered antithetical to 'family values' and to many traditional religious teachings. Some observers (Shilts, 1988) think that this consideration explains why the extraordinary levels of support needed to understand the new disease were not forthcoming during the first administration. (In the early years of the Reagan administration, CDC had to take most of the resources for work on AIDS from other on-going programmes.)

As knowledge about AIDS grew, it became apparent that the only immediately effective interventions were behavioural and social, even though 'hard' medical science might ultimately develop a vaccine. Generating specific behavioural changes in the gay community required the trust and cooperation of members of that community. Trust and cooperation in turn depended on accepting the validity and integrity of the underlying lifestyle that was so distasteful to many moral-agenda conservatives. For example, talk of a 'safe-sex' campaign seemed to many traditionalists to countenance sexual activity outside of heterosexual marriage. The Catholic Church has long opposed condoms as part of its opposition to birth control. Such spokesmen as William Bennett (who had become Secretary of Education in 1985) preached abstinence to America's teenagers in much the same way that Nancy Reagan advised them to 'just say no' to illegal drugs. He also actively supported mandatory testing as a public health measure in a controversy with Dr. Koop.

Some of those who did not object to the availability of condoms or induced changes in gay lifestyle drew the line at the enhanced sex education that became necessary if heterosexual youth in school were to be taught the dangers of unsafe sex. (Sex-education in the public schools, a major concern for many groups of fundamentalist Christians, has been one of the perennial issues that disturb local tranquility in America.)

A final issue that aroused moral-agenda conservatives was the *language* in which it was necessary to communicate. One of Koop's achievements was to mail information on AIDS to every American family; a pamphlet which required considerable rewriting and stimulated much controversy before it was approved. However a defeat for those who put public health necessity over propriety came in 1988 and 1989 when Congressional forces led by conservative Senator Jesse Helms (R-NC) frustrated HHS efforts to conduct a scientific survey to learn about sexual behaviour in the US. The survey was needed to plot strategies for the struggle against AIDS, because the last full-scale survey of American sexual habits was the celebrated work of Kinsey from 1938–52. This important, but out-dated study did not focus on the sexual practices of contemporary male homosexuals and minority groups. The Senator objected to the very idea of government surveyors asking such questions and using words that would be understood by respondents.

Although its record on AIDS is an important measure of conservative performance in a crisis, this chapter cannot undertake an evaluation of the Reagan administration's response to AIDS in any systematic way. Two facts seem indisputable. The record is clear that a shortage of resources hampered CDC's surveillance efforts in the early years of the epidemic. It is also clear that the National Institutes of Health did not assign a high priority in its research agenda to AIDS in the early years.

The Reagan administration's new federalism might have been vindicated if state and local governments had moved quickly to fill the federal gap. Unfortunately they did not. For example, the shortage of drug rehabilitation programmes that are necessary to wean heroin users and those addicted to other drugs from substances that facilitate the spread of AIDS has not been alleviated. (Drug facilities that serve those at highest risk for AIDS are usually dependent on state and local governments for funding; significant numbers of private facilities find it profitable to cater to the needs of middle class alcoholics and other substance abusers with health insurance.)

Perhaps the Reagan administration's general failure to provide *leadership* in the battle against AIDS is more significant than the failure to fund surveillance and research early in the battle. AIDS activists often point out that Reagan was well into his second administration before he even uttered the word 'AIDS'. Greater leadership might have mobilised state and local governments to deal with local transmission of the virus before so many had become infected, might have forestalled much of the prejudice and fear that has led to discrimination against persons with AIDS, and might have given direction to private-sector efforts in research and education.

Two authors present different models of how to understand the available information. Sandra Panem's *AIDS Bureaucracy* (1988) explains what others see as failures in terms of the seeming inevitability of large bureaucracies to move slowly, despite good will on the part of all involved. Her book tends to demonstrate the truth of the aphorism that to understand all is to excuse everything. AIDS journalist Randy Shilts (1988), on the other hand, documents failure after failure of leadership in the upper reaches of the Reagan administration, the health establishment, the universities, the blood banks and the gay community. He describes efforts by individuals at the lower and middle levels in these institutions and communities to take effective action.

The Second Reagan Administration

The second administration began with a number of personnel changes. Perhaps most startling was the switch between James Baker, the White House Chief of Staff in the first administration, and Donald Regan, who was the Secretary of the Treasury. Some, including Nancy Reagan (1989, pp. 312–16), blame many of the problems of the second administration on Regan's performance in the crucial job of managing the White House staff. Other changes included Stockman's resignation from the administration in 1985. By 1986 HHS had a new chief in Otis Bowen MD, a former governor of Indiana.

By 1985 the economy was in reasonable shape with inflation under control, moderate real growth in GNP and unemployment that had fallen sharply from the recession highs.[9] The tax cuts that were the centrepiece of supply-side economic policy in the first administration were in place. The major problem was that economic growth failed to generate the new federal revenues that the supply-siders had promised. Instead the federal government had given up tax revenue, which compounded the deficit problem of the Carter years. Deficits of a magnitude unprecedented in peacetime became inevitable. Administration pleas for further spending cuts ran into strengthened resistance as all the likely candidates among the discretionary spending programmes had already been cut. Yet the deficits lacked much immediately visible impact on the lives of American voters. Contrary to the predictions of knowledgeable observers, the US dollar continued to be strong internationally during most of the second administration, even as the trade deficits swelled. Economists and financiers who were not absorbed in speculative corporate buyouts expressed foreboding, but real disaster never occurred despite one scare in the stock markets. By the end of the second administration politicians had learned to live with unthinkably huge deficits in what was perhaps an analogue to the way an earlier generation had learned to live with the bomb.

With the tax cuts and PPS in place, firm Congressional resistance to significant future spending reductions and the best economic news in a decade, it seemed reasonable to expect that the second Reagan administration would begin to attend to the demands of moral-agenda conservatives. Perhaps the personnel changes were signals of the continued focus on economic matters. As the chief spokesman for the administration on economic policy, especially after the departure of Stockman and Martin Feldstein, Reagan's second CEA Chair, Baker applied his deft political touch to tax reform legislation. The complex tax-reform proposal involved lowering the marginal income tax rate for most taxpayers, exempting more low-income families, and eliminating a large number of deductions – or 'loopholes' – by which middle and upper class families reduced their tax liability. Efforts to reduce federal tax-expenditure subsidies for the purchase of health insurance were again dropped as the legislation made its way through Congress. The upshot of the focus on what was called 'tax simplification' was that moral-agenda conservatives did not receive noticeably more attention in the second administration than in the first.[10] Increasing interest in foreign affairs with the advent of the Gorbachev era also helped to keep issues favoured by moral-agenda conservatives off the action agenda.

In health care the bureaucracy was focused on implementing PPS. As success began to be achieved in holding down the rate of increase in Medicare's hospital costs, attention on Capitol Hill and in HHS began to be paid to controlling Medicare Part B payments to physicians. Congress took the lead in forcing HHS to fund research on the resource-based relative value scale (RB-RVS). In 1989 Congress passed legislation requiring Medicare to use the new scale. In time an RB-RVS may reduce variation in payments to physicians practicing different medical specialities.

Just as PPS increased direct federal intervention in hospital care across the nation, so the adoption of a national RB-RVS for paying physician's bills constitutes the first attempt to institute a uniform national payment system for physicians. Its vigorous implementation will ultimately have an impact on physicians' incomes. Those in primary care specialities expect to be helped by the legislation, while surgery and some other high-income specialities may ultimately suffer a reduction (or a relative reduction) in that portion of their income derived from Medicare.

The most dramatic health initiative in the second Reagan administration was the Catastrophic Health Protection Act of 1988. The legislation is significant as the first attempt to design major social welfare legislation in an age of governmental austerity. Its story should be a cautionary tale. It was initially proposed by Secretary Bowen, who wished to ensure that Medicare beneficiaries were fully protected from the catastrophic costs of acute illnesses. (Long-term care is too expensive to cover under any program except Medicaid.) As usual the Democrat-controlled Congress expanded the benefits proposed in the administration bill. The most expensive addition was coverage of prescription drugs. It also added a progressive feature to the funding. The second change caused the legislation's downfall.

The federal deficit had grown so large by 1986 that proponents of new proposals had to show that they were 'budget neutral'. The original Bowen proposal would achieve neutrality with a flat premium to be paid by beneficiaries. When Congress enriched the benefit package, it added a surcharge restricted to the elderly, which increased according to annual income (up to $800 in 1989). It was regarded as fair to require the class which benefits to pay for it with some reference to ability-to-pay. The compromise seemed attractive and equitable: the many elderly who have purchased expensive private 'Medigap' policies to fill the gaps in Medicare save money by paying Medicare's new tax-like surcharge and dropping private coverage; many Medicare beneficiaries would only pay the flat monthly premium of $4; and the typical surtax would amount to approximately $300 a year for most of those required to pay the additional fee. Consequently most elderly would have profited from the 'Catastrophic' legislation.

However, to the surprise of Congress, the administration and the leaders of America's largest senior citizens interest group, the most affluent elderly mobilised enough support to force Congress to repeal the legislation before it was implemented. The campaign for its repeal developed largely after the election of Bush, whose administration did not take a clear stand on repeal.

No other significant welfare legislation has been rolled back, at least since Roosevelt's New Deal. The repeal will probably make future expansions of social welfare legislation difficult to achieve unless the economy and federal deficit improve. The exercise of political muscle against catastrophic protection has cost the elderly considerable sympathy and may have postponed new programmes to deal with the difficult problem of long-term care. Since the movement to repeal Catastrophic Illness Protection blossomed, for example, there has been increasing media and political attention to the needs of poor children and pregnant women.

The defeat also suggests that the common American practice of incremental extension of existing programmes has become bankrupt. There is renewed interest in comprehensive efforts to provide access to health care and to control costs. In this context the Canadian system of health insurance received much attention in 1988 and 1989.

To counterbalance this chapter's account of the lack of national resources and leadership on AIDS, it should be emphasised that Reagan's HHS Secretary had initiated the Catastrophic Illness Protection Act and the administration agreed to Congress' expansion and changes. Medicare is a compulsory national programme; yet the Republican president who championed new federalism supported this expansion of social welfare legislation.

CONCLUSION

The conclusion will focus on the broad principles that the administration brought with it when it came to power, and the problems that it later recognised:

- Reducing the role of the federal government by increasing the responsibilities of state and local government, the private sector and individuals.
- Deregulating the health care system.

- Controlling health care costs by instituting a competitive market.
- Stopping the 'slaughter of innocent young lives'.
- Coping with AIDS by developing a vaccine.
- Protecting the elderly against Catastrophic Illness costs.

Systematic evaluation of the success of Reagan's health policy would require considerable effort in establishing criteria for judgement. In contrast the broadscale assessment that is the aim here is based largely on internal consistency. This informal exercise treats 'rhetoric' as equivalent to a promise and 'reality' as the test of its fulfillment.[11] In addition to asking if an effort was made to embody the rhetoric in 'reality', one can also ask whether both the rhetoric or the actual health policies were 'successful' in achieving specific health or political goals. Thus, for each broad health topic, the following dummy table could be completed:

Table 7.1 Health issue assessment schema

	Rhetoric	Reality
Successful		
Unsuccessful		

Reducing the Federal Role

Perhaps the clearest failure to turn rhetorical promises into reality is in shrinking the role of government. The reimbursement innovations – PPS and RB-RVS – make a giant step towards nationalising and politicising the US health system. Research efforts involving major quantitative studies to ensure that the federal government is getting its money's worth when it pays for health care will further enhance federal power. Until the courts and Congress acted, the Baby Doe rules threatened to make the federal government the final arbiter of decisions regarding treatment in local hospitals.

None of these programmes were anticipated in its rhetoric when the administration took office. Unlike the financing programmes however, the Baby Doe policy was implied by its rhetorical principles (even if it conflicted with the 'hands off' ethos of other passages in the rhetoric).

To the degree that nationalising health care (even though it was not *federalised*) was contrary to the rhetoric of the Reagan administration, there seems to be a failure in the rhetoric. Yet as policy, most observers give PPS credit for restraining some of the likely Medicare cost increases. Modest hopes for the new RB-RVS programme to control Medicare payments to physicians are also commonly expressed. Of course any careful observer will note that both programmes have created new problems and weaknesses and exacerbated old ones. The Baby Doe rules were a failure as policy (because they had to be rolled back), but ironically they may have succeeded as rhetoric. The policy has made the withholding of food, water and even treatment from newborns into a national ethical issue. It has surely had a chilling effect on parents, hospitals and doctors, who in the 1970s would more readily have considered letting similarly impaired infants die.

Early in the first administration Stockman tried to shift much programme decision-making and financing onto state and local governments, but Congress fought him to a virtual standstill on the health programmes. (In other areas he was more successful.) Thus the administration was unsuccessful in achieving the massive shift away from federal health responsibilities that was called for in its rhetoric.

Deregulation

Formal deregulation has largely been accomplished. The health planning organisations no longer receive federal money or authority, although some states have decided to continue a public planning function. A hospital's growth or stagnation is now largely determined by access to capital markets. (Thus it can be argued only half-facetiously that Moody's Investors Service and Standard & Poor's Corporation, which determine the desirability of bonds and consequently the interest hospitals must pay, function *de facto* as health planners. Of course their criteria involve financial solvency rather than population needs or optimum access for patients.) Although PSRO's, which undertook utilisation review, were abolished, Congress felt that local organisations reporting to HHS were needed to ensure against underservice in hospitals reimbursed under PPS. Despite this exceptional re-regulation, it is probably accurate to at least claim that there was no net increase in federal monitoring and regulation of day-to-day activities in the local health care system under Reagan. (I will suggest that regulation can be distinguished from control.)

As rhetoric, deregulation must be judged to be successful. The federal government is not seen to be a major player (as distinct from a major *payer*) in the governance of local health care systems. In reality the federal government exercises more direct control of local health care systems now than in the Carter presidency. This control arises from its greater grip on payments (through PPS for hospitals and the nascent RB-RVS for physicians). The federal government however lacks adequate means of direction (that is, of influencing private and nonfederal government interests) in the public interest. If cost-control is the principal health issue in the 1990s, then federal control does not effectively look after anybody's cost problem except its own.

Reforming the Market for Health Care

Although competition among doctors and hospitals is much more prevalent now than in 1980, this is not due either to government rhetoric or its actual policies. In the early years the administration pushed a procompetition bill that was never passed. After 1983 competition took a back seat to the implementation of PPS, which was only competitive in letting hospitals keep any money that they could save.

By the middle of the Reagan years, the rhetoric of regulation versus competition began to sound stale. Reality seemed to have passed these rhetorical categories by. Forces operating in the health care system generated more new forms of organisation and other arrangements than health care professionals could think up and name with new acronyms. Yet significant amounts of diffuse control have also continued. So observers now generally believe that we have both 'competition' and 'regulation' (of a nondirective sort).

Since the Reagan administration never formally instituted competition, it could hardly claim to be successful in embodying its rhetoric in reality. Instead of reforming the health care system, the federal government achieved PPS, which probably did save some federal dollars that would have been spent without it. However the federal government essentially renounced efforts to control the increase in total societal costs of health care (that is, the per cent of GNP spent for health). The larger vision of the leading market-reformers definitely included control of total health care costs. The very best gloss that can be given to the performance of the Reagan administration in this category is that the federal government has become a leader in managed care programmes for its beneficiaries and invites other groups that can maintain tight control over their members' expenditures to follow its lead.

Stopping the 'Slaughter of the Innocents'

The administration's right-to-life views functioned as 'trumps' that would override policy-as-usual when they became relevant. Thus the moral agenda played a significant part in the administration's rhetorical definition of itself, but the administration also acted on its beliefs when specific policies seemed to involve core values. Although the moral agenda included much besides the right to life, that issue is the central one in health care. Related issues like contraception, the right to die and sex education have had to take a back seat to abortion in this chapter, which reflects the relative political and media attention accorded various moral agenda concerns during the Reagan administration.

Moral agenda issues *were* raised continuously, for example, by the issue of letting severely impaired infants die; by AIDS; by foreign allies whose family planning programmes countenanced abortion; and by research involving foetal tissue. When such issues raised right-to-life issues, there was usually no doubt about how the administration would deal with the reality.

Yet moral agenda conservatives can reasonably fault the administration for not working harder to change the rules of the game (in contrast to its practice of using the trumps already held in the federal hand). In overt politics involving Congress, the states and party competition, the Reagan administration was not willing to sacrifice other political goals to achieve its moral agenda. Supporters of the administration would be justified in responding that the strategic actions of the administration are much more likely to achieve its right-to-life policy than dramatic polarising confrontations. That policy was to apply what came to be called the 'litmus test' to prospective justices of the Supreme Court, in the hope of finding appointees who would overturn the court decisions that found a woman's right to abortion implied by the US Constitution. At the beginning of the last decade of the century, Reagan administration policy appears likely – but not certain – to become successful.

Coping with AIDS

The Reagan administration never took a leadership role in AIDS and therefore did not have a clear rhetorical stance. In general it seemed to maintain that the administration was fulfilling its responsibilities and that any short-comings were the fault of states, local government and private philanthropy, the appropriate primary service providers for patients suffering from AIDS.

The one area where the federal government had undeniable responsibility was research. HHS Secretary Margaret Heckler voiced the rhetoric of the biomedical silver bullet when she enthusiastically – and unnecessarily – promised to develop a vaccine against AIDS within two years of her US announcement of the discovery of the virus. In reality the federal government was very slow and inefficient in organising the biomedical research required by this epidemic.

If the executive branch failed to perform adequately in the realm where it was clearly responsible, it was a *disaster* in responding to the broader need for leadership in a national crisis. Most political appointees never seemed to grasp that the federal government had a fundamental responsibility to mobilise the country over the problem of AIDS.[12]

Catastrophic Illness Protection

The administration did fulfill its rhetoric about protecting the elderly from very expensive health care costs that did not include long-term care. Yet the elderly revolted, forcing repeal of the programme that was supposed to benefit them. Although the administration had not proposed the progressive financing that required the more affluent elderly to pay more of the cost than low-income seniors, Reagan's assent to the legislation signalled his concurrence.

Rhetoric and policy reality – promise and fulfilment – were in synchrony on this issue. It seems to follow that both were unsuccessful in light of the repeal of the legislation. There is no doubt that the Catastrophic Protection Act of 1988 was politically unsuccessful because it provided beneficiaries with a programme that was not valued. Yet as substantive health policy the programme would have been useful even though it did not address the seemingly intractable problem of financing long-term care. Thus some blame for the failure of Catastrophic Protection can be shifted from the administration and Congress to the elderly – especially the most affluent and educated among them – who failed to comprehend their own best interests. The administration, Congress and the major elderly interest groups however failed to explain the importance of catastrophic protection to the average Medicare beneficiary and the broader public. That failure of political education and policy implementation proved to be fundamental.

Economic and Moral-Agenda Conservatisms

Because adding up some overall policy box score would be pointless, this chapter will conclude by returning to the broader question of the two types of conservatism. Traditional economic conservatism and moral-agenda conservatism were able to coexist – albeit uneasily at times – by dividing government activity into domains. Economic conservatives (who include supply-side economists for these purposes) generally had their way in matters of money, while moral issues were treated by the administration with rhetoric that was pleasing to the moral-agenda conservatives. The administration's legislative focus on tax and budget issues throughout the eight years rather deftly preempted significant legislation in support of the moral agenda. In health, the administration boasted of its support for a constitutional amendment on abortion and it did select Supreme Court Justices who could be expected to overrule abortion-rights. Yet the full force of the administration's influence was never focused on a 'do-or-die' assertion of moral-agenda issues, including the abortion amendment.

By the end of President Reagan's second term, many moral-agenda conservatives had become restive. However they lacked any viable political alternative to George Bush (at least after the Reverend Pat Robinson failed to excite voters in the early primaries). Since his inauguration, Bush appears to be trying to strengthen his bonds with moral-agenda conservatives. In one of the few instances of assertiveness in domestic policy in his first year, he vetoed a bill slightly liberalising the prohibition against paying for abortions for poor women with federal Medicaid dollars.

Notes

1. Efforts to combat the importation, sale and use of illegal substances are not considered as health policy in this essay. The rationale for this exclusion is that the federal focus under Reagan was on increased interdiction and enforcement rather than on the psychological and physical effects of substance abuse on patients. Nancy Reagan's 'just-say-no' campaign against drugs was of course compatible with the moral-agenda principles of personal responsibility and judgement.
2. The analysis of market failure in health care is much more sophisticated and comprehensive than this essay can indicate. For example, see Arrow, 1963.
3. Even today HMO subscribers amount to fewer than fifteen per cent of the population. Although it is widely acknowledged that HMOs do in fact save money, their competitive effect on the rest of the system is as uncertain as ever.
4. In this author's opinion, the only unarguable government success during the Reagan years was the grand compromise in 1983 that restored the surplus in the Social Security Trust Funds (OASDI) for the near and intermediate terms. Perhaps the fact that the Social Security problem was actually 'solved' explains why this legislation is rarely mentioned.
5. The other source of growing federal jurisdiction came from the expanding interpretation of the 'commerce clause' of the Constitution, which provided the federal government with the basic legal framework necessary to develop the integrated economy that made America a modern state. For example, federal power over the economy was used to justify national intervention to promote factory health and safety, food and drug regulation and innovations in health delivery like HMOs.
6. Part of the reason why states did not fill the gap left by federal cutbacks is that state tax revenues declined, due to the sharp economic recession induced by Washington to bring down inflation. Most states are prohibited from running deficits.
7. Perhaps the fundamental fact required for nonAmericans to understand the US health care system is that Americans insist on finding an assigned payer to bill for every episode of illness for every individual patient. In an attempt to quantify the paperwork and bureaucracy generated by this billing activity, Himmelstein and Woolhandler suggest that 'more than half of the current hospital bureaucracy could be eliminated' to save 8 to 10 per cent of total US health spending, or 29 to 39 billion dollars (in 1983 dollars) (Himmelstein, *et al.*, 1989, p. 106; Himmelstein and Woolhandler, 1986).
8. All levels of government pay about 40 per cent of personal health expenditures in the US. Federal payments constituted 41.1 per cent of all hospital revenues in 1987; the Medicare programme alone was 27.4 per cent (Letsch, Levit and Waldo, 1988, pp. 116–17).

9.   David Stockman, the architect of Reagan's economic policies during the first four years, declines to take credit for the positive economic developments: 'What economic success there was had almost nothing to do with our original supply-side doctrine. Instead Paul Volcker and the business cycle had brought inflation down and economic activity surging back' (Stockman, 1986, p. 377).

10.   Tax reform had bipartisan appeal. Senator William Bradley (D-NJ) in particular had championed tax reform for years. Although it substantially altered Administration proposals, Congress did pass 'tax simplification' that was acceptable to the President.

      Tax reform, which involved fundamental changes that at first seemed visionary, was politically possible, whereas the demands of the moral-agenda conservatives probably could not have been achieved. Democrats controlled both the House and Senate after Reagan's first Congress. For all its professions of ideological purity, the Reagan administration would have sacrificed chances of success for any legislative programme if it had actively pursued the divisive issues of those with a moral agenda. Jim Baker especially is a superb and flexible politician who understands the politics of possibility and of agenda manipulation.

11.   The assumption underlying this assessment is open to the objection that 'rhetoric', which has quite a different ontological status from 'reality', has its own highly developed and unique criteria for evaluation. If applied too simplistically, the equivalency is also liable to neglect the fact that ever-changing conditions alter what is appropriate to undertake.

12.   Surgeon-General Koop and William Bennett are possible exceptions. However their involvement in AIDS was late (in the second administration) and hardly amounted to a clarion call for federal leadership.

References

Arrow, K.J. (1963) 'Uncertainty and the Welfare Economics of Medical Care', *American Economic Review*, vol. LIII (December) pp. 941–73.

Brandon, W.P. and E.K. Lee (1984) 'Evaluating Health Planning: Empirical Evidence on HSA Regulation of Prepaid Group Practices,' *Journal of Health Politics, Policy and Law*, vol. IX (Spring) pp. 103–24.

Brandon, W.P. (1982) 'Health-Related Tax Subsidies: Government Handouts for the Affluent', *New England Journal of Medicine*, vol. CCCVII (7 October) pp. 947–50.

Bremner, R.H. (1988) *American Philanthropy*, 2nd. ed. (University of Chicago Press).

Brook, Robert H. *et al.* (1983) 'Does Free Care Improve Adults' Health? Results from a Randomised Controlled Trial', *New England Journal of Medicine*, vol. CCCIX (8 December) pp. 1426–34.

Brown, L.D. (1986) 'Civil Rights and Regulatory Wrongs: The Reagan Administration and the Medical Treatment of Handicapped Newborns', *Journal of Health Politics, Policy and Law*, vol. XI (Summer) pp. 231–54.

Council on Wage and Price Stability (1976), Executive Office of the President, 'The Problem of Rising Health Care Costs', Report to Members and Adviser Members of the Council on Wage and Price Stability, 26 April 1976, reprinted as Appendix II in *idem, The Complex Puzzle of Rising Health Care Costs: Can the Private Sector Fit it Together?* (Washington, DC: GPO).

Ellwood, P.M. *et al.* (1971) 'The Health Maintenance Strategy', *Medical Care*, vol. IX (June) pp. 291–8.

Ellwood, P.M. (1978) 'The Importance of the Market', *Journal of Health Politics, Policy and Law*, vol. II (Winter) pp. 447–53.

Enthoven, A. (1978) 'Consumer-Choice Health Plan', *New England Journal of Medicine*, vol. CCXCIII (23 and 30 March) pp. 650–8, pp. 709–20.

Enthoven, A. (1988) 'Managed Competition of Alternative Delivery Systems' *Journal of Health Politics, Policy and Law*, vol. xiii (Summer) pp. 305–21.

Enthoven, A. and R. Kronick (1989) 'A Consumer-Choice Health Plan for the 1990s: Universal Health Insurance in a System Designed to Promote Quality and Economy', *New England Journal of Medicine*, vol. CCCXX (5 and 12 January) pp. 29–37, 94–101.

Gibson, R.M. (1979) 'National Health Expenditures, 1978', *Health Care Financing Review*, vol. I (Summer) pp. 1–36.

Gibson, R.M. (1980) 'National Health Expenditures, 1979', *Health Care Financing Review*, vol. II (Summer) pp. 1–36.

Glaser, W.A. (1987) *Paying the Hospital: The Organization, Dynamics, and Effects of Differing Financial Arrangements* (San Francisco: Jossey-Bass).

Goldfarb v. Virginia State Bar (1975) 41 U.S. 773.

Gottlieb M.S. *et al.*, 'Pneumocystis Pneumonia – Los Angeles', *Morbidity and Mortality Weekly Report*, vol. XXX (5 June) pp. 250–2.

Green, M. and R. Nader (1973), 'Economic Regulations vs. Competition: Uncle Sam the Monopoly Man', *Yale Law Journal*, vol. LXXXII (April) pp. 871–89.

Greenberg, W. (ed.) (1978) *Competition in the Health Care Sector: Past, Present, and Future* (Germantown, Md.: Aspen).

Havighurst, C.C. (1973) 'Regulation of Health Facilities and Services by "Certificate of Need"', *Virginia Law Review*, vol. LIX (October) pp. 1143–232.

Havighurst, C.C. (1977) 'Improving the Prospects for Innovation in Health Care Financing and Delivery', paper prepared for the conference on Antitrust Laws and the Health Services Industry sponsored by the American Enterprise Institute for Public Policy Research, December.

Havighurst, C.C. (1978) 'Professional Restraints on Innovation in Health Care Financing', *Duke Law Journal* (May) pp. 303–87.

Havinghurst, C.C. (1982) *Deregulating the Health Care Industry* (Cambridge, MA: Bollinger)

Himmelstein, D.U. *et al.* (1989) 'A National Health Program for the United States: A Physicians' Proposal', *New England Journal of Medicine*, vol. CCCXX (12 January) pp. 102–8.

Himmelstein, D.U. and S. Woolhandler (1986) 'Cost Without Benefit:

Administrative Waste in U.S. Health Care', *New England Journal of Medicine*, vol. CCCXIV (13 February) pp. 441–5.

Keeler, Emmett B. *et al.* (1987) 'Effects of Cost Sharing on Physiological Health, Health Practices and Worry,' *Health Services Research*, vol. XXII (August) pp. 279–306.

Letsch, S.W., K.R. Levit and D.R. Waldo (1988) 'National Health Expenditures', *Health Care Financing Review*, vol. X (Winter) pp. 109–22.

Miller and Byrne, Inc. (1977) *Final Report: Evaluation of the Impact of PHS Programs on State Health Goals and Activities*, Office of Planning, Evaluation and Legislation, Health Resourses Administration, DHEW, DHEW Pub. No. (HRA) 77–604 (Washington, DC: GPO, May).

Nozick, R. (1974) *Anarchy, State and Utopia* (New York: Basic Books).

Panem, S. (1988) *The AIDS Bureaucracy* (Cambridge, MA: Harvard University Press).

Pifer, A. (1984) 'The Quasi Nongovernmental Organisation', in his *Philanthropy in an Age of Transition: The Essays of Alan Pifer* (New York: The Foundation Center) pp. 19–30.

Reagan, N. (1989) *My Turn: The Memoirs of Nancy Reagan* (New York: Random House).

Roe v. Wade (1973) 410 U.S. at 113.

Salamon, L.M. (1987) 'Partners in Public Service: The Scope and Theory of Government-Nonprofit Relations', in W.W. Powell, (ed.) *The Nonprofit Sector: A Research Handbook* (New Haven: Yale University Press) pp. 99–117.

Sardell, A. (1988) *The U.S. Experiment in Social Medicine: The Community Health Center Program, 1965–86* (University of Pittsburgh Press).

Shilts, R. (1988) *And the Band Played On: Politics, People, and the AIDS Epidemic* (New York: Penguin).

Stevens, R. (1971) *American Medicine and the Public Interest* (New Haven: Yale University Press).

Stockman, D.A. (1986) *The Triumph of Politics: How the Reagan Revolution Failed* (New York: Harper and Row).

Webster v. Reproductive Health Services (1989) 109 S.Ct. 3040.

Weidenbaum, M.L. (1975) *Government-Mandated Price Increases: A Neglected Aspect of Inflation*, Government Affairs Study 28 (Washington, DC: American Enterprise Institute).

Weidenbaum, M.L. (1988) *Rendezvous With Reality: The American Economy After Reagan* (New York: Basic Books).

8 Health Policy under Conservative Governments in Canada

Pranlal Manga and Geoffrey R. Weller

INTRODUCTION

In Canada, the rise of Conservative governments seems to have coincided with a decline in the number of political scientists analysing health care policy. There never were very many political scientists who published in the health policy field, despite its size and importance, but now there are even fewer. Far more attention is accorded the field these days by economists and sociologists. In fact most of the political scientists in Canada left in the field are members of the Canadian Health Economics Research Association (CHERA). It may be for this reason that the difference between the rhetoric and the reality of the recent wave of Conservative governments has not been clearly delineated.

The few political scientists who still concern themselves with matters of health policy in Canada seem to have lost much of their separate identity and have concentrated their efforts on a small set of largely economic issues such as physicians extra-billing. This has been partially a reflection of the relative rise in influence of health economics, but it is also a reflection of a seemingly persistent inability to fully break with political science's traditional focus on pressure group type analyses of the health field, namely the concentration on the major group actors in the policy field, such as physicians.[1] Perhaps this is political science's equivalent of the problem health economists are perceived to have, that is a focus on a small set of issues and especially upon micro-economic appraisals.[2] This concentration on the small scale is one reason that the larger issues seem not to be analysed to any great extent.

Furthermore, preoccupation with the micro curiously mirrors the shift in the scene of the action in health policy from the macro, the

207

federal or national level, to the micro, or the provincial and territorial level. The steady Balkanisation of the health care system in Canada has led to the realisation that Canada has many different health care systems, and that little is known about the dynamics of health policy within each. The focus in the past has been upon the interactions between the federal government and the provinces on health policy matters.[3] This shift to the provincial sphere is an invitation for political analyses in health to also become Balkanised and micro rather than macro in scope. This is perhaps especially the case as provincial politics is not itself a major area of concentration in Canadian political science and much preparatory groundwork has yet to be undertaken.[4] The analysis of provincial political patterns and policies is often regarded as somewhat parochial and therefore of lesser value and interest, and this may also explain why some political scientists have moved away from the health care field entirely.

Another reason why the gap between the rhetoric and the reality of recent Conservative governments in Canada has not been much commented upon by political scientists in Canada is that there seems to have been a trend to a return to an avoidance of values or value-laden issues. Whether this is anything inherent in political science in Canada or merely a reflection of the strong influence of health economics on political scientists is difficult to detect. Whatever the reason it is a disturbing trend to have developed just when policy actors in health care are engaged in conflict over the future direction of health care policy. This debate reflects considerable differences in basic values towards health and health care delivery. Political scientists and, to a lesser degree, health economists are not contributing a great deal that is useful to the debate, and the centre of new thinking seems to be shifting out of academia and into the governmental, bureaucratic and pressure group arena, that is to those who are directly engaged.

Another part of the reason why the rhetoric–reality gap among recent Conservative governments in Canada has not been the subject of much attention on the part of academic political scientists, is the consensus of point of view or values that seems to exist among them on the macro issues. There are a few who want to see 'market forces' have a greater influence, but in Canada that greater influence is advocated very much on the margins of the existing system, and normally not in such a way to threaten the basic structure. There are virtually none who advocate more than marginal changes in the direction of greater public influence, although there are many who would like to see a return to the situation that existed a few years ago in terms of the degree of public intervention. There is an overwhelming consensus on the point of view that the essentials of the current system must be preserved. Those who wish to return to a situation of a very much larger private sector do not get much of a hearing and neither do those, like ourselves, who have argued that a large move should be made in the other direction, by taking extensive actions on the supply side of the medical marketplace by policies such as manpower substitution, new community based comprehensive delivery mechanisms, salary and capitation methods of paying doctors, effective utilisation review committees and formal and strict mechanisms to control the diffusion of medical technology. What the private sector advocates want raises the spectre of the health care mess in the United States and what the public sector advocates want raises the spectre of 'socialism', whether the measures are motivated by socialist ideology or not.

In this chapter we shall attempt to analyse the broader sweep of events in the politics of the health policy field in Canada in recent years, and look at the macro value-laden issues that have been raised or are likely to be raised as a result of these events. We shall begin by briefly describing the nature of conservatism and the recent rise in influence of Conservative governments in Canada. This will be followed by an analysis of the rhetoric of Conservatives on health policy matters in Canada and of how this rhetoric compares with Conservatives in other nations, but especially in the United States and the United Kingdom. We shall then examine the reality of health policy outputs by the Canadian Conservative governments at both the federal and provincial levels. We address the question of whether or not the gap we observe between rhetoric or reality is what it seems, or if there may be a hidden agenda possessed by these governments. We conclude by arguing the case that Canada is at a critical juncture in the health policy field, and political scientists in Canada would be well-advised to pay greater attention to the situation if they are not to have events outrun analysis.

CONSERVATISM AND CONSERVATIVE GOVERNMENTS IN CANADA

By the early 1980s in Canada, the long dominance of the Liberal Party, both at the provincial and the federal level, had been broken and the Progressive Conservative Party emerged triumphant at both levels. Its rhetoric was much like that of the Conservative Party in Britain and, especially, that of the Republican Party in the United States under Ronald Reagan. Conservatives in Canada were impressed by the approach and, as time went by, the actions of their perceived colleagues in the United Kingdom and the United States. However the Progressive Conservative Party was a very different party from the Republican in the United States and the Conservative in Britain, and the rhetoric has largely not translated into reality to the same extent or in the same way as has been the case in the other two nations. This is probably more so in the case of the health policy field than in any other. Before analysing the rhetoric and the reality, the special and distinctive nature of conservatism in Canada will be discussed.

At the federal level the Conservative Party led by Brian Mulroney won a huge victory in 1984. Of the 282 seats in the House of Commons it took 211, while the Liberals won only 40 and the New Democratic Party (NDP) 30. At the time of this victory seven of the ten provinces had conservative governments, while one was Social Credit, one NDP and one Parti-Quebecois. The Social Credit government was an essentially conservative one, indeed it was one that professed to be more conservative than the Conservatives. The impressive size of the federal victory and the strength of the party throughout the country led many to think that Canada was on the threshold of the 'Mulroney revolution' and changes similar to those introduced by Reagan and Thatcher would soon be introduced. While some efforts were made to begin such a process, as will be observed later, nothing really similar occurred, partly because of the nature of conservatism and Conservative political parties in Canada and partly because of the nature of the Canadian political system itself.

The Progressive Conservative Party in Canada is a far less ideologically motivated party than is the case of the Republicans under Reagan or the Conservatives under Thatcher. It is a party motivated far more by the need to obtain electoral success than it is by the need to persuade the society of the truth of its ideas. In Canada the gaining of electoral success is a complicated matter because of the regional diversity and the ethnic and racial mix of the population. Electoral dominance can only be achieved by aggregating a vast range of ethnic, regional and other interests. This means that the two major political parties have to operate very regionalised campaigns based on broadly integrating themes such as personality and leadership ability, and the avoidance of solid issues. The two major parties therefore vie for the centre of the political spectrum in an attempt to aggregate the widest range of support and thus they 'could (and sometimes do) exchange large parts of their party programmes with no visible effect'.[5]

While most members of the Progressive Conservative Party would no doubt have a difficult time articulating a clear and coherent definition of what they believed conservatism to be, the traditions of their party indicate a hangover of an older form of conservatism that never did really exist in the United States and which, under Thatcher, is losing its influence in Britain. This refers to a true conservatism, as opposed to the liberal-individualism which the United States has oddly and not a little perversely labeled conservatism and which the British Conservative Party has adopted with such a vengeance, seemingly not caring that it is changing the meaning of the word as it has been understood in its own tradition. The origins of the Progressive Conservatives lay with those who rejected the liberal beliefs in individualism and freedom, like the Loyalists who fled the United States and came to Canada to avoid the impositions of a society based on such beliefs. They had a belief, as did many coming to Canada from Britain, in collectivism, privilege and the inadvisability of revolutionary change. This was rooted in the idea that individuals were the ultimate value in and of themselves and could be perfected by societal artifice in the form of pieces of paper called constitutions.

The history of conservatism in Canada has been one of a long, slow and losing battle to resist what has happened in Britain, that is the imposition of the American definition of the word, and thereby a conversion to liberalism by default. The American definition of conservatism is nowadays largely reduced to meaning a desire to return to the earlier days of unrestricted business activity and associated individual freedoms without government intervention; that is, a return to a more pure form of liberalism. In Canada Conservatives returning to their older and root beliefs would be returning to loyalty to the crown, a belief in the importance of privilege, strong nationalism and a strong and intrusive central government which would place the group over the individual and the primacy of politics over that of economics.[6] The lack of success that the Progressive Conservative Party has had in resisting Americanisation is most clearly indicated by the fact that it is now the strong proponent of the current free trade agreement with the United States, whereas free trade was one of the parties' biggest fears until well into this century.

Despite being the proponent of free trade with the United States, the Progressive Conservative Party in Canada is still not as ideologically strident as its counterparts in the United States and Britain. This may well be because it does not have the same fundamentalist religious element as the Republicans seem to have these days, nor does it feel it is heavily engaged in a class war as the British Conservative Party appears to believe. Certainly the history of the Progressive Conservative Party actions indicates that it has not been reluctant to exercise state power and create many nationalised industries, or 'crown corporations' as they are called in Canada. It is often pointed out that it was a Conservative federal government which created Canada's largest crown corporation, the Canadian National Railways (CNR), and a Conservative government in Ontario which established many large provincial crown corporations.

In the realm of health policy Conservatives in Canada often seek to associate themselves with the current system, which remains very popular with the public, by indicating that they were responsible for some of the more important stages in its development. The first two steps in Canada were taken by a 'socialistic' New Democratic Party government in the province of Saskatchewan. These were public hospital insurance in 1944 and medical care insurance in 1963. The Liberal Party claims responsibility for introducing similar federal schemes in 1957 and 1968. The Progressive Conservatives indicate that it was a Conservative Premier of Ontario who called for hospital insurance and started the process that led to the enactment of the Hospital and Diagnostic Services Insurance Act of 1957. They also indicate that it was they who were responsible for establishing the Royal Commission (the Hall Commission) that led to the Medical Care Act of 1968.[7]

THE RHETORIC

Most of the Conservative governments in Canada in the early 1980s were caught up in the general rhetoric of conservatism of the day, the major elements of which could be said to comprise a general intention to reduce the role of government in Canadian society. They were also caught up in a more specific rhetoric about health care, largely amounting to a belief that the perceived major problem of cost escalation was consumer not supplier induced, and therefore actions would have to be taken that were aimed at consumers. While the rhetoric was there it was much less virulent than in the United States or Britain. Moreover, as we shall later observe, few actions resulted from the rhetoric. The more general and then the more specific health aspects of the Conservative rhetoric will be dealt with in this section.

The general rhetoric of the Conservative governments in Canada in the early 1980s very much reflected that of the United States and Britain. It had as its root the belief that governments in general were wasteful and inefficient whereas private enterprise was cost-effective and efficient. Hence many anticipated that the Canadian Conservative governments would have privatisation as a major thrust, and this was certainly indicated at least in their election statements. Another part of the general rhetoric was that since governments were wasteful and inefficient there could easily be spending reductions without there being large service level reductions. This, it was felt, would also make it possible to achieve another one of the objectives inherent in the general rhetoric, namely that government deficits should be significantly reduced. A further element in the rhetoric was that governments were overly intrusive and complex. Thus a stated objective was to simplify taxation and reduce the degree of regulation government imposed. The general rhetoric of the Conservative governments also reflected a belief that Canada had become too much of a welfare-state and that there should be significant cuts in social spending over and above the reductions that might be necessary for deficit reduction. While these key elements of the general rhetoric existed in the United States, Britain and Canada they were stated with less ideological fervour in Canada.

The specific rhetoric related to health care used by Conservative governments in Canada is based upon the belief that a rapid increase in demand for health services in response to the introduction of public insurance has caused rapid cost escalation and that consumers are responsible. Hence the correction needed is to take actions aimed at consumers. Evans refers to this as the 'naive medico-technical model' and accuses those who hold this view of not recognising that no big jump in demand occurred after the introduction of the public insurance schemes. Instead the trends in demand that were well underway long before the introduction of the insurance schemes merely continued.[8] The Conservative rhetoric conveniently overlooks the fact that cost increases have a great deal more to do with the supply side (providers) than the demand side (consumers). Supply side phenomena such as the increase in the supply of physicians, the retention in Canada of the fee-for-service system, the nearly unchecked profusion and diffusion of technology, inefficient institutions and delivery mechanisms, unnecessary hospitalisation and surgery, and the rapid rise in all health workers' incomes seem not to be seriously considered as major causes of cost escalation.

The Conservative governments' reform agenda in response to the escalation of health care costs favoured certain solutions. One solution was the imposition of user fees so that consumers would 'feel' the results of their actions and therefore act more responsibly. Thus user fees and premiums were to be either introduced or increased, and physician extra-billing of patients was looked upon with equanimity if not favourably. This went under the title of enhancing 'patient responsibility'. Also looked upon favourably were measures that were intended to increase the influence of the market in the health care sector by such mechanisms as having hospitals contracting out certain services, including the management function.[9]

Both the general and specific rhetoric were to be provided with substance and result in concrete policies as a consequence of the Nielsen Task Force. This Task Force was established only one day after the government was sworn in on 17 September 1984 and was given the job of reviewing over one thousand government programmes to see if they could be better managed or the service provided at lower cost. It did this by establishing 22 study teams overseen by three key cabinet Ministers (Crosbie, Wilson and de Cotret) all under the leadership of Erik Nielsen, the Deputy Prime Minister. The Task Force was given five months in which to complete its task. This approach to reviewing government programmes reflects the influence of the Reagan Administration's way of doing things on the Progressive Conservative Party in Canada. The Nielsen Task Force approach was partly inspired by President Reagan's appointment of J. Peter Grace to lead the President's Private Sector Survey on Cost Control (PSSCC).[10] To some degree the influence of the Seldon group which advised Margaret Thatcher can also be seen.

However the conversion of the specific rhetoric to health policy was impeded by two things, the first being a preemptive strike on the part of the Liberals at the federal level just before they were defeated, and the second was the rather surprising (to some) conclusion of the Nielsen Task Force Report on Health and Sports.[11]

The preemptive strike of the Liberals consisted of their successful passage of the Canada Health Act in April 1984.[12] The Liberals were to some degree aware of the fact that they were heading for a very tough election in 1984, and wished to fight that election partially on the grounds that they were the defenders of Canada's publicly popular health care system. They did this by preventing extra-billing and reaffirming and strengthening the system's basic principles. In the late 1970s and early 1980s, there was a dramatic rise in the phenomena of opting out and extra-billing by physicians. Opting out involved leaving a provincial plan and billing separately; extra-billing meant staying within a plan but levying additional charges directly against a patient. The cause of the rush of opting out and extra-billing was largely the holding down of fee increases for physicians by provincial governments trying to contain costs. Opting out and extra-billing were clearly actions by physicians intended to circumvent this and increase their incomes.

The federal government, and those who supported the principles of Medicare, saw both phenomena as a threat because they thought they would lead to a two-class health care system by reducing accessibility to health care services for low income patients. They also thought the two practices violated the principle of portability. In addition they raised the issue of consumer risk-bearing relative to a system of universal first dollar insurance coverage. Opting out and extra-billing transferred the burden of health care costs from the general taxpayer to the sick and were thereby inequitable. The Canada Health Act was intended to both reaffirm the basic principles of Canada's health care system and impose financial penalties on those provinces that allowed extra-billing or imposed hospital user fees. The Progressive Conservative Party, aware that an election was in the offing, at first seemed ready to oppose the bill, then for a long time seemed uncertain of what to do and finally decided to come out in favour of the legislation, no doubt largely because it did not want to give the Liberals a major issue with which to fight the forthcoming election.[13] This agreement to the legislation has obviously limited the range of possible actions in the health care field by the Progressive Conservatives now that they form the government. Indeed the Canada Health Act was unanimously supported by every member for all three political parties in the House of Commons. Any significant move against the basic principles, or move to allow extra-billing, would be blatantly hypocritical in view of their support for the Canada Health Act.[14]

The rather surprising conclusions of the Nielsen Task Force Report on Health and Sports has been another limiting factor for the Progressive Conservative government. The report might have been used to form a basis for something of a retreat from the stand of support for the Canada Health Act if it had been markedly critical of the existing health care system. However the report was not overly critical of the health care field. For instance, on the critical area of privatisation the report said nothing definitive and simply stated that a report done for the Minister of Health and Welfare in 1985 'found no significant support for privatisation of the health care system from providers or consumers'.[15] Moreover the extent of the general changes in all fields recommended by the Task Force was regarded as disappointingly small by many Progressive Conservatives. Many of those changes that were recommended were blocked in Parliament and the whole process largely fizzled out.[16]

THE REALITY

The reality of the situation since the federal election of 1984 is that there has been relatively little action on the health policy front in Canada. Few actions that imply a major attack on the current Canadian health system have been taken by Conservative governments at either the provincial or the federal level. It is clear to the Conservative governments that there would be a great deal of public resistance to any significant changes. It is also clear that if the federal government undertook major initiatives they would be resisted by the provinces, even many of those governed by Conservatives. In any event it is evident that in view of lack of action at the federal level against the whole basis of the system, the scene of the action, so to speak, has shifted to the provinces, which have largely been attempting to come to grips with the health care cost escalation problem.

The first reality that struck home after the election of 1984 was that rather than moving forward with preferred conservative policies there was, from the Conservative point of view, a step backward. This was the steady progression among the provinces to the outlawing of extra-billing as a direct result of the passage of the Canada Health Act. The process caused a lot of hard feeling between some provinces and the federal government, especially when both were Conservative, but the federal government had to impose the penalties called for in the Act, especially since they had supported it. The process also caused a great deal of antagonism between provincial governments and the medical profession.[17] The clearest example of this was the bitter strike in Ontario over the issue.[18]

The hard feelings between the provinces and the medical profession have been exacerbated by the other actions of the provincial governments in their post-1984 attempts to hold down cost escalation. These actions have mainly related to limiting the supply of physicians, holding down the rate of fee schedule increases for physicians, limiting the growth of hospital budget levels, limiting the spread of high technology, and limiting the cost of pharmaceuticals.

In an attempt to hold back the escalation of health care costs, the provincial governments, regardless of partisan stripe, have been trying to limit the number of doctors for more than a decade. They have done this via a variety of measures, including the cutting of the supply of immigrant doctors, freezing the number of places in medical schools, and restricting the number of residencies available. These actions have however been a dismal failure. The supply of physicians has risen sharply in most provinces. All that can be said about the actions taken is that the situation would have otherwise been much worse. The failure to limit supply has been exaggerated or compounded by the fact that even with an increasing supply of physicians there has been no success in getting them to spread out into the underserviced areas of the north, rural regions and inner city cores – thus negating one of the major arguments for maintaining a large supply of physicians.[19]

Most Canadian provinces have tried to limit the payments to physicians for their services, that is, they have tried to limit physicians' incomes. This was and still is done largely by restraining the increases in the fees paid to doctors for the various types of services they provide. The Conservative provinces clearly thought that allowing extra-billing would relieve the pressure on them, but after the Canada Health Act that avenue was denied. The pressure on fees continued to be applied with the very predictable result that physicians, denied the chance to get their desired income level by charging patients, simply increased the number of patients they saw or the frequency with which they saw them and billed the provincial governments.[20] The provincial governments now have to contemplate placing volume controls on physicians.

Attempts to hold down health care cost escalation by limiting the growth of hospital budgets have also not been very successful. A good part of the problem is that even now there are relatively few financial incentives built into the provincial health care systems to limit hospital stays, to limit expensive tests and treatments, or to reduce unnecessary admissions. In part this is because the provinces have for years allowed hospitals to overspend with virtual impunity. Ontario, until recently, so regularly permitted hospital cost overruns that it even had a special allowance in the regular budget for the estimated overrun. So far the provinces have not made any moves to truly tackle this problem.[21]

Very few provinces have yet to place restrictions on the introduction and use of high technology advances in the health care field, even when the supposed benefits from the advance of technology are either dubious or marginal. As medical technology advances, more problems are diagnosed and more solutions found, usually at high cost. The problem then becomes the political and ethical one of deciding when and how to limit the diffusion of medical technology. Apart from anything else nobody seems to want to make the decision. Physicians certainly do not, and in any event their training and ethic tends to breed the attitude that whatever can be done should be done for the patient and that costs are not directly their concern. While provincial governments might want to limit these costs, it is politically unpopular to do so and if such efforts were made they would face a strong lobby from what has been termed the 'medical-industrial' complex.[22]

Yet another cause of the rapid escalation of health care costs in Canada in recent years has been the rise in the cost of pharmaceuticals. In Ontario the rise has averaged 21.3 per cent per annum for the past decade.[23] Few serious actions have been taken by provincial governments in relation to drug costs. This was clearly revealed in Ontario when Dr. George Carruthers, the chairman of the Minister of Health's Advisory Committee on Drugs, resigned – severely criticising government inaction in the field as he did so.[24]

Thus the reality is that Conservative governments have found themselves boxed-in in the health policy field since 1984. They have been unable to undertake their preferred policies because of the passage of the Canada Health Act and their support of it, as well as the negative public reaction that would result if they did undertake those policies. They have been forced in some instances to take the type of actions against health care suppliers that they really do not prefer, so this has been done rather half-heartedly and certainly not effectively. The preferred policy is, as we noted, to take action on the demand and not the supply side of the equation. Since the preferred policies cannot be undertaken up-front, so to speak, there appears to be a hidden agenda on the part of Conservative governments to obtain what they want via the back door or to avoid the problem altogether. It is to this hidden agenda that we now turn.

A HIDDEN AGENDA?

Unable to undertake their preferred policies in a direct fashion, largely through fear of alienating Canadian voters, Canadian Conservative governments have attempted to make the consumer of health care services pay an increasing share of the burden by promoting 'lifestyle' health, volunteerism and philanthropy. The federal government has also shifted the burden onto consumers indirectly in another sense, by devolving authority over health care to the Territories (the Yukon and the Northwest Territories) and attempting to do so to native self-government authorities, largely in the provincial northern regions. In addition there are those who think that what the Conservative governments could not do via the front door they hope to do via the back, by obtaining a free trade agreement with the United States.

In Canada, as in many other countries, there have been moves to place greater emphasis on health promotion. This involves three things: self-care, namely the decisions and actions individuals take in the interest of their own health; mutual aid, the actions people take to help each other cope; and healthy environments, the creation of conditions and surroundings conducive to health.[25] While these are certainly good and advisable things to do it is the context within which they are done which is critical. The problems are threefold. Firstly, self-care can be used as a justification for reducing the level of the types of health care services currently emphasised. Secondly, it is likely to distract attention away from structural analyses and solutions to the social, political and economic aspects of ill health. Finally, the concept brings with it the potential for victim blaming.[26] Illness can be blamed on personal failure of behaviour rather than occupationally induced causes. Unfortunately the efforts to promote self-care – or more generically, health promotion – are not coordinated at the structural level with changes in the professional or traditional health care sector, or policies intended to produce healthy social and physical environments.

Much the same kind of argument can be made in relation to the promotion of volunteerism or philanthropy in health. While not in itself a bad thing to encourage, it is a mechanism of privatisation if governments promote it in order to lessen reliance on public funding of health services. Canadian governments are actively promoting philanthropy and volunteerism, and indeed arguing that where volunteerism involves mutual aid it may well be a preferred form of care giving. But this active encouragement may be counter-productive. It complicates the structure of the health care system and it means that governments may lose some control over, for example, the purchase of advanced equipment by hospitals, thus limiting control over the diffusion of technology and the increased costs that it brings.[27]

The Conservative federal government is following a policy of shifting the burden in a somewhat different sense by its policy of devolving authority over health care to the Yukon and the Northwest Territories, as well as the native groups south of the Territories. Again this could and may be a very laudable objective if the prime objective is indeed devolution of power and true self-control by native groups. However there is the suspicion that it is partly just an off-loading of expensive burdens, because it is very uncertain that the fiscal transfers to be made to the newly responsible units will be adequate. The fear is that the federal government will treat them like the provinces; that is, they will cap federal expenditures or transfers to them at a level related to the growth of federal revenues rather than at a level related to the real growth in the cost of health care services or health care needs of native populations. Since neither the Territories nor the native groups have much or any fiscal capacity themselves, service levels would in such circumstances necessarily decline.[28]

Canada has negotiated a bilateral free trade agreement with the United States. Many groups have suggested that the trade agreement poses a serious long term threat to the existing health care system in Canada. The Liberal and NDP trade critics have argued that Chapter 14 of the agreement, which is merely entitled 'Services', will seriously undermine Canada's system and result in a trend towards a private pay-as-you-go health care system.[29] Moreover there is the fear that equitable access will be destroyed and that it will be an early casualty of the invasion by private enterprise, domestic as well as foreign, of the health care system.[30]

The Conservative government argues that these fears are groundless and that its intent is not to subvert the principles of Medicare and introduce a privatised health care system by the back door. Health Minister Jake Epp has indicated that the federal government has all along assured Canadians that social programmes were not at risk in the free trade agreement and that 'our own brand of health care is fundamental to our sovereignty and way of life'.[31] The Minister even went so far as to say that 'I am convinced that closer ties in trade will increase Americans' knowledge of Canadian health care. This in turn may lead to the United States adopting Canada's approach, because I think our system is better!'[32] Mr. Epp's opponents remain unconvinced and fearful.

CONCLUSIONS

It seems odd that at a time when the fate of Canada's health care system or some parts of it may be hanging in the balance because of the free trade deal, Canadian political scientists are not paying a great deal of attention to the health policy field in general, let alone the specific issue of whether or not there is indeed a hidden agenda. There is a very clear danger that events will outrun analysis. It is certainly the case that Canadian political scientists are not involved in the process of setting the agenda.

Both the debate over and actions related to health policy seem strangely frozen in Canada. The Conservatives appear to have been unable to effect a major move toward their objective of making consumers directly pay a far greater share of health care costs. The opponents of the Conservatives have dug themselves into a position of defending the existing system, and regard any suggestion of change as an almost traitorous act. This leads them to overlook or ignore the fact that the present system is not a particularly efficient one and could do with a great deal of change. The tendency is to argue that Canada should not become the expensive mess represented by the American health system or the perceived penurious system of the United Kingdom.

In our view it is inadvisable to defend too strenuously a flawed system even if it is better than others. The attack on that system by Conservative governments in Canada has largely failed, and while there may still be a 'hidden agenda' lurking behind the signing of a free trade agreement, there is no real excuse to resist quite valid and needed changes. If anything it might be a suitable time to initiate far more strenuous measures on the supply side, to redesign and restructure it and impose a number of regulatory and control devices, as suggested earlier in this chapter. Since it seems likely that the only way to increase economic efficiency and maintain a semblance of equity is not to follow the Conservative route of enlarging the private sector but to move in the other direction, then this should be done sooner rather than later by the non-Conservative provincial governments. Those provincial governments should take back the increasing amounts of the power they earlier delegated to the dominant professionals and their associated institutions, and use that power to effect strict cost controls and a shift towards less expensive forms of delivery, and away from doctor-dominated, technologically oriented, high cost medicine. It should be a true shifting of resources and restructuring of the health care delivery system and not merely an additional system added to the present one.

Notes

1.　　See Geoffrey R. Weller, 'From Pressure Group to Medical-Industrial Complex: The Development of Approaches to the Politics of Health', *Journal of Health Politics, Policy and Law*, vol. 1, no. 4 (Winter 1977) pp. 444–70.

2.　　See A.J. Culyer, 'Health Economics: The Topic and the Discipline' in John Horne (ed.) *Proceedings of the Third Canadian Conference on Health Economics* (Winnipeg: The Department of Social and Preventive Medicine, The University of Manitoba, 1987) pp. 1–17.

3.　　The focus of this attention was on the lead up to, and then the effect of, the Established Programs Financing Act of 1977.

4.　　We indicated that it would be increasingly important to understand the particular nature of the political cultures and policy process of each province in Geoffrey R. Weller and Pranlal Manga, 'The Development of Health Policy in Canada', in Michael M. Atkinson and Marsha A. Chandler (ed.) *The Politics of Canadian Public Policy* (Toronto: University of Toronto Press, 1983) p. 242.

5.　　Robert J. Jackson, Doreen Jackson and Nicholas Baxter-Moore, *Politics in Canada* (Scarborough: Prentice-Hall Canada, 1986) p. 475.

6.　　See Chapter IV of W. Christian and C. Campbell, *Political Parties and Ideologies in Canada*, second edition (Toronto: McGraw-Hill Ryerson Limited, 1983).

7.　　See Geoffrey R. Weller and Pranlal Manga, *op. cit.*

8.　　R.G. Evans, 'Supplier Induced Demand: Some Empirical Evidence and Implications' in M. Parkman (ed.), *The Economics of Health and Medical Care* (London: MacMillan, 1974).

9. See Geoffrey R. Weller and Pranlal Manga, 'The Push for Reprivatisation of Health Care Services in Canada, Britain and the United States', *Journal of Health Politics, Policy and Law*, vol. 8, no. 3 (Fall 1983) pp. 495–518.

10. President's Private Sector Survey on Cost Control, *A Report to the President* (2 vols) (Washington DC: Government Printing Office, 1984).

11. The Task Force on Program Review, *Improved Program Delivery: Health and Sports* (Ottawa: Supply and Services Canada, 1986).

12. See Pranlal Manga and Geoffrey R. Weller, 'The Canada Health Act of 1984 and the Future of the Canadian Health Care System'. A paper delivered at the 1985 annual meeting of the Association of Canadian Studies in Ireland (Cork, Ireland, April 12–13, 1985).

13. *Ibid.*, p. 19.

14. The battle over the Canada health Act is detailed in Monique Begin, *Medicare: Canada's Right to Health* (Montreal: Optimum Publishing International Inc., 1987).

15. The Task Force on Program Review, *op. cit.*, p. 32.

16. See V. Seymour Wilson, 'What Legacy? The Nielsen Task Force Program Review', in Katherine A. Graham (ed.), *How Ottawa Spends* (Ottawa: Carleton University Press, 1988) pp. 23–47.

17. See S. Heiber and R. Deber, 'Banning Extra-Billing in Canada: Just What the Doctor Didn't Order', in *Canadian Public Policy*, vol. XIII, no. 1 (1987) pp. 62–74.

18. See Carolyn J. Tuohy, 'Medicine and the State in Canada: The Extra-Billing Issue in Perspective', *Canadian Journal of Political Science*, vol. XXI, no. 2 (June 1988), pp. 276–96, especially pp. 287–96.

19. See M.L. Barer, 'Regulating Physician Supply: The Evolution of British Columbia's Bill 41', *Journal of Health Politics, Policy and Law*, vol. 13, no. 1 (Spring 1988) pp. 1–25.

20. The year after the strike in Ontario, physicians using this method increased payments by OHIP by its biggest single jump ever, namely 17 per cent or $500 million. See *Toronto Star*, 6 April 1988, 'Our Ailing Health System Needs Care'.

21. See Thunder Bay *Chronicle-Journal*, 14,June 1988, 'Using Hospitals'.

22. See Barbara Ehrenreich and John Ehrenreich, *The American Health Empire: Power, Profits and Politics* (New York: Random House, 1971).

23. See Ontario Hospital Association, *Focus, 1988–89 Provincial Budget* (Toronto: O.H.A. 22 April 1988) p. 7.

24. See Thunder Bay *Chronicle-Journal*, 12 April 1988, 'Caplan's Mistakes'.

25. Jake Epp, *Achieving Health For All: A Framework for Health Promotion* (Ottawa: Health and Welfare Canada, 1986) p. 7.

26. See B.S. Bolaria, 'Self-Care and Lifestyles: Ideological and Policy Implications', in J.A. Frey (ed.), *Economy, Class and Social Reality* (Toronto: Butterworths, 1979) pp. 350–63.

27. Pranlal Manga, 'Privatisation of Health Care Services in Canada: Reform or Regress?', *Journal of Consumer Policy*, vol. 10 (1987) p. 15.

28. See Carl Baker, 'Presentation to the Devolution Workshop'. Paper presented to the Devolution Workshop, Carleton University, 4 and 5 June 1988.

29. As reported in the Thunder Bay *Chronicle-Journal*, 19 July 1988.

30. Sean Usher, 'Health Care Endangered', in Ed Finn (ed.) *The Facts on Free Trade* (Toronto: James Lorimer, 1988) pp. 68–71.

31. Jake Epp, 'Health Care Reform: The Challenges for North America', Speech to the America's Society (Plaza Hotel, New York City November 18–19) 1987, p. 3.

32. *Ibid.*, p. 4.

9 Health Policies in the Conservative Transition to Democracy in Brazil

Sonia Maria Fleury Teixeira

INTRODUCTION

The inclusion of the Brazilian case in a survey concerning the new political conservatism, which emerged during the 1970s in the wake of an economic crisis in all industrialised nations, calls for some qualification. This is particularly so since the country is now undergoing a process of transition towards democracy. This chapter will analyse the strategies adopted by the sanitary (in most countries known as public health) movement to alter policy networks established during military dictatorships, and the constraints imposed by both the present economic crisis and the conservative nature of the transition in Brazil. Although this process is still in progress, some results can already be identified, underlining the distance between intention and action, or rather, between rhetoric and reality.

From 1964 until the mid-1980s Brazil endured 21 years of conservative military governments, who abolished many democratic mechanisms of political representation in favour of highly centralised decision-making processes. Military dictatorships replacing populist governments generated a new political order: the authoritarian-bureaucratic regime. This new order was characterised by the political and economic exclusion of lower sectors of society, the demobilisation and depolitisation of society as a whole, a transnationalisation of the country's productive framework and the institution of a civil and military technocracy enjoying enormous freedom in decision-making.

The economic success which the early military governments obtained has led to the consolidation of an associative process between transnational and national monopolistic capitals, with a repressive and entrepreneurial state increasingly playing the role of an intermediary. This combination produced a pattern of development characterised by high rates of economic growth marked by an ever stronger participation of foreign capital in the production as well as in the financing of public investments. The outcome of this policy has been a greater concentration of income in the hands of a few, while the living conditions for over half of the population have considerably worsened. In addition Brazil has incurred a tremendous indebtedness in foreign money-markets.

While the values behind economic policies of the authoritarian governments were originally liberal, in reality the organic weakness of the Brazilian bourgeoisie and the conditions imposed by international lenders have generated an unprecedented expansion of state intervention in every field of productive as well as social activities. On the other hand, such liberal economic values as the support of the free market, coincided with an extremely repressive political orientation towards civil society, in itself one more reason for the increase of state intervention.

The exclusion of workers from this new power pact, and their demobilisation by means of violent repression exerted over their organisations, had its reflections upon the mechanisms of social policy, with the state intervening to varying degrees in the welfare system, and the workers being consequently withdrawn from its management.

As concerns the dominant sectors, the closure of democratic channels of representation entailed the creation of substitutive 'bureaucratic rings' (Cardoso, 1975), that is, forms of interest articulation which involve both public (civil and military) bureaucracies, with private interest being inserted and organised in the context of state machinery.

In the Brazilian case, starting from the early 1970s, the following trends in the organisation of health services are particularly outstanding:

- The expansion of coverage under social security to include almost the entire urban and part of the rural population.
- The reorientation of national health policy toward curative medicine stressing specialisation and sophistication but deemphasising preventive and collective public health measures.
- The development of an entrepreneurial organisational pattern of medicine centered on profit, through the preferential allocation of security funds for the payment of services rendered by private individuals.

– The establishment of a medical and industrial complex, as a result of both an expanded technological infrastructure of a service network and the consumption of drugs.

A by-product of these changes was the administrative and institutional modernisation of governmental instruments of social policy, greater specialisation of each agency and increased centralisation and concentration of institutional resources.

By the end of the decade, the enormous inadequacies of this approach in addressing the sanitary conditions in the country manifested themselves. On the other hand, the process of redemocratisation brought about new political imperatives to solve the enormous social debt accumulated in previous years.

A number of economic, political and social questions have manifested themselves in the recent redemocratisation process experienced by different Latin American countries. First, the transition occurs simultaneously with a frightening indebtedness of the regional economies and with the pernicious effects of recessive policies over public expenditures, especially fragile social service expenditures. It is well known that the institution and expansion of welfare states in the developed countries are part of the rising cycle of the economy, Keynesian economic policy and the predominance of social-democratic ideology. The recent economic crisis in Brazil indicates the close connection between economic, political and social phenomena. In the case of Latin America, creating universal mechanisms of social policy and granting citizenship has become a necessity exactly at a time when economic conditions are extremely adverse.

Second, we must bear in mind structural problems intrinsic to dependent and laggard processes of capital accumulation in which great restrictions in the saving capacity coexist with an enormous working force outside the ordinary labour market. These two factors alone demonstrate that resources for financing the establishment and expansion of social policies are limited and that they cannot follow the model applied in the developed countries.

Politically the process of democratisation presently under way underlines the constraints now imposed on the relationships between the state powers and a strengthened Executive during monopolistic stages of capitalism, as well as the increasing bureaucratisation of society. These are demonstrating the impossibility of control by the state using the political tools of the last century (Cardoso, 1974). Moreover, as stressed by Bobbio (1983), technological advances, characteristic of industrial societies and increasingly implying technical solutions for all problems, added to the process of 'massification' endured by large societies and represent current limitations to democracy.

The revival and strengthening of urban social movements as a form of popular organisation to stress people's consumption needs, express new routes to be followed by democracy, by taking the State as their target, and tinging again the question of citizenship with political colours. Urban social movements of today are an undeniable phenomenon for the democratisation of the state machinery and for the universalisation of citizenship towards thousands of underemployed Latin-Americans. Other significant experiences in this direction must also be taken into account, such as the rise of middle class trade-unionism, resulting from a tendency to subject intellectual production to the capitalistic process of accumulation.

In addition, in the Brazilian case the peculiarities of the country's transitional process which started in the late 1970s, when military governments proved their incapacity to sustain the high rates of economic development and thus achieve legitimacy for the power they exercised, must be taken into consideration.

O'Donnell (1988) perceives two types of transition to democracy in Latin American countries. The first involves the authoritarian–bureaucratic regimes which have been economically destructive and highly repressive and thus have progressively come to corrode their bases of political support, which finally collapsed. In those cases of *transition by collapse*, the authoritarian state is incapable of controlling its transactions with the forces of opposition and so, in spite of economically extremely unfavourable conditions, the new democratic regimes achieve relatively high degrees of freedom for action. The second case includes authoritarian–bureaucratic regimes which, as in Brazil, enjoyed some economic success and used repressive measures less extensively and less systematically. Economic success is of benefit to the middle class and industrial areas favoured by military governments. Thus civil and military elites find themselves as leaders of a *transition by agreement*, forcing their viewpoints in the ensuing negotiations upon the opposition.

The model of transition by agreement can be understood as a *conservative transition*, since it recreates obsolete political relations between social classes, political elites and the state. On the other hand, this type of transition underscores the knife's edge of freedom for action of democratic governments which is insufficient in itself to change the dramatic social panorama consolidated through many years of discriminating development.

Within this context what are the perspectives of the sanitary movement (solidly organised since the mid-1970s), engaging academic groups, professionals, segments of the bureaucracy, people's and syndicalist organisations in the struggle for guaranteeing a universal right to health and the establishment of a unified and official system of health services? These goals are firmly stated in the proposal for a broad Sanitary Reform, but they are restricted by the very nature of the conservative transition.

POLICY NETWORKS

Up until the military coup of 1964, the public health sector[1] in Brazil had been controlled by the Ministry of Health. Services were rendered by service networks under the jurisdiction of different Social Security institutions. The Ministry of Health was responsible for preventive measures, and also for formulating national health policies. In addition the Ministry was also accountable for confinement institutions or asylums, for people afflicted by mental or contagious diseases, such as tuberculosis and so on. Curative medical care was rendered through its hospitals and attendance units and was in the realm of Social Security, covering only the insured urban population. Outside the public sector, health assistance was supplied by religious orders caring for the destitute, and private medicine was available only to a very limited number of persons.

In the beginning, the military governments' social welfare policy aimed to unify the Institute of Social Security, and to exclude the employees – employers' representatives of these Institutes from the new and centralised administrative board. However the 'liberal' ideology inspiring these governments progressively impacted upon the institutional framework of the health sector by including private medical care. This process involved the following:

– The budgetary resources of the Ministry of Health were considerably reduced, thus rendering the networks of public services obsolete, especially those concerned with preventive care. They lacked physical, material and human resources. The Ministry's responsibility in the formulation and coordination of national health policy became an unfulfilled written promise

given its declining influence within the organisational structure of
the state.
- The Social Security system strengthened curative medical services. This development was favoured both directly, through the
extension of social security benefits to sectors of the working class
which until then were excluded from the system (elderly people
without income, domestic servants, independent professionals,
peasants); and indirectly, due to the significant weight of the
Social Security budget in the complex formed by the organisations rendering social services. Although the amount contributed
by the Federal Government equals only approximately 5 per cent
(to help finance a system which includes such benefits as
retirement pensions, health services, and social welfare), the
resources from employees' and employers' contributions made it
the second largest budget in the country, surpassed only by the
federal budget.
- Finally, the building up and maintenance of a system of private
hospitals, which had received a greater part of public resources
for health, became evident.

This latter point will be more carefully addressed because of its
importance for effectively achieving a policy of privatisation at the
service level, and consolidating a highly concentrated and exclusive
power structure and decision-making process. This policy network
resulted from the private sector oriented health policy of previous
military governments. It has formed the nucleus of great resistance to
change during the democratic transition, as we shall see later.

The first obstacle to an effective policy of privatisation in the health
area was the absence of a private network of health services (namely
hospitals and outpatient units – a consequence of intrinsic market
conditions and the limited purchasing power of the majority of the
population). This in itself was a serious impediment to the development of an active private sector for the delivery of health services.

During the 1960s, in reality the majority of the existing hospitals
were public or operated by philanthropies. However, once a special
governmental fund to offer highly subsidised financing for the
construction of mental health units was established – and which was
used almost entirely for private hospitals – the situation was
completely reversed. Add to this situation the obsolescence forced
upon public services and the lack of support for the philanthropic
services 20 years later. Any health policy concerning nosocomial

infections depended on the private sector for implementation.

In the early 1980s, the private hospitals' network already surpassed that of the public service. The beds in the private network represented 80.43 per cent of all beds in the country, reflecting over 90 per cent of hospital admissions reimbursed by Social Security during the preceding decade.

Health services however did not become private in an indiscriminate way, but only in those activities where profit was guaranteed. Consequently businessmen interested in the health area concentrated on hospitals, while prevention and the provision of outpatient care were left to the public sector. Hospitals, besides the delivery of specialised and more sophisticated services, have also been directly involved in the production and consumption of products, such as technological equipment and pharmaceutical products. The profit rationale underlying health policies resulted in a high concentration of private hospitals (72 per cent) in the most affluent parts of the country, with only scant public hospital services in the poorer areas.

The growth of private networks of the existing hospital capacity in both absolute and relative terms resulted from public financing for modernisation and expansion, and from Social Security contracts and covenants which governed the reimbursement of hospital services. We shall proceed to analyse each one of these forms and their consequences for the delivery of services.

To purchase medical services from the private network, Social Security established a system of contracts which reimbursed each medical act separately. The value of each one was calculated in accordance with a Table of Units of Service (the USs). In consequence, each medical act, taking into account the level of sophistication and complexity, would correspond to a certain number of USs. The effects of this fee-for-service compensation of private services reimbursed by the Social Security system were soon to make themselves obvious.

To start with, it led hospital entrepreneurs eager for profit to adopt a number of practices, such as: multiplying and duplicating medical procedures; resorting to more expensive types of treatment; emphasising surgery; and paying low salaries to professional personnel who were, in many instances, in short supply. Those trends are manifest in the diversity of conditions prevailing in hospitals belonging to Social Security and in those under contract; for example, in 1970, the percentage of births through Caesarean operation (the more lucrative type) was about 10 per cent in the public service while hospitals under contract performed more than 30 per cent of the same operation.

Secondly, it is necessary to stress the financial consequences of such a system of payment; in addition to the incentive given to highly sophisticated and, therefore, expensive procedures, it created a serious, twofold problem for the Social Security budget. Any planning became impossible and the costs of medical care increased tremendously. Retrospective reimbursement of services was like a blank cheque assigned by Social Security to each hospital and to be honoured at the end of each month. Moreover this reimbursement system led to such an increase in fraudulent actions that it became necessary to set up sophisticated and expensive mechanisms of control.

The emphasis on private hospital services to the detriment of public-network ambulatory services led to a complete overhaul of the rational delivery of services, thus creating a system which stressed expensive tertiary over primary care. The same phenomenon can be observed in relation to the distribution of manpower, which produced a large concentration of specialists and a limited use of general practitioners as well as nursing personnel. The very success of the policy of privatisation has provoked the crisis of the health care model, because extensive utilisation jeopardises the financial structure of Social Security in Brazil and raises fundamental questions about its practicability as the sole alternative for expanding medical coverage.

New relationships between Social Security and private providers, that is, group practices or 'medical enterprises' modeled after health maintenance organisations, developed by means of a covenant among three institutions: an enterprise or industry x, Social Security, and the medical enterprise. The latter would receive a lump sum for the contract (the cost was to be calculated on the basis of the number of persons employed by industry x). It was also agreed that the medical enterprise would initially assume complete responsibility for the provision of services to the group of workers employed by industry x.

The services are bought with the payment of a fixed amount for each worker, regardless of the care that he will receive. Thus the simpler the medical acts performed, the greater the profit will be, because this type of medical care uses primary attention of limited technology and is rendered by less specialised professionals. Nevertheless this approach remains restricted to a special segment of the labour force in large monopolistic enterprises in sectors of advanced technology with high levels of productivity and also high levels of salary. This segment is generally known to be a low risk group.

Some diseases, notably those which are likely to become chronic, have proved to be nonlucrative. This includes alcoholism, mental diseases, and illnesses which require complex surgeries. The new covenants explicitly excluded these non-profitable illnesses. An afflicted person, although he was insured, had to go back to the public network, which in turn became unduly overburdened, and an unrealistic alternative to the covenants governing hospital services.

After a few years, during which the policy of privatisation was implemented, the power structure in the health sector was clearly established and a decision-making process on health policies was in place, which clearly involved highly exclusive administrative and institutional mechanisms. The bureaucracy played a significant role during the authoritarian-bureaucratic regime. Its alignment with the vested interests of the industrialists on the one hand, and the absence of social control on the other, have created conditions that render privatisation in medical care viable.

In other words, in contrast to the nations where a policy of privatisation has been rhetoric rather than action, the Brazilian case shows that the military dictatorships have indeed enforced it without any need for a strong ideological tenet. Public funds were channeled into the private sector and the effectiveness of these measures resulted from the lack of opposition from other actors concerned with defining health policies. This absence was due to the prevailing repression and disruption of democratic mechanisms of interest representation.

It should be pointed out that the liberal model of medicine was not considered because it was almost completely extinct as a consequence of doctors having become salaried employees in the face of the entrepreneurship and the constraints imposed upon the exercise of their profession in hospitals. In sum, the state, here represented by the Ministry of Social Security, became the protagonist in the decision-making arena of health policy, creating a situation of mutual dependence between the business sector and the bureaucracy of Social Security. For its legitimation the authoritarian power also depended on the growing expansion of the coverage for social services, which in turn became unfeasible because of the tremendous growth of the costs resulting from the deprivatisation policy.

These contradictions were greatly stimulated by the financial crisis faced by the system of Social Security in the early 1980s, although the origin of these difficulties cannot be found in the model adopted for the provision of health services. This financial crisis indeed reflected the general economic crisis which brought about higher rates of unemployment and a corresponding reduction of most salaries. As the system relied on contributions based on salaries as the main source of revenue, it became extremely vulnerable to the economic recession. What happened then was a drastic reduction from 30 per cent to 19 per cent of total Social Security resources available for the provision of health services.

To this financial crisis (which has persisted into the early 1980s) endured by the Social Security should be added other political factors which have also pushed for changes in the privatisation model.

STRATEGIES OF REFORM

To understand the strategies for change, put together nowadays under the umbrella of the Sanitary Reform, one must understand the constitutive process of the sanitary movement, the reform's leading agent. It started back in the first years of the military dictatorship, when almost all channels of political expression were barred and the university became the main bastion for contesting the authoritarian government. With the recommendation of the Pan-American Health Organisation, departments of preventive medicine were created in the Schools of Medicine, which reintroduced a liberal policy for medicine and required a change of attitude on the part of the professionals. A new scientific paradigm began to be developed and to introduce social disciplines in the analysis of the health–illness process. These disciplines introduced the historical-structural method in the health field in an attempt to understand processes such as the social determination of disease and the social organisation of medical practice.

Although the sanitary movement was originally confined to the community, it did not limit itself to the production of new knowledge; on the contrary, one of its consistent aims has been to connect scientific knowledge with a search for new political practices and to diffuse a new health awareness. Within the academic arena, through the development of projects for 'community medicine', alternatives to the prevailing health practices have been created. Along the same lines, and through agreements between Secretaries of Health in the states and international organisations, experimental projects for regions of great poverty were developed.

These projects were all marked by their experimental character and their marginality to the health system in which the above mentioned privatisation policy dominated. However it was with such projects that the sanitary movement could experiment with an alternative policy for the health sector, trying to develop a more rational and more adequate system which took into consideration the epidemiology situation and the country's availability of resources. Although these projects were identified as 'providers of second class medical care for second class citizens', they constituted the laboratory in which directives for reversing the prevailing model have been tested. These directives included the development of a public network capable of providing complete care, from preventive measures to complex surgical treatment; the establishment of a system of referrals to and from various units; the use of planning instruments in the administration of services; and finally, the creation of forms of participation for users and professionals alike in the management of health services.

These projects obviously could only start the process, since they faced chronic problems ranging from lack of financial resources and administrative discontinuity to strict limitations of medical services. This was so because they could not involve other sectors in the health field, such as the production of inputs, the development of technologies, sanitary surveillance and control of working environments.

On the political–ideological side, the movement looked for mechanisms for diffusing a new health awareness. At the same time it hoped to build up a much needed network to organise and orient the different forms of opposition to the official policy of health. The Centro Brasileiro de Desudos de Saude – CEBES (Brazilian Centre for Health Studies) – was created. It started by editing a review, *Saude em Deabte*, and a collection of books published in an editoral line under the same name. Through the articles written by the intelligentsia of the sanitary movement, and the diffusion of books by foreign authors and former health professionals (persecuted by the military government), it provided the specialists in the area with a new vision not only of the health-illness process but also of the health policy applied by the authoritarian regime.

Through this Centre, its publications and the events it sponsored – lectures and so on – a new organisational proposal for the health system was disclosed. It was embedded in the general struggle for the nation's democratisation. At the same time a web of relationships, involving intellectuals, segments of the bureaucracy, popular and unionist leaders, professionals from the health service and others, had been firmly established. The sanitary movement was clearly linked to progressive forces in a coalition to fight for the democratisation of the country. Nonetheless it always preserved its own independence from parties and embraced different classes, an essential condition for maintaining political unity.

Starting around 1975, when the failure of the economic model adopted by the military governments spilled over to the political process (the opposition had won the elections of 1974), the whole of society began to be mobilised and organised in its struggle for redemocratisation. The first professional sector to challenge the military government and to go on a general strike for better wages was the medical class. As previously mentioned, the privatisation and concentration of the services have required the employment of numerous salaried health professionals with a consequent loss of status and socio-economic position. It is important to stress that the dissatisfaction was channeled into strengthening a medical trade union, its leaders making demands which included a more democratic health system, or rather a health system less dependent on business interests and better equipped to serve the population. In addition, they insisted on better working and remunerative conditions for their professionals.

The incorporation of medical trade unions in the sanitary movement, which was still only composed of intellectuals, gave a rare political dimension to demands for changes in the health system in several ways. Firstly, strikes discontinued services and challenged the policy of health. Secondly, this discussion was taken to the federations of workers. Finally, the doctors' movement materially and politically gave support to the first steps of enabling people to participate in questions of health.

The new visibility which health problems gained was also expressed in the National Congress where important symposia were held, in association with CEBES, and health policies discussed. Given the state of powerlessness to which military governments had reduced the legislative instances, the most important role played by these was in promoting meetings in which the various protagonists in the health sector – businessmen, bureaucrats, the sanitary movement – were able to face one another on the same footing. Until then the sanitary movement had been treated, and identified itself, as a subversive group, while the businessmen established invisible connections –

bureaucratic rings – with the bureaucracy of Social Security. Therefore the symbolic value of the debates which took place in the Health Symposia was to underscore the contrasting views in the area of health policy in a democratic arena. This move most certainly contributed to a change in political self-image and the true identity of the different groups. The sanitary movement then started to seek beyond the ideological level for a way to explicitly present its pragmatic proposals for the restructuring of the health system.

It is true that this process of forming a movement and developing a reform project did not occur without contradictions, since different political groups with distinctive interests belonged to the same opposition forces. However unity was guaranteed by the more comprehensive purpose of creating conditions for the effective democratisation of Brazilian society. In the early 1980s, when the financial crisis of Social Security became evident and the crisis of the model itself was disclosed, because the privatisation of the sector could not be continued on the same basis, the sanitary movement was the only group which was able to offer a concrete alternative for reforming the health system.

In the preceding years the movement had been slowly building this condition, consolidating a technical and political project which was clearly formulated around a body of directives and principles conducive to the organisation of a public, universal and comprehensive system of health care. A complex web of political relations had simultaneously been woven, which, although external to the leading organism in the execution of health policies, namely Social Security, gradually gave more significant signs that it could no longer be ignored in the process of formulating and implementing these policies.

The weakness of the sanitary movement resulted mainly from its inability to enlarge its supportive bases in such a way as to include those circles supposedly most interested in a change of health policy, that is, the segment of the population disinherited by the (highly concentrative) economic model enforced by the authoritarian governments. In fact the poor, beside being concerned with problems of immediate survival, could hardly be said to be organised, and they participated little in the political process. Only a small group in this politically unprepared mass distinguished itself, due to its adherence to the *Comunidades Eclesiais de Base* (Ecclesiastic Community Cells). These bodies are connected with the Progressive Catholic Church, which has embraced the theology of liberation. In this case however, a radical ideology which rejects any possible alteration in public policy as a strategy for social change usually prevails.

The health sector, although in need of substantial support from the users of the health system, did not give up its strategy for bringing politics into the discussions on health. In addition to organising a block of opposition forces around a project of reform which became increasingly more detailed and comprehensive, it progressively occupied political space as it was eventually made available. In view of the crisis, some theorists who are clearly associated with the reform project have been called to fill top positions in the bureaucracy of the Social Security system. This decision is an attempt to solve the impasse confronted by the policy of health.

Since then the centre of the struggle for changing health policy has transferred from the outside to the inside of the main organisation responsible for health care. In other words, the Social Security bureaucracy, functioning as a political actor during the more repressive and centralising phases of the military governments, has been transformed into a political arena, where conflicting interests confront each other in efforts to define a policy of health.

Open discussions of reform proposals and rational measures to curb public expenditures all have the potential to preserve the existing power structure in the health sector. However in introducing this approach there is also a chance that demands of the sanitary movement, which transcends rational measures and which intends to bring about a change in the structure of power and the organisation of the health system, may also be included. There is a tension between two opposing paths inside the bureaucracy of the health sector, and it is gaining momentum as the sanitary movement has been able to influence many other areas as a consequence of the process of democratic transition.

CONSTRAINTS AND OUTPUTS

The first civilian government after 21 years of military dictatorship resulted from a coalition of opposition forces to the authoritarian regime, and segments of the business community who were dissatisfied with the failure of economic policy and the elimination of political channels for interest representation. Thus the civilian government did not have a clearcut ideological profile, since the democratic alliance comprised political viewpoints ranging from a typical liberal orientation to curb state intervention, to social-democratic views aiming at a more equitable and egalitarian distribution of national resources.

The composition of the civil transitional government reflected the strength of each group within a broad alliance of democratic forces. Broad consultations with the military and the business elites, who were connected to the authoritarian government in the past, are still necessary.

As concerns the health sector, and given the organisational strength of the opposition in the health movement and the elaboration of a project to introduce consistent sectorial changes, it was possible to demand that the movement's leadership be present in top managerial positions and responsible for health policy. The proposal for a universal right to health was advocated by that group and was increasingly perceived as an alternative to the previous situation. It clearly contradicted the set of liberal ideas agreed upon between the international financing agencies and the indebtedness of the Third World.

From 1985, at the beginning of the transitional government, measures had been taken to change the privatisation policy in health and also to strengthen and make the public sector responsible for medical care. They were taken in three basic directions: to give a political dimension to health; to alter the constitution; and finally, to change the institutional framework and practices. We will briefly consider each one of them, stressing nevertheless their concomitancy and mutual influence.

The inclusion of a political dimension in the debate on health was one of the first goals to be achieved, in order for people's awareness of health to be improved, and in order for it to become visible and thus justify the inclusion of its demands in the governmental agenda. In addition it was necessary to organise the democratic forces to secure the political support required to implement the changes that would have to face the vested interests which had existed inside the health sector for a long time.

These goals were basically achieved through the Eighth National Conference of Health, which was summoned by the Ministry of Health. The Ministry used an entirely new procedure, in comparison to procedures followed in the preceding meetings. Previous conferences had a strictly technical character, assembling the state bureaucracy and some reputed professionals only in order to discuss a few documents and elaborate recommendations concerning health policy. It can be said that the seven previous gatherings had no impact whatsoever on such policy.

The Eighth Conference however was innovative; its comprehensive agenda included subjects transcending both the health sector and the technical milieu itself, such as a right to health, the health system, and financing. Moreover, ten months of preparation preceded the holding of the Eighth Conference. These themes were discussed in each territorial unit of the Brazilian Federal Republic by health professionals, users, intellectuals, political parties and trade unions. These debates finally culminated in the Eighth Conference, which assembled approximately 5000 participants chosen as delegates in their original institutions, and secured an equal number of representatives of the states and the citizenry. This democratic process reached its goal in bringing the debate on health to the heart of society in an unprecedented mobilisation of all groups concerned. This was previously unrecorded in Brazilian history. The Final Report of the Conference, which was thoroughly discussed and finally approved by the plenary, represented a technical advance and was a political pact largely legitimised by the social forces represented in the event.

There is no doubt that the history of health in Brazil was deeply affected by the process and the approval by the Eighth National Conference on Health, which defined and formulated a real programme for the Sanitary Reform. The mobilisation which was achieved for the Conference was later channeled into organising lobby groups, which have been active at all stages of elaborating the new democratic Constitution.

Previously all constitutions enforced in Brazil have addressed the health question in a superficial and discriminatory way, leaving responsibilities and sources of financing undefined on the one hand, while granting the right to health services only to the users of Social Security on the other. In elaborating the present constitutional provisions there has been consensus on the need to detail each subject area. This has been necessary in light of the transitional situation in which the Constitution emerged, which not only would have to face the *status quo*, consolidated during 21 years of dictatorship, but also promote the necessary and nondelayable changes.

In the National Constituent Assembly the many health interests faced each other and progressively organised themselves into two diametrically opposed factions: the business group headed by the

Federação Brasileria de Hospitais (Brazilian Federation of Hospitals), which was deeply entrenched in the private sector, and the *Associação de Indústrias Farmacêuticas* (Association of Pharmaceutical Industries) representing the multinational concerns and the forces fighting for the Sanitary Reform, led by the Plenary of Health Entities. This body assembled almost two hundred entities from the sector, such as trade unions and syndicalist organisations, professional and cultural associations, political parties, popular movements, users' associations and others.

The Plenary was able to achieve its objectives so efficiently because it used valuable weapons. It had the technical capacity to prepare a clear and coherent project of constitutional provisions beforehand. It exerted constant pressure on the constituent representatives and, finally, it mobilised society around the constitutional process. The fighting style of business interests reflected the usual practices of the sector in which group pressures are combined with different forms of bribery.

The final text of the Constitution, which was approved after a series of political agreements, responded to the majority of the demands made by the sanitary movement. It frustrated the more egotistical interests of hospital entrepreneurs, but it did not at all alter the situation of the pharmaceutical industry. The major points approved in the new Constitution include:

– A universal right to health and the responsibility of the State to guarantee it, thus eliminating the discrimination between insured–non-insured and urban–rural.
– Health services and actions in the health field are now considered of public importance, and as a consequence the government has become responsible for regulating, financing and controlling the health sector.
– A single system of health has been established, which integrates all public health services into a network organised along hierarchical lines. The system has been regionalised and decentralised, and includes comprehensive medical care and allows for community participation.
– The private sector participates in the health system in a complementary way, preferably through philanthropic entities. The allocation of public funds to subsidise for-profit institutions is prohibited. Contracts signed with private service entities will be governed by public law, which gives the State the right to step in

when these entities do not abide by contractual provisions.
– The sale of blood and other by-products is prohibited.

The approved constitutional text follows many of those proposals advocated for some time by the health movement, although the movement did not obtain complete satisfaction of its demands in light of the more powerful industrial and–or governmental interests. As a consequence, important points concerning the financing of the new system were not clearly defined, such as the percentage of the budget allocated to health. With regard to drugs, there is little evidence that the system can actually control their production and consumption.[2] In the area of workers' health some proposals were not approved; for instance, the right to refuse to work in places found to be unhealthy, the right to be informed about toxic products handled whilst at work, and other rights.

All constitutional provisions must now be translated into institutional norms and procedures so that the relevant rights can be enforced. However the alteration of institutional practices has been in progress for several years – since the end of the dictatorial regime. This has resulted in stressing the policy of privatisation and, as a consequence, the financial crisis of Social Security. Increasingly these institutional changes have included the following objectives:

– The strengthening of the public sector through the integration of different entities, thus creating embryonic elements of a future unified health system.
– A reduced role for the private sector in rendering health services; greater monitoring of accounts, and new forms of relationships.
– The political and administrative decentralisation of the decision-making process in health and services performed at local levels, thus enhancing social control.

Since the beginning of the transitional government in 1985, and the appointment of personnel from the sanitary movement to top governmental positions, especially in the most important institutions in the Social Security sector, it has been possible to carry out many measures conducive to achieving these objectives.

A programme for the integration of public health institutions was created. Instead of expanding the scope of coverage through contracts with private entities, the Social Security would get the same result through agreements with the network of Secretaries of Health. This network was for outpatients and was located throughout the needy regions, providing health care for the entire population indiscriminately. As a consequence of the previous policy of privatisation and the lack of financial resources to be allocated to the Ministry and the Secretaries of Health, this public network was obsolete and ineffective and rendered services of bad quality.

Given the agreements with the Social Security, the re-equipment of the network became a possibility; it was now in a position to offer conditions which may revert the model of privatisation. Its major limitation however is the absence of hospital units. This in turn makes the network dependent on the private sector.

To get an idea of how efficacious these measures are, we have to look at the distribution of Social Security resources allocated to health. In 1974, 63 per cent of all funds were allocated to the private sector under contracts. In 1988 however this percentage had dropped to 39 per cent.

Another strategy was to distinguish between philanthropic and profit institutions in the private sector. The previous practice transferred the profit motivation to philanthropic services, while the adoption of differential treatment shifted the philanthropic services' approach to the public services. The measures which were implemented in the private profit sector primarily sought to control the delivery of services and enhance accountability. Instead of paying hospital bills at face value, Social Security started to define parameters for hospital admissions and surgeries. When these limits were surpassed, detailed auditing would take place before any payment was made. This in turn significantly reduced the number of hospital admissions.

Another important measure was to change the fee-for-service reimbursement scheme, thus reducing abuses in the delivery of contract services. Several attempts at establishing a standard public law contract were also made, but private hospitals resisted this measure strongly. Only after the Constitution took effect did it become possible to achieve this objective. In order to minimise the power of veto of private hospitals over these new policies, a strategy of introducing new actors – such as the philanthropic network, secretaries of health administration in member-states, health professionals and users – in the decision-making process was adopted.

CONCLUSION

All these measures of change converge in a strategy of decentralisation of the health system that is now under way. This process makes it possible to effectively dismantle the centralised framework inherited from authoritarian governments. Moreover it allows for the creation of collegial management bodies in which professionals and users participate. The purpose is to reduce possible clientelism in the handling of social resources. It is true that the risk of co-option is always present, but Brazilian society will have to pay this price on its march towards democracy.

The health sector is undergoing a rather complex process which in part reflects the economic regression which the country is currently experiencing in its democratic transition. As policies are adopted to establish a more egalitarian and equitable society, they jeopardise the interests of the dominant elite, who continue to be firmly entrenched in the process of transition, hence reactivating conservative forces.

Just as the progressive forces succeeded in imprinting their mark on the new Constitution, the Chief Executive unexpectedly resorted to reactionary measures and dispensed with the collaboration of its members, who by their very combativeness and strong social-democratic views had obtained their positions in the new civil government. In the health sector almost all heads of service who espouse such views have been removed from office, so the continuity of the Sanitary Reform remains to be seen in light of:

- The fragility of reform measures now in progress.
- The ineffectiveness of the public sector, which jeopardises the entire project.
- Tension among health professionals who are asked for more professional devotion and commitment.
- Diminishing popular support in view of missing results concerning people's health.
- A revival and reorganisation of counter-reform forces.

The limits imposed upon the process of change in the health sector are fairly clear, and it is dependent on the reform forces to envisage new strategies in order to carry on with their project.

Notes

1. The health sector is composed of federal institutions, such as the Health Ministry and Social Security Ministry, and by their correspondents in the state and municipal levels (Health Secretaries – whether state or municipal).
2. Control in the sense of quality, prices, hazardous medicine, prescribed medicine and publicity.

References

Bobbio, N. (1983) *Qual Socialismo? Discussão de uma Alternativa* (RJ, Paz e Terra).

Cardoso, F.H. (1974) 'La Sociedad y el Estado' in, *Pensamiento Ibero Americano – Revista de Economia Política*, Cepal, no. 5, 5ª Enero–Junio.

Cardoso, F.H. (1975) *Autoritarismo e Democratização* (RJ, Paz e Terra).

O'Donnell, G. (1988) 'Hiatos, Instituições e Perspectivas Democráticasa in *A Democracia no Brasil, Dilemas e Perspectivas*, (SP, Vertice).

Further Reading

Fleury Teixeira, S.M. (1989) *Reforma Sanitária: Em Busca de uma Teoria* (SP, Cortez).

Oliveira, J.A.A. and S.M. Fleury Teixeira (1985) (Im) *Previdência Social – 60 Anos de História da Previdência no Brasil* (RJ, Vozes).

Nunes E.D. *et al.* (eds.) (1986) *Ciencias Sociales y Salud en la America Latina* (Montevideu: OPS, CIESU).

10 Medical Care Security and the 'Vitality of the Private Sector' in Japan

William E. Steslicke

As Japanese health policy-makers look ahead to the 1990s, they realise that the imperatives of 'economic restructuring', 'globalisation', and a 'rapidly aging society' will affect the way in which health care is organised, delivered, and financed. This will provide both opportunities and challenges for them. Although they can take some pride in the accomplishments of the 1980s, they know that the Japanese health care system has not reached a state of perfection (Koseisho, 1989; Ministry of Health and Welfare, 1988, pp. 14–19). Not only is there much room for improvement in the quality of health services, but a good deal of readjustment of organisation, delivery and financing of services, in keeping with the changing domestic and international environment of the 1990s, will also be necessary (Economic Planning Agency, 1988, p. 5). Health care is not an area in which Japanese national policy-makers can afford to relax or simply follow business-as-usual.

Of course health care is not the only determinant of health status, a host of other social, economic, and political factors – largely outside the direct control of health policy-makers – are equally or even more important in promoting individual health and welfare (OECD), 1987; Steslicke, 1987; Masaki and Koizumi, 1987). For example; there are no guarantees that the relatively high health status of the Japanese people will survive the generally affluent life-style that has developed in the past few decades. The emergence of the so-called 'advanced country diseases' (cerebrovascular disease, hypertensive disease, neoplasms, heart disease, and cirrhosis of the liver) as leading causes of death is especially worrisome in that regard (JICWELS, 1983). Moreover the nature of the public policy-making process, as well as the priorities assigned to various other domestic and international issues and problems on the national agenda, are also basic constraints over which health policy-makers have relatively little control. They

247

must coordinate and accommodate the health policy agenda to reflect the broader national policy agenda and its emphasis on 'Economic Management within a Global Context' (Economic Planning Agency, 1988).

If there are many uncertainties in looking ahead, health policy-makers also realise that Japanese health care institutions are basically sound and, in spite of a certain amount of discontent, enjoy both popular and elite acceptance and support. This is especially true with respect to the system of medical care security, which has become institutionalised during the past century and which is now undergoing a 'rationalisation' process as a result of public policies initiated in the early 1980s. It is a mixed public–private system that offers a measure of medical care security to Japanese citizens which is as high or higher than any in the world – and for much less than is expended in most other industrial nations. In 1987 total health expenditures were estimated to be 6.8 per cent of Gross Domestic Product (GDP) as compared with 11.2 per cent in the United States, 9.0 per cent in Sweden, 8.6 per cent in Canada and France, 8.27 per cent in Germany, and 6.1 per cent in the UK (Schieber and Poullier, 1989, p. 170). Nevertheless the medical care security system has not been exempted from the intensive scrutiny and serious reevaluation that was applied to other areas of Japanese life during the 1980s (Inoguchi, 1987; Kumon, 1987; Noguchi, 1987).

As in other areas, health policy-makers have been urged to exploit the 'vitality of the private sector' (*minkan katsuryoku* or *minkatsu* for short) in adjusting the medical care security system to meet the needs and priorities of the 1990s. One response to *minkatsu* has been the opening of the health insurance market to both domestic and foreign private insurance products. However this has led neither to 'disman-tling' of the public components of the medical care security structure, nor wholesale or indiscriminate 'privatisation' of the overall system. Indeed such privatisation as has taken place thus far appears quite marginal and has not *fundamentally* altered the already blurred public–private balance – even through there has been some important cost-shifing within the medical security system.

The Japanese state remains deeply involved in the medical care security system, as it has been for the past century, and it is unlikely to 'wither away' in the years ahead. However state power is diffused and fragmented in contemporary Japan, and national policy-making usually involves considerable competition and struggle between various public and private stakeholders within particular policy networks – what has been aptly referred to as 'patterned pluralism'. During the 1990s, health policy-makers will continue to function in the kind of 'patterned pluralism' that has characterised Japanese national politics in the 1980s, in which 'the government and its bureaucracy are strong, but the boundaries between state and society are blurred by the integration of social interest groups with the government and by the intermediation of political parties between social interest groups and the government' (Muramatsu and Krauss, 1987, p. 537). In the Japanese case, 'the government is not weak, but it is *penetrated* by interest groups and political parties (*Ibid.*, p. 537).

Health policy-making during the 1980s has tended to reflect the pervasiveness of 'patterned pluralism' in Japanese national politics, as well as the national policy priorities that have been articulated through that process (Steslicke, 1987; 1982c; Calder, 1988, pp. 369–438). It has also reflected the more general pattern of 'rhetoric and reality' in contemporary Japanese politics.

MEDICAL CARE SECURITY IN JAPAN: IDEAS AND INSTITUTIONS

The term 'medical care security' (*iryo hosho*) is used in Japan to refer to one of three functional categories of the contemporary social security system. The other two categories are income security and public welfare services. The former includes employment insurance, workmen's accident compensation insurance, and seven public pension programmes. Included in the latter (public welfare services) are programmes based on the Public Assistance Law of 1946 and 1950, the Child Welfare Law of 1947, the Law for the Welfare of Physically Handicapped Persons of 1949, the Law for the Welfare of Mentally Retarded Persons of 1960, the Law for the Welfare of the Aged of 1963, the Law for Maternal and Child Welfare of 1964, and the Social Welfare Service Law of 1951. Although there is considerable overlap between and within these categories, each program also has its distinctive features and clientele (Japanese National Committee, 1986).

This is also true with respect to 'medical care security'. In its narrow usage, it includes six basic medical insurance schemes and the Health and Medical Services for the Aged Act of 1982, as well as public assistance medical services and medical services related to the Infectious Diseases Prevention Act, the Tuberculosis Prevention Act, and the Special Assistance Act for the War Wounded. Used more broadly, 'medical care security' also includes the pluralistic medical services delivery system (Steslicke, 1989; Ohnuki-Tierney, 1984).

In this paper 'medical care security' will be used in the broader sense to include organisation, delivery, and financing of personal health services (or medical care) as well as relevant public health services. However the major focus will be on financing of medical care services in contemporary Japan and on the impact of recent conservative government efforts to emphasise the 'vitality of the private sector' in that area. It will be seen that the emphasis on *minkatsu*, as well as various examples of 'privatisation' in medical care and in other public services, has a distinctive Japanese flavour and should not be confused with neo-conservative agendas and programmes in other OECD nations. This refers to both 'rhetoric' and 'reality'.

A brief description of some of the major institutions in the Japanese medical security system will provide a better picture of the 'reality' under discussion here, and also help to place the health policy developments of the 1980s in historical, ideological and international perspective (Frenk & Donabedian, 1987).

Physicians and Government

Within the Japanese system of 'biomedicine' that was first established in the 1870s, provision of medical services has been restricted and regulated according to national laws. Currently there are 13 separate statutes covering 21 different types of medical care personnel. The statutes address education, licensure, examination, responsibilities, and other matters related to individual delivery of medical services. From the beginning the physician has been authorised to dominate the division of labour (Long, 1987; Steslicke, 1982a).

According to the Medical Practitioner's Law of 13 July 1948, only 'duly licensed' individuals may use the title *ishi* (doctor) and 'take charge of medical treatment and guidance of health, and contribute to the improvement and promotion of public health in order to secure the healthy life of the people'. Organisational and technological changes in medical practice are affecting physician dominance in Japan as in other nations. However the combination of traditional deference to physician authority and continued state support for the 'take charge' role inhibit substantial redistribution of power (Long, 1987). The fact that only physicians may serve as heads of medical care organisations, and that physician ownership of facilities is also extensive, further reinforces physician dominance.

In 1984 there were 181 101 duly licensed physicians (150.6 per 100 000 population) and this number is expected to increase rapidly in the future. The issue of physician supply and distribution has been on the health policy agenda for several years and it seems clear that the regulatory mechanisms that are already in place will be more fully utilised to address the problems.

Of the total physician population in 1984, 95.8 per cent were actually engaged in clinical practice, and of that number 65 740, or 36.6 per cent, were owners of hospitals or clinics. Another 107 712 physicians, or 59.4 per cent of the total, engaged in clinical practice and were therefore salaried employees. There has been a steady trend toward salaried status in recent times that is likely to continue into the foreseeable future as the physician supply increases. While difficult to document, it seems that Japanese physicians are well rewarded by international standards and that medical practice offers an attractive career. Nevertheless the status and role of the Japanese physician within the medical care system as well as within society in general is changing. 'Doctor knows best' is no longer the unquestioned rule among patients, insurers, and public policy-makers (Steslicke, 1987; Takahashi, 1986).

Professional Associations

Nowhere is the changing status and role of Japanese physicians better reflected than in the organisation and activities of the Japan Medical Association (JMA). During the 1960s and 70s, the JMA was frequently compared with its American counterpart in terms of its influence on national health policy. Although the JMA was never able to initiate important policy changes, even at the peak of its power, it was nevertheless a force to be contended with and could often veto the best laid plans of others in the health policy arena. Under the leadership of Dr. Taro Takemi, who was president from 1957 to 1980, the JMA was the major voice for Japanese physicians in general, even though it more clearly reflected the interests and concerns of self-employed, owner-managers than of salaried physicians. Dr. Takemi, popularly known as *kenka Taro* ('contentious Taro'), enjoyed celebrity status in Japan and was also well-known and respected in international medical circles. Since his retirement and death in 1982, JMA political influence has declined as a consequence of a number of factors – some related to the internal politics of the organisation itself and others related to the changing nature of national health policy priorities and processes (Takahashi, 1986).

Although the JMA remains the largest and most influential of the various physicians' organisations at the national or regional levels, its membership has declined from well over 90 per cent of all Japanese physicians thirty years ago to under 60 per cent at present as newer, more specialised associations have been formed and as the JMA itself has failed to appeal to younger salaried physicians in particular. Thus the role of professional associations in Japanese medical care remains strong in several dimensions (economic, occupational, social, educational, technological, philosophical, and political), even though the JMA is itself undergoing substantial change and can no longer mobilise Japanese physicians as it once did (Steslicke, 1972b; 1973; 1982; Takahashi, 1986).

Medical Care Facilities and Government

As in the case of medical care personnel, organisation of medical facilities in Japan is governed by national law. The basic governing statute is the Medical Service Law of 30 July 1948 that distinguishes between hospitals and clinics. Hospitals have 20 or more beds and must meet specified criteria relating to personnel and equipment in order to obtain approval of the prefectural governor of the area in which the facility is located. Those hospitals with 100 or more beds which offer internal medicine, surgery, obstetrics and gynaecology, ophthalmology, and ENT services, and which also have research, library and laboratory facilities, can qualify as 'general hospitals' if approved by the prefectural governor. Clinics, according to the Medical Service Law, are organisations with 19 or fewer beds and which are restricted to a length of stay of 48 hours. The Law reinforces the dominant role of the physician by requiring both hospitals and clinics to be managed by physicians.

In 1985 there were 9608 hospitals and 1 495 328 beds, 8527 of which were general hospitals with 1 080 419 beds, as indicated in Table 10.1. There were also 78 927 clinics with 283 390 beds. Table 10.1 also indicates the number of hospitals and hospital beds by type of hospital (mental, TB sanatoria, leproseria, infectious diseases, and general) and type of ownership. The categories are not entirely clear, but if we take public ownership to mean those facilities included in

Hospitals

	Total	State MOHW	State Other	Prefecture	Municipality	Japan Red Cross	Saiseikai, Hokkaido Social Activities Assoc.	Organisations	Companies	Public Corporations	Schools and other Corporations	Medical Care Corporations	Independents
Total	9 608	255	156	307	768	97	76	89	261	390	353	3 450	3406
Mental Hospitals	1 026	3	—	40	11	—	1	—	2	64	14	586	305
Tuberculosis Sanatoria	27	—	—	2	1	—	—	—	1	6	—	9	8
Leproseria	16	13	—	—	—	—	—	—	—	2	1	—	—
Hospitals for Infectious Diseases	12	—	—	1	11	—	—	—	—	—	—	—	—
General Hospitals	8 527	239	156	264	745	97	75	89	258	318	338	2 855	3 093

Beds

	Total	State MOHW	State Other	Prefecture	Municipality	Japan Red Cross	Saiseikai, Hokkaido Social Activities Assoc.	Organisations	Companies	Public Corporations	Schools and other Corporations	Medical Care Corporations	Independents
Total	1 495 328	107 170	55 580	83 780	155 406	37 723	19 888	15 866	74 504	87 450	87 439	506 500	264 022
Mental Beds	334 589	6 967	2 323	17 134	8 029	1 802	538	308	3 883	27 664	8 231	195 512	62 198
Tuberculosis Beds	55 230	19 829	1 592	5 192	7 235	1 757	453	245	3 246	3 893	1 674	6 553	3 561
Leprosy Beds	10 471	10 314	—	—	—	—	—	—	—	125	32	—	—
Beds for Infectious Diseases	14 619	1 163	140	2 203	8 101	915	192	114	1 193	258	126	214	—
General Beds	1 080 419	68 897	51 525	59 251	132 041	33 249	18 705	15 199	66 182	55 510	77 376	304 221	198 263

Source National Federation of Health Insurance Societies (KEMPOREN) (Tokyo: KEMPOREN, 1987) p. 181.

the state, prefecture, and municipality categories, with all others as private, then clearly the majority of Japanese hospitals and hospital beds are in the private sector. In fact it is estimated that about 79 per cent of hospitals and 60 per cent of hospital beds, plus more than 90 per cent of clinics are 'privately' owned and operated. If one were able to delve more deeply into public financing and subsidisation of ostensibly private sector medical facilities however, the picture would be even more cloudy – but the basic point would still obtain; that is, medical services in contemporary Japan are delivered mainly through non-government providers.

There is an important caveat. The figures show that direct governmental provision of medical services is substantial. Indeed public hospitals are of generally high quality and prestige. Historically they have played a leadership role in education, research, and technological development – and they have also demonstrated that they can be effective competitors in the medical care marketplace (to the chagrin of non-governmental providers). During the next few years there will be some trimming of public facilities and services, especially those under national government auspices, but the 'privatisation' impulse will not result in major surgery (Koseisho, 1989).

Financing Mechanisms: Blurring of Public and Private

When we look at the way in which Japanese citizens pay for medical care services, the distinction between public and private becomes even more blurred. Japan has a system of compulsory, universal, and comprehensive sickness insurance that covers virtually the entire population. It is based on the contributory principle and includes premiums, co-payments, and taxes for the vast majority of insurees under one of the several insurance schemes. Because the system is quite complex, it is impossible to describe in detail here. However the main features of the system are indicated in Table 10.2.

Note that the employee based component has three major subdivisions. The first, based on the Health Insurance Law of 1922 as amended, offers coverage to both regular and temporary workers. The former are organised into government managed groups (for which the national government serves as insurer), and into 1777 privately managed health insurance societies that serve as insurer-managers. The second major subdivision for seamen is the smallest of the three employment based schemes and national government

Table 10.2 Japanese health insurance system in 1987

Scheme	Insurer (as of March 31, 1987)	Number of Insured Persons (As of March 31, 1987) insured persons / dependents — Unit: 10,000 persons	Insurance benefits — Medical care benefits: Medical benefits	Dependents' medical expenses	High-cost medical expenses	Cash benefits	Financial resources insurance Contribution	National government subsidy for medical care benefits costs	Percentage receiving health and medical services for the aged (%) (as of March 31, 1986)
Employee's Health Insurance — Health Insurance — Regular Employees — Government-Managed Health Insurances	National Government	3,262 / 1,543 / 1,719	90%, 80% from day following Diet approval	• Inpatient 80% • Outpatient 70%	Patient maximum deductible: ¥54,000 (¥30,000 for low income persons)	• Injury and sickness allowance • Maternity allowance • Delivery expenses, etc.	8.3%; Special insurance contributions 1% (Since March, 1986)	16.4% of benefits costs	4.2
Society Managed Health Insurances	Health Insurance Societies 1,777	3,005 / 1,302 / 1,703	Same as above (additional benefits available)	Same as above (additional benefits available)	• Total medical expenses per household (When 2 or more payments exceeding ¥30,000 each (¥21,000 each for low income households) are made, benefits cover the total expense.)	Same as above (additional benefits available)	8.103%. (Average for all societies, as of March 31, 1987)	¥6,700 million as benefit cost assurance (Fiscal 1987)	2.8
Day Labourers Health Insurance	National Government	23 / 15 / 8	*Deductible will be ¥100, ¥200 or ¥800 depending on cost of medical treatment provided at desired medical facility, total bill not to exceed ¥3,500.	• Inpatient 80% • Outpatient 70%	Same as above	Same as above (additional benefits available)	Grade I ¥840 per day; Grade II ¥1,970 per day (Since April, 1986)	14.4% of benefit costs	14.3
Seamen's Insurance	National Government	54 / 17 / 37	Same as above	Same as above		Same as above (additional benefits available)	8.2% (Since April, 1981)	None	5.4
Mutual Aid Association Insurance — National Public Service MAAs (27 MAAs) — Local Public Service MAAs (54 MAAs) — Private School Teachers and Employes MAA (1 MAA)		1,235 / 520 / 715 (As of March 31, 1986)		Same as above (additional benefits available)	Abatement to households with repeated application (Patient deductible is lowered to ¥30,000 (¥21,000 for low income households) from the 4th application made in 12 months.)	Same as above (additional benefits available)	6.50 – 11.014% (As of March 31, 1987)	None	3.8
National Health Insurance — Agricultural Workers, Self-employed, etc.	Cities, towns, villages 3,270; National Health Insurance Associations 167	4,529	70%		Abatement for patients suffering from diseases requiring costly treatment (Patient deductible is ¥10,000 for hemophilia and those suffering from chronic insufficiency of the kidneys requiring regular dialysis.)	• Midwifery expenses • Funeral expenses • Nursing allowances, etc. (Optional)	Contributions based on individual income, assets etc.	50% of benefit costs; 32% – 52% of benefit costs	12.4
Retirees from Employees' Insurance	Cities, Towns, Villages — National Health Insurance Associations 297 (As of March 31, 1986)		Insured person: 80%, Dependents: inpatient 80%, outpatients 70%			Provided by each insurer of health insurance		None	
Health and Medical Services for the Aged (End of fiscal 1987)	[Operating entity] Head of city, town or village	5,312 — Employees Insurance 1,883 — National Health Insurance 3,429	Patient cost sharing Outpatient: ¥800 per month Inpatient: ¥400 per day (¥300 per day maximum two months for low income persons)				[Share of costs] National government 2/10; Local governments 0.5/10, 0.5/10; Insurers of each health insurance 7/10		

Source Ministry of Health and Welfare (KOSEISHO) 1988; Health and welfare services in Japan, 1988 (Tokyo: Japan International Corporation of Welfare Services) p. 45.

serves as insurer-manager. The third subdivision includes three categories of mutual-aid associations (MAAs), as indicated in Table 10.2, that serve as insurer-managers for their respective members. Note here that there were 27 MAAs for national public employees, 54 MAAs for local public employees, and 1 MAA for private school teachers and employees.

Roughly 62 per cent of the Japanese people are covered by statutory, employment based insurance. Of that percentage, about 43 per cent are part of what might be considered *public* schemes and 25 per cent are part of *private* schemes. Historically those employees and dependants covered by privately managed health insurance societies and mutual-aid associations were favoured both in terms of benefits and costs. This was often pointed to as one manifestation of Japan's 'dual economy' (Steslicke, 1982a) but the disparity has lessened in recent years.

Table 10.2 indicates the medical care and cash benefits to which workers and dependants covered by employment based insurance are currently entitled. Especially noteworthy is the 'high-cost medical expenses' feature that applies to all schemes. In effect it establishes an individual and household monthly cap on insuree cost-sharing of either 54 000 yen or 30 000 yen, depending on an income of 10 000 yen per month for insurees requiring continuous and expensive treatment for long periods of time. Regardless of the remaining disparities in cost-sharing and benefit structure between the various schemes, this feature is quite generous by international standards and greatly reduces the risk of sickness-related poverty for Japanese citizens. Employees and dependants covered by Seamen's Insurance and by the various mutual-aid societies, as indicated on Table 10.2, also enjoy entitlement to the high-cost feature and benefits and costs similar to those provided for in the Health Insurance Law.

Japanese citizens not covered by one or another of the employment based schemes are entitled to coverage under the National Health Insurance Law of 1958 as amended. A revision of the original National Health Insurance Law of 1938 that applied mainly to the rural population, the new law required every city, town, or village in Japan that had not already done so to institute an insurance scheme for residents by 1 April 1961. This meant extending health insurance coverage to 25 million persons (or roughly 30 per cent of the total population) not previously covered, including agricultural workers and the self-employed. Foreigners are also eligible for coverage, as are retirees from employment based insurance schemes. As Table

10.2 indicates, in 1987, 3270 cities, towns and villages under 167 National Health Insurance Associations covered over 45 529 000 self-employed, agricultural workers, and dependants as well as over 2 970 000 retirees. This totalled over 37 per cent of the population covered by National Health Insurance. The benefit structure is similar to that of employment based schemes with one notable exception. Whereas the cost-sharing for the former is 30 per cent of charges, it is 10 per cent (but soon to be 20 per cent) for the latter. Thus, in terms of a rough public-private distinction, in 1987 about 75 per cent of the population was covered by sickness insurance that was publicly based.

Administrative–Policy Network

Under all health insurance schemes, medical care providers are reimbursed on a fee-for-service basis in accordance with national fee schedules determined annually by the Ministry of Health and Welfare (MOHW), in consultation with the Central Social Insurance Medical Council composed of provider, consumer, insurer, and government representatives. The detailed fee schedules assign points for different services and medications (each point is worth 10 yen) and providers are reimbursed for total points. The current schedules were established in 1958 and were revised upwardly every two or three years during the 1960s and 70s. During the 1980s however, annual increases were slight (0.3 per cent in 1983; 2.8 per cent in 1984; 3.3 per cent in 1985; and 2.3 per cent in 1986). Provider claims submitted to insurers are reimbursed through the Social Insurance Medical Care Fee Payment Fund, with branches of the Prefectural Federation of Health Insurance Association located in each prefecture, which are authorised to review and adjust claims. As part of its cost containment effort, the MOHW encouraged more stringent auditing of provider claims during the late 1980s. The health insurance administrative process and the relationship between contributions, benefits, and payments, as well as the major agencies involved, are depicted in Figure 10.1.

Of course it is the MOHW that assumes major responsibility for administration of the medical security system at the national level, and for health and welfare matters in general. It oversees the administrative and programmatic activities of prefectural and local governments in that regard and is headed by a minister of cabinet rank. The nine bureaux, two departments, separate Social Insurance

258

Figure 10.1 Japanese health insurance administrative process

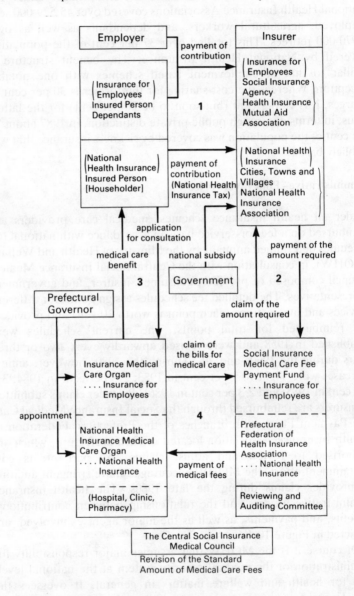

Source Social Insurance Agency, Japanese Government; *Outline of Social Insurance in Japan, 1987* (Tokyo: Social Insurance Agency, 1987) p. 120.

Agency, nineteen affiliated agencies, and the various regional and local branch offices that comprise the MOHW play the major role in health and welfare policy planning and administration, but they also share jurisdiction and compete with a number of other powerful national government agencies. These include the Ministry of Finance, the Ministry of Education, Science and Culture, the Ministry of Labour, the Ministry of Construction, the Ministry of Home Affairs, the Economic Planning Agency and the National Land Agency. Also, the Social Security System Council, attached to the Office of the Prime Minister, and the Economic Council of the Economic Planning Agency participate in the health and welfare administrative–policy network, as do a number of advisory councils attached to the MOHW itself (for example, Social Insurance Council, Central Social Insurance Medical Council, Central Pharmaceutical Affairs Council, Medical Service Council, Medical Service Facilities Council, Public Health Council, and others).

This complex administrative–policy network functions within the broader context of Japanese national government, which greatly resembles that of European parliamentary systems (Baerwald, 1986). Since 1955 the conservative Liberal-Democratic Party (LDP) has held a majority of seats in both houses and has been one of the dominant forces in Japanese politics and administration in general, as well as in the medical security arena (Sato and Matsuzaki, 1986; Hrebenar, 1986).

The medical security administrative–policy network is thus part of a broader network of governmental institutions and agencies that is not always easy to sort out. Among the non-governmental partici-pants in the network are about fifty national associations representing provider, consumer, insurer, business and management, labour, and other interests as well as many academic, professional, journalistic, and other consultants and 'experts' who interact with the appointed and elected government officials and interest group representatives in the kind of policy community or network that is both 'patterned' and 'pluralistic' (Steslicke, 1987, 1982). It also tends to be a relatively stable community of full-time professionals who see each other in Diet committee meetings, advisory council sessions, public and private study groups – of which there are many – task forces, seminars and social gatherings, and various other institutionalised channels for communication and decision-making. Informally, it is something of an 'old-boy' network, in which there are few strangers and few surprises, and in which the *amakudari* ('descent from heaven') practice tends to be followed (retired MOHW officials, for example, are able to find positions in the Diet or with various interested associations on whose behalf they deal with former associates and subordinates in the ministry).

Although this is the more or less normal, or routine, administrative–policy network – the 'mainstream' through which most health and welfare related actions have flowed during the 1980s (including the 'rationalisation' policy developments to be described later) – 'privatisation' initiatives in the medical security arena did not follow the same course. As will be seen, the opening of the private health insurance market emerged from a quite different administrative–policy network with the Ministry of Finance and the private insurance industry as the major actors. The result has been an uneasy convergence of two separate policy streams in which the direction of future policy flows is uncertain.

Public and Private Sectors in Modern Japan

Japan has become one of the leading members of the advanced, industrial, capitalist club of nations. However its membership is relatively new and Japan is regarded as a 'late moderniser' in comparison with the leading Western members of the club. Although 'late', Japan's development and modernisation were 'rapid' and membership was achieved in less than a century. In retrospect, it seems quite remarkable that Japan was able to overcome numerous obstacles both foreign and domestic – especially those present in the early days of modernisation. How and why Japan was able to overcome those early obstacles is subject to different interpretations. According to one major interpretation: 'With the Meiji Restoration (1868), Japan came to be governed by a political elite convinced that rapid, state-directed industrialisation was the key to national survival, and that ultimately this would provide the basis on which to build an internationally powerful Japan' (Pempel, 1984, pp. 47–8). Even if the members of the Meiji political elite had a socialist model before them, it is unlikely they would have opted for it. Capitalism as they observed it in the West was not only the most plausible model available to them but it also seemed most consistent with their own values. However, they were not impressed with the 'night watchman' theory of the capitalist state. In effect, what they and their successors saw as most appropriate for Japan was what Pempel refers to as 'state-led capitalism'. Thus, during the past century, 'capitalism' has held sway in Japan but the state has continued to play a major role in directing economic development (Johnson, 1982). State intervention has varied from time to time in keeping with changing domestic and international circumstances but 'state-led capitalism' persists. The recent emphasis on utilising the 'vitality of the private sector' is not inconsistent with that historical pattern. Moreover contemporary 'privatisation' of public services has precedents in modern Japanese history. It should be viewed from that peculiar national historical perspective as well as in the broader, international context of deregulation and privatisation developments in other major industrial nations during the 1980s.[1]

'Privatisation' of Public Services in Contemporary Japan

To say that Japan's national policy-makers discovered the 'vitality of the private sector' in the early 1980s would be absurd. Private production and distribution of goods and services for profit have been the major forces in Japan's modern economic development. Also, as in other capitalist nations, private investment decisions have had a substantial impact on Japanese political development. Several generations of the nations' political leaders have been committed to nurturing conditions favourable to the success of Japan's corporate community and have been rewarded for their efforts in various ways. Recently the reciprocal relationship has been referred to pejoratively as 'Japan, Inc.' (Pempel, 1987).

Nevertheless, the slogan 'vitality of the private sector' has been ubiquitous in national policy pronouncements during the 1980s as though it had indeed been newly discovered. For example, in the national economic and social plan adopted by the Japanese Government in 1983 (Outlook and Guidelines for the Economy and Society in the 1980s) that embraced the goal of 'building a creative and stable society', it is also emphasised that the Japanese government 'should try to build up an environment in which the private sector can be brought into full play and the whole nation can display its creative ability amid new changes and respond positively to the new requirements of the economy and society' (Economic Planning Agency, 1983, p. 10).

Although such pronouncements served rhetorical or symbolic purposes and offered reassurances to the Japanese business community regarding the importance of their contributions to the economy and the society, the fact is that the renewed emphasis on the 'vitality of the private sector' has also led to many significant tangible and instrumental changes in various policy sectors. While this wave of privatisation is by no means a case of history repeating itself, and the 1980s were quite different from the 1880s, there is at leat one similarity to the experience of the past. In both periods, 'privatisation' was undertaken by the Japanese government for apparently pragmatic political and economic reasons – to promote efficiency whilst also reducing the size of government as well as national budget deficits – and not for what could be termed mainly *ideological* reasons. More specifically, it is difficult to see recent governmental actions as primarily an expression of the kind of 'neo-liberalism' that has been so influential in Great Britain and the United States during the 1980s. This is not to say that there have not been strong advocates and admirers of such tendencies in Japan (Takenaka, 1987). Ronald Reagan and Margaret Thatcher have had many avid admirers in Japan, including former Prime Minister Yasuhiro Nakasone (Pyle, 1987). However, the Japanese-style neo-liberals seem not to have been as influential in Japanese national policy circles as elsewhere. More important, the concept of a 'Japanese-style welfare society' remains a basic component of LDP social policy rhetoric, as well as part of the reality of everyday life in the polity they hope to continue to manage (Jiyu-Minshuto, 1989, pp. 337–61).

THE 'JAPANESE-STYLE' WELFARE-STATE AND THE CONSERVATIVE PARTY STRATEGY

At the time of its establishment in 1955, the LDP declared itself to be among other things 'a force aiming for the realisation of a welfare state' (Kishimoto, 1988, p. 96) and its initial platform called for the construction of a welfare-state (*fukushi-kokka*) in Japan (Jiyu-Minshuto, 1988). In 1957 Prime Minister Tanzan Ishibashi called for the construction of a Japanese welfare-state and the immediate extension of health insurance coverage to the whole population. His successor, Nobusuke Kishi, assumed responsibility for the implementation of the LDP sponsored programme of 'Health Insurance for the Whole Nation' (*Kokumin kai-hoken*) as well as enactment of other welfare-state measures. Under the leadership of Prime Minister Hayato Ikeda in 1960, the LDP adopted a new platform that declared:

The expansion of social security is an important pillar of the new policy. With the aim of building a welfare state (*fukushi-kokka*), our party has provided health insurance for the whole nation as well as national pensions, but as part of the new policy, an epoch-making expansion of social security will be carried out so as to guarantee that there will not be a single hungry or poverty-stricken person in the nation (Jiyu-Minshuto, 1961, p. 657).

Although Ikeda did not preside over 'an epoch-making expansion of social security' during his time as Prime Minister, he and his immediate successors continued to support the concept of a welfare-state for Japan. The social policy measures instituted in the 1950s provided the foundation for renewed efforts in the early 1970s that did culminate an 'epoch-making' growth that closed the gap between welfare-state rhetoric and reality. Of course the LDP's commitment to the Japanese welfare-state was consistent with its support for Japanese capitalism and the prosperity of a business community that would continue to fund the Party's electoral success (Calder, 1988).

It was also consistent with what has come to be known as the 'conservative party line' (*hoshu honryu*) that has served as the general political strategy of the ruling LDP since at least the mid-1950s and been followed, though by no means uniformly, by a succession of Japanese prime ministers beginning with Shigero Yoshida. MacDougal points out that:

The trajectory of postwar Japan was to an extraordinary extent set during Yoshida Shigeru's tenure as Prime Minister (22 May 1946 to 20 May 1947 and 15 October 1948 to 7 December 1954) and maintained on its course by his chosen political successors, who dominated the leadership of the ruling party and the government for over two decades from 1960 (1988, p. 55).

The 'Yoshida vision' that subsequently became institutionalised as *honshu honryu* 'gave the conservatives an identity based on pragmatism, economic priorities, and flexibility, rather than on traditional values or an inflexible symbolic ideology' (Muramatsu and Krauss, 1987, pp. 521–2).

Indeed, economic priorities have driven the national policy agenda in contemporary Japan. However it is important to note that *honshu honryu* also emphasised political and social stability as an intrinsic aspect of the conservative strategy and accepted that the emergence of a 'Japanese style' welfare-state would further the LDP's interrelated economic, political and social goals. In other words, 'growth Japan' would also mean development of 'welfare Japan'.

The medical security system became the foundation for that development, and social insurance became the major instrument for implementing social policy in general. Public health programmes were also fostered by national, regional, and local governments, and such programmes were of great importance in the immediate postwar period and contributed to the Japanese 'health miracle' (Steslicke, 1987). However it was the medical care security system and its perceived relationship to economic productivity, as well as enhanced political and social stability, that elicited greater support from Japan's conservative political elite, including both management and labour organisations.[2]

MEDICAL CARE SECURITY POLICY OUTCOMES: 'RATIONALISATION ' AND 'PRIVATISATION'

Although Japan was regarded by many as a welfare 'laggard' during the first two decades after World War II, the fact is that significant welfare-state measures were introduced during that time, including the establishment of the universal, comprehensive, and compulsory health insurance system in 1961. With the subsequent economic growth came demands for expansion of social benefits and amenities that could not be ignored by conservative policy-makers who wished to remain in power. In 1973, generally referred to in Japan as 'the first year of welfare' (*fukushi gannen*), the LDP responded to a combination of mass-media and grass roots pressures as well as intra-party rivalry that led to the institution of the truly 'epoch-making' programme of virtually free medical care for the elderly (Campbell, 1984).

This provides a good illustration of what Calder refers to as 'strategic benevolence'.[3] According to Calder, 'Many of the policy decisions, such as that regarding free medical care for the aged, were made in late 1971 and early 1972 in response to previous moves by progressive local governments and in anticipation of upcoming national elections where LDP success was problematic'. He goes on to note that decisions to further expand various welfare measures were also taken in 1973 'as the LDP's political plight and the strength of the Left became dramatically clear' (1988, p. 372). Calder writes:

New welfare policies emerging during this period included the Children's Allowance (implemented during January 1972–April 1974), free medical care for the elderly (January 1973), indexation of welfare pensions to the inflation rate (1973), sharp increases in both Employees' Pension and the National Pension (1973), major increases in reimbursement provisions under National Health Insurance (October 1973), and provision of intracorporate retraining subsidies to reduce economic pressures to lay off employees (December 1974). Together these measures brought per capita entitlement standards for many Japanese welfare programs close to Western European levels and introduced several programs, such as the children's allowance, which did not exist in the United States (1988, pp. 372–3).

Although some complained that Japan was becoming a 'welfare superstate' and warned of the dangers of incipient 'English disease', the welfare-state measures cited by Calder were also seen as a way to stimulate domestic demand at a time of growing surpluses in Japan's international payments balance following the 1971 'Nixon shock'. The new welfare-state measures also had popular support and the LDP's 'strategic benevolence' was rewarded at the polls accordingly.

As it turned out however, Japan's 'first year of welfare' was soon being thought of as possibly 'the last year of welfare'. Even before the second oil crisis of 1979, the increased costs of the new welfare-state measures, as well as what was seen as an inequitable distribution of costs and benefits in health and welfare programmes, generated discomfort in the high-level, conservative political and business community. Free medical care for the elderly proved especially worrisome, and both national and local government finances were strained by the rapid growth in population of those aged 65 and over which nearly doubled between 1960 and 1980. During the same period, medical care costs increased by 29 times and the ratio of medical care costs to national income rose from 3.1 per cent to 6.0 per cent. As might have been expected, the increased medical care costs of the elderly were striking; a sixfold increase between 1973 and 1981 (Ishimoto, 1989). Thus it was that the medical care security system came to be viewed as problematic by national policy-makers along several dimensions – but especially the financial!

As Japan entered the 1980s, the environment of the medical care security system had also changed dramatically (Lincoln, 1988; Yashiro, 1987). The combination of international and domestic economic circumstances, demographic changes, national fiscal distress, new ideological currents in Japan and abroad, plus the internal organisational and financial problems within the medical care security system itself, stimulated a sense of malaise and of the need for curative state intervention. For some Japanese policy-makers, deregulation and 'privatisation' appeared to be an approach whose time had come. For others, state initiated 'rationalisation' seemed more appropriate. It will be seen that state intervention in the Japanese medical care security system during the 1980s followed both approaches and resulted in a *convergence* of two initially separate policy-making networks – what might be thought of as a 'rationalisation stream' and a 'privatisation stream'.

The 'Rationalisation' Policy Stream

Medical care security policy outcomes flowing from the 'rationalisation' stream during the 1980s addressed both demand and supply issues. Ministry of Health and Welfare (MOHW) officials have navigated a course through sometimes murky and generally turbulent waters. Moving in the direction of the goals articulated by Japan's conservative political and business leaders in various national policy pronouncements during the decade, they appear to have enhanced their potential for influencing the course of medical care security policy development during the 1990s. Although still very much in the water, the JMA was not able to prevent enactment of various measures it opposed during the early 1980s, and is now riding in the wake generated by the MOHW's policy crew (Takahashi, 1986; Fujii and Reich, 1987).

Much of the MOHWs course had been charted and many of the crew assembled by 1982, when the Health Care for the Aged Law was enacted and Japan's experiment with free medical care for the elderly came to an end. Taking their cue from the concerns being expressed over governmental spending by top political and business leaders, MOHW officials seized the initiative by establishing a Medical Insurance for the Aged Policy Headquarters within the Ministry in June 1980 to draft a bill that would reorganise financing and delivery of medical care services for the elderly. The MOHW bill was endorsed by the Cabinet and sent to the Diet in May 1981 and, after heated debates and some delays, was passed in August 1982. In addition to instituting a small co-payment for those 70 years and older (disabled and bedridden of 65 years and older) for medical care services, significantly the law provided for the institution of various health promotion and health education programmes for the elderly, as well as a plan to integrate medical and social welfare services. Most important perhaps, it instituted a cost-sharing mechanism requiring contributions to the new scheme from existing employment-based insurance schemes. (Campbell, 1989; Steslicke & Kimura, 1985).

In a richly detailed study of the series of events leading to enactment of the new law and of subsequent MOHW activities, Campbell emphasises the emergence of Ministry leadership in the health policy arena *vis-à-vis* both the JMA and the LDP, as well as other organisations active in the health policy community. MOHW officials acted quickly to maintain their momentum and to stay on their charted course. According to Campbell:

> Welfare Ministry actions following passage of the Health Care for the Aged Law were consistent with an interpretation that officials were following a conscious strategy of reshaping the health care system. It created a new agency, quickly moved to bring local government in line, forced a radical reform in hospital administration, and in 1984 managed to pass – against tough opposition – a major reform of the overall health insurance system which included an extension of the logic of cross-subsidisation in health insurance to a new group. The process of top-down, bureaucratic-dominated policy change was continued (1989, IX–12).[4]

Actually two new agencies were created. One was the Health Care for the Aged Deliberation Council under the jurisdiction of the MOHW, and the second was the Headquarters for Promoting Comprehensive Measures for National Medical Care Costs Rationalisation withih the MOHW. Established in October 1982 and headed by the Vice-Minister, the Headquarters were designed to serve as the 'nerve-centre' for the rationalisation strategy. They quickly formulated a short-term and long-term agenda related to both supply and demand issues (JICWELS, 1983, pp. 17–18).

That agenda was incorporated into the 27th Annual Report on Health and Welfare, published in October 1983 and appropriately subtitled, 'The Trend of a New Era and Social Security'. Taking note of past developments of the social security system during the period of high economic growth, and the fact that Japan had become 'an affluent society' that accounted for 10 per cent of the world's GNP, the Report announced to the Japanese people:

The first basic proposition of this Annual Report is that in Japan, which has now become an affluent society, the future course for social security shall no longer follow the same trends as hitherto. The era of extending the social security system and simply seeking quantitative improvements is probably at an end (p.1).

In a chapter titled 'Medical Care Security to Comply with the Times', the implications of 'the first basic proposition' were spelled out in considerable detail with respect to such medical care supply-side factors as personnel, facilities, new technology, drug production and distribution, emergency medical services, the relationship of medical treatment, prevention and rehabilitation services, and 'systematisation of medical care services in the regions'. With respect to the latter, it was pointed out that the MOHW had drafted an amendment to the Medical Services Law (that had already been presented to the Diet) which called for the formulation of regional medical plans within each prefecture dealing with distribution and coordination of medical personnel and facilities.

This was a bold revival of the kind of regional planning that the MOHW had long favoured and that the JMA had long-opposed. it further underscored the Ministry's determination to push its reform programmes forward. The Report itself was both a public expression of the determination as well as an effort to gain the kind of public understanding and support necessary to continue navigation in the increasingly turbulent 'rationalisation stream'. Noting that,

> whereas some are pursuing only expansion of benefits based on the recognition that the social security in Japan is lagging, others are voicing concern about the present situation and future prospects in the light of the long-term economic stagnation in the Western advanced countries.

The MOHW concluded:

> The course for social security for the future must be to aim for *the creation of a solid and vigorous welfare society* consonant with the new directions taken by the economy of the affluent society (p. 126, emphasis added).

Clearly, the 1983 Report does not anticipate dismantling of the Japanese welfare-state (in another passage, the Report refers to the 'consensus within the society as a whole in pursuit of a 'welfare state') and makes only passing reference to the 'vitality of the private sector'.

The next major medical care security policy outcome of the rationalisation process involved what Campbell refers to as 'an extension of the logic of cross-subsidisation in health insurance to a new group'. Once again MOHW officials quickly initiated actions leading to the modification of the National Health Insurance scheme to include a special plan for retirees not yet eligible for coverage under the Health Care for the Aged Law. Such individuals and their dependants (who were no longer eligible for benefits under prior employment-based health insurance coverage) had become a strain on the financial resources of the community-based National Health Insurance programmes. MOHW officials devised an amendment to the law calling for mandatory contributions from health insurance societies to the special plan for retired persons. As passed in August 1984, the amendment also allowed health insurance societies to continue coverage for employees after retirement and to have their contributions to the National Health Insurance-based scheme for retirees reduced accordingly. This was generally regarded as another significant cost-shifting, cost-containment measure sponsored by the MOHW to bolster its image and influence in the health care policy community – at the expense of the JMA and others.

Moreover it paved the way for termination of the Day Labourers Health Insurance scheme (that had also been consistently in the red) which was also absorbed into the newly subsidised National Health Insurance scheme and, with the strong support of the Ministry of Finance, the LDP and the business community in 1984, the institution of a 10 per cent co-payment for employment-based insurees. This was another example of the 'extension of the logic of cross-subsidisation' to one more new segment of the insured population.[5] All this time the MOHW was also using its regulatory authority, under the various health insurance laws, to monitor provider reimbursement more closely and thereby discourage many of the inflated claims and outright fraud that had been overlooked in the past. Although they were unhappy, providers seemed to respond by exercising greater self-restraint in filing reimbursement claims.

The crowning achievement for MOHW officials in the sequence of new medical care security policy outputs was the December 1985 enactment of the amendment to the Health Services Law mandating formulation of regional medical care plans by prefectural governments. This was first introduced into the Diet in 1983 and vigorously opposed by the JMA ever since. Following this major victory in the rationalisation process, the MOHW once again established a new internal agency (the National Headquarters for Comprehensive Medical Care Measures) in January 1987 to reassess the progress that had been made and to devise a long term plan to guide the continuing journey in the 'rationalisation stream'. Actually a revised set of long term goals had already been articulated with the MOHW (Koseisho, 1985; Saguchi, 1985, p. 286) and the new Headquarters was expected to reaffirm those goals and develop a more concrete implementation plan. An interim report was prepared by the Headquarters and was published by the MOHW in June 1987 (Ministry of Health and Welfare, 1988, pp. 14–15).

Interestingly it was at that high point in the 'rationalisation stream' in 1985 that MOHW officials moved closer to the *minkatsu* movement underway in other national policy sectors (as described earlier), with the strong support of conservative political and business leaders as well as influential national bureaucrats in the Economic Planning Agency (MITI) and the Ministry of Finance. Perhaps it is straining the metaphor (Kingdon, 1984) but what seemed to happen in 1985 was a convergence of the 'rationalisation stream' with one important tributary of the 'privatisation (main)stream'. Even though the preceding description has not captured the dynamics of the medical care security policy rationalisation process in depth, and has omitted mention of several important policy outputs related to hospitals, long-term care, drugs, medical technology, and health promotion programmes (not to mention concurrent developments related to rationalisation of the national pension system), it would be useful at this point to turn to a description of what was happening in the 'privatisation stream'.[6]

The 'Privatisation' Policy Stream

Both in terms of international standards and its role in the domestic economy, the Japanese private insurance industry is definitely 'big business'. Historically its products have been designed mainly for domestic consumption and it has been the beneficiary of a tightly protected market. This has allowed the industry to become a major player in the Japanese financial and investment capital marketplace, and recently to extend its investment activities abroad. During the past decade it has also been a major investor in Japanese government bonds, the issue of which has contributed to worrisome and controversial national deficits.

In addition to tending to the insurance business, it is well organised for dealing with the Japanese state. Among the numerous associations that provide representation for the industry, the two peak associations are the Marine and Fire Insurance Association of Japan and the Life Insurance Association of Japan. These associations have operated quite effectively in the political arena on behalf of the industry. Nevertheless it is currently facing the challenge of heightened domestic competition by foreign companies as a result of the high priority 'structural adjustment' policies being pursued by the Japanese government.

Foreign insurance companies have been trying to crack the Japanese market with relatively little success since the end of World War II (Murray, 1987) but they now find themselves with a window of opportunity. Several have already managed to set up business in Japan (Seki, 1982) and others are making plans for doing so. However it seems unlikely that the Japanese government and the powerful Ministry of Finance (MOF) will allow itself to be overwhelmed by foreign competition. In short the private insurance industry and the Japanese government seem to agree on the importance of the industry's role in the political-economic structure, and that the industry's capacity to compete in both domestic and foreign markets should be enhanced by a combination of judicious regulation and deregulation – administrative guidance and private sector vitality. The medical care security market provides one arena for the implementation of this strategy (Seki, 1986a, 1986b).

During most of its hundred year history, the Japanese private insurance industry has been closely regulated by the national government. The basic statute regulating the industry, the Insurance Business Law, was enacted in 1939 and has been supplemented by numerous amendments, laws, cabinet overs, ordinances, and other administrative instruments, including the Law Concerning Foreign Insurers of 1949. A key provision of the Insurance Business Law states: 'Insurance business . . . may not be carried on unless and until a license from the competent Minister has been obtained', (Article 1). The Minister of Finance has been designated the 'competent Minister' and a complex administrative apparatus for implementing this and other provisions of the law has evolved within the Ministry.

A second major provision states 'No insurance company may carry on life insurance and insurance against loss concurrently' (Article 7).

In effect this means that the private insurance industry in Japan, as in many other nations, has been divided into separate life and non-life components. Similar provisions are stated in the Law Concerning Foreign Insurers. The implications of these two provisions of the statutes as they relate to the medical security market require further discussion.

The Regulatory Nexus

MOF regulation of the private insurance industry is justified in terms of the public interest, and its authority is quite extensive. It should be noted that the Ministry has been one of the strongholds of Japanese national government for decades (Tsuji, 1984). Its officials are highly respected and manage to find choice post-retirement positions in business and politics. Naturally the private insurance industry has become the post-retirement home for many MOF officials, and their expertise and contacts have been an invaluable resource for the industry. It is an institutionalised communication and cooperation network that has facilitated 'administrative guidance' by MOF officials, as well as judicious use of their regulatory authority, with the result that the industry has been allowed to grow and prosper since World War II.

In addition to the licensing of both domestic and foreign companies, the MOF is authorised to issue notifications, instructions, recommendations, advice, information and encouragements related to practically all aspects of company operations, including investments. It is also authorised to require full information regarding company activities and to conduct unannounced inspections. During the immediate postwar era, such authority was fully utilised and the industry was among the most highly regulated in Japan. However there were trade-offs for the industry in what amounted to an 'escorted convoy' system that offered MOF protection against both foreign and domestic market threats. This was generally accepted as legitimate and proper within the industry until the late 1970s when a growing desire for greater 'flexibility and freedom' emerged. It included a desire to expand the very limited involvement in the medical security market and to develop other new products and investments. Generally the Ministry was sympathetic and responsive to industry desires and a liberalisation of administrative control in various areas was implemented. it was not simply a matter of bowing to the industry; there was also a growing concern regarding increased medical expenditures, rapidly aging society, cost containment and so on, and the realisation that the private insurance industry could play a more positive role in supplementing the social insurance system. One of the complicating factors was the ambiguous legal definition of the 'insurance business' and what was seen as a 'grey area' between the life and non-life components of the industry with respect to sickness insurance, among other matters.

The Life and Non-Life Insurance Business

As indicated, the Insurance Business Law requires national licensure and prohibits concurrent engagement in life and non-life insurance business. Article 5 of the Law provides that 'An insurance company may not carry on any other business'. Since the Law does not specify just what the 'insurance business' is, it is not clear what constitutes the 'other business' that is prohibited. Nor does the Law clearly specify the difference between 'life' and 'non-life' insurance. The legal ambiguity has persisted over the years while the operational distinction has been subject to 'administrative guidance' by the MOF. In other words the MOF has been in a position to say who could do what, when, and how with respect to the private insurance business. Although problematic, this was generally acceptable within the industry until recent times. However as the need for diversification and development of new products, in what had become a largely saturated domestic market, was recognised by both government and the industry in the late 1970s, the problem was intensified. One of the issues related to who should be allowed to do what, when and how in the medical security market. By the early 1980s the life and non-life components of the industry were in open conflict over that issue, among others, and were demanding a clarification that would permit them to compete for survival while also fulfilling the new expectations regarding their role in the economic restructuring process. For the most part they were eager to supplement the social insurance system but had vague and conflicting notions as to how to proceed. Major clarification was provided by the MOF Insurance Council in 1985 (The Life Insurance Association of Japan, 1986; The Marine and Fire Insurance Association of Japan, 1986).

The Insurance Council and Private Health Insurance

The Insurance Council was established by Cabinet Order in 1959 as an advisory body to the MOF. Members are appointed for two-year terms by the Finance Minister and may be reappointed. There are twenty members selected from among 'persons of knowledge and experience concerning insurance' and an unspecified number of temporary members who may be appointed by the Finance Minister from among 'persons of technical knowledge concerning insurance'. Of course the private insurance industry is well represented in both groups. Other members include academics, journalists, bureaucrats, business executives and 'public interest' representatives.

Since its establishment the Council has produced numerous reports and recommendations. For present purposes the Council's report of 5 May 1985 is of greatest significance. In that report the Council strongly endorsed the need for diversification and flexibility, deregulation and internationalisation, computerisation, and the development of new products related to medical and welfare services and annuities. The Council emphasised that such products should supplement the social insurance system and deal with cost sharing and other gaps in coverage (Seki, 1986a). This reinforced the position that the MOF and the private insurance industry had been moving towards. Although there was some resistance within the Ministry of Health and Welfare at first, by the end of the month the Council's report had been endorsed by the Minister and other leading members of the health policy community. The MOHW now takes the position that private insurance companies can make a valuable contribution in dealing with medical security problems in Japan's rapidly aging society by offering products that will supplement the social insurance system (Koseisho, 1989).

By the time that the 10 per cent cost-sharing provisions of the 1984 Health Insurance Law amendment were enforced (April 1, 1986), 73 private insurance companies had secured MOF and MOHW approval for new health insurance products that were then put on the market. Twenty-six life insurance companies were authorised to sell group policies to private corporations, labour unions, various government offices and other groups and associations. Those policies offered medical treatment, hospitalisation, private nursing care, and death benefits to supplement social insurance coverage for employees and their dependants. Forty-seven non-life insurance companies (21 domestic and 26 foreign) were authorised to sell both group and individual policies covering extra room and nursing charges, certain high-tech medical treatments specified by the Health and Welfare Ministry and excess medical expenses incurred during hospitalisation and not covered by social insurance.

Although private health insurance has not become the bonanza many in the industry hoped it would be, by 1988 the life insurance companies had over 30 million hospitalisation benefit riders in force and over 7 million riders related to degenerative disease benefits. Also over 12 million independent medical benefit policies of various types were in force. The non-life insurance industry had also issued over 17 million policies providing various types of medical benefits (Koseisho, 1989, p. 151). Even though most companies currently do not regard health insurance as a major product, they are optimistic regarding future developments and the probable emergence of an expanded market of elderly and middle-aged customers looking for luxury benefits not offered through the social insurance system, such as private hospital rooms, special meals and nursing expenses, extra charges for dental care, expensive high technology medical care services and home health care services. Increased patient cost-sharing under current health insurance schemes would also offer an expanded market for private health insurance products of special interest to the non-life insurance industry.[7]

CONCLUSIONS: JAPAN'S MIXED PUBLIC-PRIVATE MEDICAL CARE SECURITY SYSTEM

Döhler has pointed out that 'During the post-war decades conservative governments contributed to an almost comparable degree as social-democratic or socialist governments to the expansion of the welfare-state' (1987, p. 1). In Japan of course there have been no social democratic or socialist governments and conservative policy-makers have played *the* major role in building the Japanese welfare-state. Döhler also notes:

Since the first oil-price shock in 1973, conservatives started to rethink their commitment toward the welfare-state. During the 1970s a process of programmatic modernisation has taken place inside conservative parties which culminated in more or less radical anti-welfare state programs at the end of the decade (1987, p. 1).

A good deal of rethinking regarding the welfare-state and its alleged 'crisis' also took place in Japan but it did not culminate in 'more or less radical anti-welfare-state programmes'. Japanese conservatives have not sought to dismantle the structure of their welfare-state or to weaken its basic components. Indeed they have not hesitated to express their commitment to their vision of a 'Japanese style' welfare society – one that is based very heavily on the system of medical care security and health insurance developed by conservative governments in the post-war era.

To be sure, the medical care security system in general and the health insurance system in particular have been sources for concern within elite conservative circles in recent times, and a number of important 'reforms' were instituted during the 1980s. Even though there has been substantial cost-shifting within the system, such changes have not resulted in drastic cutbacks in the levels of financing or services previously established. Nor has there been notable 'privatisation' of what have come to be regarded as legitimate state interventions in the medical care security system. Instead conservative policy-makers have taken advantage of the impressive state capacity to intervene in the medical security system in order to initiate a series of incremental adjustments in response to their perceptions of the fiscal and demographic constraints associated with the new era of slower growth and the rapid aging of Japanese society. 'Rationalisation' and not 'privatisation' is a much better way to characterise the process (JICWELS, 1983).

Ideological considerations have not been absent during this time, but they have not blunted the basically pragmatic edge of Japanese conservatism (Curtis, 1988). This more or less 'realistic' approach to public policy-making, with a strong emphasis on 'practicality first' (Takeshita, 1988, p. 20), that has been embraced by their conservative predecessors since the end of World War II, has also been advocated by recent prime ministers (Kaifu, 1982) and was reflected in the development of medical care security policies during the 1980s. It is an important aspect of what Pempel has termed 'creative conservatism' and what Calder refers to as 'strategic benevolence'.

As a result of the application of this approach to health policy development during the 1980s, the Japanese government and the private insurance industry are providing the Japanese people with a mixed public–private medical care security system based on the social insurance model that has been incrementally developed since the 1920s. Although it is too early to evaluate, the most recent *rationalisation–privatisation* increments do not appear to be a step backward. In fact they may prove to be an enhancement of the already high degree of medical care security available to the Japanese people. So far they appear to have gained popular acceptance as well.

Notes

1. For historical analysis concerning government activities, see Smith, 1955; Pempel, 1982, p. 48. On strategic considerations, see Norman, 1975, pp. 232–4. For historical analysis of privatisation debate, see Norman, 1975, pp. 234–5; Pempel, 1982, p. 49.
2. Calder aptly notes: 'In common with conservative patterns in Germany and France, Japanese welfare policy has given early precedence to accident and health insurance, which enhances the prospect of a health work force. Although more than a generation behind Bismark, Japanese conservative leaders of the early twentieth century were influenced by his example in giving precedence to programmes which both reinforced industrial potential and indicated state concern for the rising working class. Early policy in conservative Third Republic France, like that in Japan, also broadly followed German priorities but failed to move significantly beyond the area of health policy' (1988, p. 352).
3. According to Calder, 'Welfare policy patterns, like their counterparts in the agricultural, small business, and regional policy areas, show the sensitivity of the Japanese state to grassroots pressures, especially once a critical threshold of public pressures is achieved. They also indicate the contrasting tendency toward inaction or retrenchment during periods of relative political stability. Expansion in welfare's share of the Japanese national budget has come in sudden surges during major periods of flux in national politics. Indeed, 95 per cent of the increase in welfare's budget share since the late 1940s came in six crucial years. In well over half the noncrisis years since 1949, welfare's share in the general account budget has actually declined, although the magnitude of retrenchment has not been sufficient to prevent a gradual ratcheting up of welfare budget shares due to the large increases during crisis years. Declines in welfare shares of the national budget occurred in seven of the ten years from 1976 to 1986, despite the steady aging of Japanese society during that period (1988, pp. 350–1).
4. He also notes: 'It is interesting, in fact, that unlike Britain and the United States, free-market ideology plays little role in the Japanese discussions of health care in this period. The sections on health care in the various Rincho reports could have been written by Welfare Ministry bureaucrats themselves (and in effect probably were). They included no evocations of free competition as a route to efficiency and no calls for a shift to private insurance' (1989a, IX-221).
5. Fujii and Reich conclude that: 'By reforming the health insurance system in 1984 and the pension system in 1985, Japan took two

important steps towards assuring the future stability of its social security system' (1988, p. 18). With respect to the 10 per cent cost-sharing amendment, they write: 'During parliamentary review of the amendment, the health consequences of cost sharing were widely debated. Despite opposition to the amendment from both the Japan Medical Association and the opposition parties, the proposed amendment passed the Diet with exceptional speed in August 1984. The Nakasone cabinet gave the amendment high priority, as an important step towards political stability. In order to remain as Prime Minister, Nakasone sought to demonstrate strong leadership within the Liberal Democratic Party and also against the opposition parties. Passage of the amendment also allowed the Health and Welfare Ministry's budget for the coming year to be reduced to the level required by overall austerity measures' (p. 18).

6. For the definitive treatment of pension reform in Japan, see Campbell (1989, pp. X-X-28). See also, Reed (1989); Rose & Shiratori (1986).

7. Ishimoto calls attention to another important facet of 'privatisation' in the medical care sector that has not been discussed in this paper. He points out that, in addition to private health insurance, 'the government has now recognised the advantages in using the private sector for business related to medical care. These include hospital management consultation, services consigned by hospitals (meal supply, cleaning, accounting), domiciliary medical care services (selling and renting nursing apparatus, provision of food materials for those with geriatric diseases, and medical care information services). While these services relating to medical care have only just started, if they effectively supplement the public-sector medical care and medical insurance services in responding to the needs of the public, their share of the total business will no doubt expand. It therefore follows that cooperation between the public and private sectors will be an important factor in medical care policy' (1989, p. 501).

References

Baerwald, H.H. (1986) *Party Politics in Japan* (Boston: Allen and Unwin).

Calder, K.E. (1989) *Crisis and Compensation: Public Policy and Political Stability in Japan, 1979–86* (Princeton University Press).

Campbell, J.C. (1989) *Policy Change: the Japanese Government and the Elderly* (Unpublished Ms.).

Choy, J. (1985) 'Japanese Public Corporations: New Tricks for Old Dogs', *JEI Report*, 26A, pp. 1–9.

Curtis, G.L. (1988) *The Japanese Way of Politics* (New York: Columbia University Press).

Döhler, M. (1987) 'Politics versus Institutions: Comparing Health Policy under Neo-Conservative Governments in Britain, the United States and West Germany', Paper prepared for the meeting of the 'Study Group Comparative Health Policy' of the International Political Science Association, Birmingham, England, 27–29 July.

Economic Planning Agency (1983), Japanese Government, 'Outlook and Guidelines for the Economy and Society in the 1980s (Tokyo: Ministry of Finance).

Economic Planning Agency (1988) Japanese Government, 'Economic Management within a Global Context' (Tokyo: Ministry of Finance).

Frenk, J. and A. Donabedian (1987) 'State Intervention in Medical Care: Types, Trends and Variables', *Health Policy and Planning*, no. 2, pp. 17–31.

Fujii, M. and M.R. Reich (1988) 'Rising Medical Costs and the Reform of Japan's Health Insurance System', *Health Policy*, no. 9, pp. 9–24.

Hrebenar, R.J. (1986) *The Japanese Party System: from One-Party Rule to Coalition Government* (Boulder and London: Westview Press).

Inoguchi, K. (1987) 'Prosperity without the Amenitites, in K.B. Pyle (ed.) *The Trade Crisis: How Will Japan Respond* (Seattle: Society for Japanese Studies) pp. 61–70.

Ishimoto, T. (1989) 'Japan's Medical Care Security System – Present Situation and New Policies, *Hogaku Kiyo*, no. 30, pp. 500–532.

Japan International Corporation of Welfare Services (JICWELS) (1983) 'Trends of Policies of Health Care Services in Japan: Rationalising Medical Care Costs,' (Tokyo: JICWELS).

Japanese National Committee (1986) International Council on Social Welfare, 'Social Welfare Services in Japan 1986' (Tokyo: JINCOSWO).

Kaifu, T. (1982) 'Liberal Democratic Party', in R. Shiratori (ed.) (Tokyo: Kodansha International) pp. 211–18.

Jiyu-Minshuto (1961) Sosenkyo No Iei To Shinseisaku No Gaihyo ('Meaning of the General Election and Comments on New Policy') in Kokkai Nenkan 1961 (Diet Yearbook 1961). (Tokyo: Kokkai Nenkan Hakkokai) pp. 657.

Jiyu-Minshuto Koho Iinkai (1988) '*Waga-to No Kihon Hoshin*' ('Our Party's basic policies') (Tokyo: Jiyu Minshuto).

Jiyu-Minshuto Koho Iinkai (1989) '*Jiyu-Minshuto: Seisaku No Kaisetsu*' (Liberal Democratic Party: policy commentary) (Tokyo: Jiyu-Minshuto).

Johnson, C. (1982) *MITI and the Japanese Miracle: the Growth of Industrial Policy, 1925–1975* (Stanford University Press).

Kingdon, J.W. (1984) *Agenda, Alternatives, and Public Policy* (Boston: Little, Brown).

Kishimoto, K. (1988) *Politics in Modern Japan: Development and Organisation*, (Tokyo: Japan Echo).

Kosei Tokei Kyokai (1986) '*Kokumin Eisei no Doko*' ('Trends in National Public Health') (Tokyo: Kosei Tokei Kyokai).

Koseisho (1985) '21 *Seiki Ni Mukete no Iryo Seido no Arikata ni Tsute*' ('The Medical Care System for the 21st Century') (Tokyo: Kosei Tokei Kyokai).

Koseisho (1989) '*Kosei Hakusho 63*' ('Welfare White Paper 1988'), (Tokyo: Kosei Tokei Kyokai).

Kumon, S. (1987) 'Dilemma of a New Phase: Can Japan Meet the Challenge?' in K.B. Pyle (ed.), *The Trade Crisis: How will Japan Respond?* (Seattle: Society for Japanese Studies), pp. 229–40.

Life Insurance Association of Japan (1986). 'Life Insurance Business in Japan' (Tokyo: Life Insurance Association of Japan).

Lincoln, E.J. (1988) *Japan Facing Economic Maturity* (Washington: The

Brookings Institution).

Long, S.O. (1987) 'Health Care Providers: Technology, Policy and Professional Dominance', in E. Norbeck and M. Lock (eds), *Health Illness and Medical Care in Japan: Cultural and Social Dimensions* (Honolulu: University of Hawaii Press) pp. 66–88.

Long-Term Outlook Committee (1983), Economic Council, Economic Planning Agency, *Japan in the Year 2000: Preparing Japan for an Age of Internationalisation, the Aging Society and Maturity* (Tokyo: The Japan Times).

MacDougall, T.E. (1988) 'Yoshida Shigeru and the Japanese Transition to Liberal Democracy', *International Political Science Review*, no. 9, pp. 55–69.

Marine and Fire Insurance Association of Japan, Inc. (1986) *Fact Book: Non-Life Insurance in Japan* (Tokyo: The Marine and Fire Insurance Association of Japan, Inc.).

Masaki, M. and A. Koizumi (1987) 'Increase in Life Expectancy at Birth in Japan: Some Implications for Variable Patterns of Decrease in Mortality', *Health Policy*, no. 7, pp. 41–8.

Murray, A. (1982) 'Foreign Non-Life Offices Find Regulations Too Restrictive – Forty Hold only 3% Share of Domestic Market', *Japan Insurance News*, no. 1, pp. 14–21.

Ministry of Health and Welfare (KOSEISHO) (1988) 'Health and Welfare Services in Japan' (Tokyo: Japan International Corporation of Welfare Services).

Ibid. (1983) 'Annual Report on Health and Welfare for 1983: the Trend of a New Era and Social Security' (Tokyo: Japan International Corporation of Welfare Services).

Muramatsu, M. and E. Krauss (1987) 'The Conservative Policy Line and the Development of Patterned Pluralism', in J. Yamamura and Y. Yasuba (eds), *The Political Economy of Japan: the Domestic Transformation*, vol. 1 (Stanford University Press) pp. 516–54.

National Federation of Health Insurance Societies (KEMPOREN) (1986) 'Health Insurance and Health Insurance Societies in Japan', (Tokyo: KEMPOREN).

Noguchi, Y. (1987) 'Public Finance', in K. Yamamura and Y. Yasuba (eds), *The Political Economy of Japan: Domestic Transformation*, Vol. 1 (Stanford University Press), pp. 186–222.

Norman, E.H. (1975) 'Japan's Emergence as a Modern State', in J.W. Dower (ed.), *Origins of the Modern Japanese State: Selected Writings of E.H. Norman* (New York: Pantheon Books) pp. 109–316.

Ohnuki-Tierney, E. (1984) *Illness and Culture in Japan: an Anthropoligical View* (Cambridge University Press).

Organisation for Economic Cooperation and Development (OECD) (1987) 'Financing and Delivering Health Care' (Paris: OECD).

Organisation for Economic Cooperation and Development (OECD) (1988) 'OECD Economic Surveys: Japan' (Paris: OECD).

Pempel, T.J. (1982) *Policy and Politics in Japan: Creative Conservatism* (Philadelphia: Temple University Press).

Pempel, T.J. (1987) 'The Unbundling of "Japan, Inc.": The Changing Dynamics of Japanese Policy Formation', in K.B. Pyle (ed.) *Trade Crisis:*

How Will Japan Respond? (Seattle: Society for Japanese Studies), pp. 117–52.

Pyle, K.B. (1987) 'In Pursuit of a Grand Design: Nakasone Betwixt the Past and the Future', in K.B. Pyle (ed.) *The Trade Crisis: How Will Japan Respond?* (Seattle: Society for Japanese Studies), pp. 5–32.

Reed, S.R. (1989) in J.P. De Sario (ed.), *International Public Policy Sourcebook: Health and Social Welfare* (New York: Greenwood Press), pp. 255–72.

Rose, R. and R. Shiratori (eds.) (1986) *The Welfare-State East and West* (New York: Oxford University Press).

Saguchi, T. (1985) '*Nihon no Iryo-Hoken to Iryo Seido*' ('Japan's Health Insurance & Medical Care System'), in Tokyo Daigaku Shakai Kagak Kenku-jo (eds), *Fukushi Kokka 5: Nihon no Keizai to Fukushi* (The Welfare-State 5: Japan's Economy & Welfare) (Tokyo: Daigaku) pp. 239–87.

Sato, S. and T. Matsuzaki (1986) *Jiminto Seiken (LDP Power)* (Tokyo: Chuo Koronsha).

Schieber, O.J. and J.P. Poullier (1989) 'International Health Care Expenditure Trends: 1987', *Health Affairs*, 8, 3, 169–77.

Seki, K. (1986a) 'Life Insurance Industry Must Respond to Greying Society', *Business Japan*, no. 1, pp. 49–51.

Seki, K. (1986b) 'Non-life Insurance Gaining Ground in Japan', *Business Japan*, no. 1, pp. 55–6.

Seki, T. (1982) 'Selling a Foreign Product in Japan: Cancer Insurance', (Tokyo: Sophia University Institute of Comparative Culture Business Series Bulletin No. 85).

Social Insurance Agency (1987), Japanese Government, 'Outline of Social Insurance in Japan', (Tokyo: Social Insurance Agency).

Smith, T.C. (1955) *Political Change and Industrial Development in Japan* (Stanford University Press).

Steslicke, W.E. (1972a) 'Doctors, Patients, and Government in Modern Japan', *Asian Survey*, no. 12, pp. 913–21.

Steslicke, W.E. (1972b) 'The Political Life of the Japan Medical Association, *The Journal of Asian Studies*, no. 31, pp. 841–62.

Steslicke, W.E. (1982a) 'Development of Health Insurance Policy in Japan', *Journal of Health Politics, Policy and Law*, no. 7, pp. 197–226.

Steslicke, W.E. (1982b) 'National Health Policy in Japan: From the "Age of Flow" to the "Age of Stocks"', *Bulletin of the Institute for Public Health*, no. 31, pp. 1–35.

Steslicke, W.E. (1982c) 'Medical Care in Japan: the Political Context', *Journal of Ambulatory Care Management*, no. 5, pp. 65–77.

Steslicke, W.E. (1987) 'The Japanese State-of-Health in the 1980s: a Political-Economic Perspective', in E. Norbeck and M. Lock (eds) *Health, Illness and Medical Care in Japan* (Honolulu: University of Hawaii Press) pp. 24–65.

Steslicke, W.E. (1989) 'Japan', in J.P. de Sario (ed.) *International Public Policy Sourcebook: Health and Social Welfare* (New York: Greenwood Press) pp. 89–116.

Steslicke, W.E. and R. Kimura (1985) 'Medical Technology for the Elderly in Japan', *International Journal of Technology Assessment in Health Care*, no. 1, pp. 27–39.

Takahasi, M. (1986) '*Nihon Ishikai no Seiji Kodo to Ishi Kettei*' (Political Activities and Decision-Making of the Japan Medical Association), In Minoro (ed.), *Nihonkei Seisaku Kettei no Henyo* (Transformation of Japanese-Style Policy Making) (Tokyo: Toyo Keizai Shimbunsha) pp. 237–66.

Takahashi, T. (1989) 'Jiyu-Minshuto no Iryo Seisaku' (The Liberal Democratic Party's Medical Care Policy', *Iryo*, 89, 5, p. 16.

Takenaka, I. 'New Growth through Privatisation', *Japan Echo*, 14, 4, pp. 47–52.

Takeshita, N. (1988) *For a Humanistic and Prosperous Japan: the Furusato Concept* (Tokyo: Simul International).

Tsuji, K. (1984) *Public Administration in Japan* (Tokyo University Press).

Yamamura, K. (1987) 'Shedding the Shackles of Success: Saving Less for Japan's Future', in K.B. Pyle (ed.) *The Trade Crisis: How Will Japan Respond?* (Seattle: Society for Japanese Studies) pp. 33–60.

Yashiro, N. (1987) 'Japan's Fiscal Policy: an International Comparison', *Japanese Economic Studies*, no. 16, pp. 34–59.

11 Conclusion: Grains Among the Chaff – Rhetoric and Reality in Comparative Health Policy

James W. Björkman

INTRODUCTION

The industrialised democracies of the world confront a complex dilemma. A seemingly insatiable demand for health care is outstripping supply, despite a relentless increase in the latter's share of national budgets and family incomes. Yet there is little corresponding rise in general health indices, or even in human happiness about the quality of medical services. The inability of health services to deliver greater health for more money has ironically not blunted the public's appetite for them; rather it has perversely increased it. Among the evident reasons for this paradox are that affluent humanity is less prepared than ever before to suffer minor ailments without drugs or other medical help; that demand for health care has been further stimulated both by new treatments for curable diseases and by expanded coverage throughout the poorer levels of society; that new cures for old diseases come with ever higher price tags for their sophisticated technology, so that much additional spending still saves few lives; and that the elderly, whose relative numbers in society are growing, require more routine medical care than the young. Clearly health services in the developed North are victims of their own successes.

The Third World also confronts dilemmas in health care but for different reasons. There, insufficient resources are allocated to developing human capital, while the scanty resources available are often consumed by capital-intensive, high-technology, low-productivity investments. Health services and facilities are undervalued in national development plans. Rhetoric notwithstanding, health service systems in the underdeveloped South are patterned after the urban-oriented preferences and requirements of former metropoles.

Without doubt health care has become a major component of the contemporary state. In every industrialised society it consumes significant proportions (6 per cent–12 per cent) of the Gross National Product, as well as placing increasing stress on government budgets. In developing countries, where it is estimated to consume 2 per cent or less of the GNP, health care must compete (usually unsuccessfully) for finance as a basic human need. Yet in all societies the health sector is a major source of employment and also affects the lives of all citizens. With so much at stake, arrangements for planning, financing, and operating health service systems have increasingly come to be regarded as important political issues. Of course politics permeates the very definition of health care *per se*, which can run from services provided by physicians to self-care, preventive medicine, nutrition, housing, even employment. However common usage equates health care with medical services provided through clinics and hospitals, a justifiable usage since medical services account for most health expenditures.

The political importance of health care derives partly from the evident contribution of adequate health services to the quality of human life, and so it is sought by both developed and developing societies. Political importance also derives partly from the increasing costs of these health services, a problem which is compounded because the direct contribution of health services to prolonged life expectancy, reduced morbidity, or other indicators of improved health in Western countries is increasingly marginal. Even in the Third World, investments in sanitation and clean water supplies yield greater direct benefits than the construction of more clinics and hospitals or the deployment of additional highly-trained medical personnel. Since all societies face limitations on resources and competing priorities about their allocation, the politically embarrassing fact has emerged that patients are receiving fewer unambiguously beneficial results despite higher expenditure.

This chapter summarises an explanatory political model that lies behind these dilemmas; reports some salient findings of field research in both the North and South; and discusses several methodological issues that confront comparative health policy research. The chapter ends with some speculation on the inherent problems of technological complexity and methodological mires in similar policy fields, and it suggests some lessons about the conduct of comparative field studies.

EXPLANATORY MODEL

The political elements in health care policy derive from an observation that the health sector has historically been a 'private government'. With few exceptions (confined to European countries in the last several centuries), the provision of medical services has been a private matter between supplier and consumer, between doctor–shaman–expert and patient–peasant–client. Power (the ability to change patterns of behaviour, to make others do what they would rather not do – or not do what they would rather do) over 'well-being' or personal health status was exercised by an active agent with specialised knowledge over a passive recipient without such knowledge or expertise. The concept of self-care obviously lies outside this political framework, although one might argue that the very act of removing oneself from a dyadic relationship is itself a political act.

The novel change in recent history has been the willingness, the readiness of governments to enter the domain of hitherto private relationships in order to regulate the behaviour of both sets of actors (providers and patients). The political mandate of proactive governments (howsoever elected, selected, ascertained) is exercised through their administrative machinery. In the present era, government agencies take the form of bureaucracies comprised of specialised roles based on the division of labour, which in turn are hierarchically arranged and accountable both within the organisation and, sometimes, externally to political leaders.

Consequently there are four broad categories of relevant actors in the health sector of contemporary nation-states. These categories are (1) the political leaders (or politicians) who represent (whether badly or adequately) the views and preferences of the 'people'; (2) the administrators (or bureaucrats) who serve (whether badly or adequately) the political leadership; (3) the professionals who, based on their expertise and training, provide the health care (usually medical services *per se*); and (4) the patients or clients who receive and–or consume these health services. Since all flesh is mortal and subject to disability, decay and ultimately death, this fourth category subsumes all previous three categories at some time or another in the lifecycle. Hence the fourth category is also equivalent to the public who comprise the whole population. Automatic constraints or liabilities of attentiveness (distraction) and size (disorganisation) relegate this fourth category to a residual in the political model of the health sector.

Given the pre-existing condition that all humans have health needs at one time or another in their lives, each of these broad categories of actors has specific roles (that is, expectations as well as patterns of behaviour) attached to it. The politicians set the stage by choosing among alternatives (if any) in order to establish the goals for health care; they thereby legitimate the system of health services. Politicians also raise and allocate resources (financial, material, human) to the health sector – which necessarily competes with other sectors of government for these resources (for example, transportation, defence, agriculture, education and so on). Politicians can set the stage by inaction as well as action, since the former either acknowledges and reinforces the status quo or by default delegates the decision-making to other actors in the system. By their actions in seeking help, members of the public can influence the patterns of health services; they can also raise some resources independently of the government (for example, voluntary labour or direct payment). Sometimes however the government and the public are at logger-heads in that the former tries to change the latter's behaviour. My guiding presumptions are that (a) for a variety of reasons most of the public acquiesce to government decisions although they do not necessarily support them actively, and (b) if the political leaders in government exceed the limits set by an acquiescent people, then those leaders will be replaced. In the relatively democratic polities under consideration, these assumptions seem viable.

The roles of the bureaucrats are somewhat simpler, although they too can by default resemble those of the politicians. That is, while a bureaucracy is expected to carry out the orders of the government (themselves based, however tenuously, on public mandates), the bureaucrats also can and often do pursue political roles. The study of implementation in the policy process has clearly suggested that even more political activity occurs within the bureaucracy and among administrators in relation to their peers and outside pressures (for example, interest groups) than occurs in the phase of policy formulation and legislative legitimation. Aspirations among bureaucrats and administrators to obtain recognition as professionals further complicate their roles in a health system.

The professionals who provide health (medical) services have critical roles in the whole health system. As long as health care remains invasive, based on specialised knowledge and the product of dyadic (one-to-one) relationships, medical professionals will continue to influence (if not, indeed, dominate) the health sector. Some providers of health care are 'less professional' in the sense that they have less training and greater interchangeability; but all providers aspire to, if they are not already recognised as holding, professional status; and they furnish the point of first contact for patients in the health system. That is to say, whether curing or helping or even just caring, the health provider sits at the centre of the system. Try as they will, politicians and bureaucrats cannot replace the functions of the health professionals; and this centrality of function is a source of power over all other actors. To be sure various sanctions, penalties, incentives and rewards exist which can be used to channel and direct the behaviour of health providers. But – to belabour the obvious – one cannot provide personal health services without providers. Only the patients themselves have the power to by-pass the professionals by taking care of themselves; and such self-care, while possible through publicly shared and disseminated knowledge, can only supplement the direct provision of health services. One cannot perform an appendectomy on oneself – at least within the confines of any commonly acknowledged parameters of human behaviour. Health professionals remain crucial or, as Fuchs puts it in a gamesman's metaphor, 'the physician is captain of the team.'

Finally, the residual roles of the public are germane to the health system. General habits and attitudes toward health care do shape health behaviour – though sometimes to the chagrin, lament, and disgust of professional providers, bureaucrats, and politicians alike. Hence health care patterns must be understood and appreciated in a psycho-social (cultural) context, whether one looks at single case studies or compares them. Given constraints of time and topic of course, this rich range of nuanced health behaviour by the public cannot be addressed here. But the caveat must be made explicit that, as with all model-testing and theorising, the previous three categories and their roles are limited, partial players in the system.

The one subset of patients or consumers of health care that does merit special attention includes those who organise themselves into self-conscious, energetic groups. Each of the preceding categories (politicians, bureaucrats, professionals) can also be internally divided into competing parties, associations, or interest groups; and such organisation (usually) increases the power of these actors in the health system. Among the general public however, the incidence of organised consumer groups is relatively rare and requires only occasional monitoring. Patterns of performance in any health system can best and most efficaciously be described and predicted through the activities of relatively few active elite players operating within the contexts of culturally prescribed human behaviour.

Initially, in order to explain outcomes in health policy, the primacy of political leaders in directing (or redirecting) health policy was assumed. This assumption was predicated on the legitimate control that democratically elected governments wield over their citizens, and on the likelihood that the closer decision-making over health care came to the public (who presumably are all concerned at one time or another about the lives and well-being of themselves and their loved ones), the more input the lay sector would wield over the behaviour and performance of health professionals. In short, government works best when the political directives are clear and immediate and when they emanate from decentralised sources. On matters as important as life and death and well-being, health care had better not be left to the professionals. Also, in a Millsian sense, participation is in itself a good thing and can direct resources and efforts toward ends that are immediately relevant to the people. This was unabashedly a utilitarian argument of the greatest good for the greatest number, as self-determinedly as possible.

Over time in field experiences however, evidence emerged to counter and in a sense reverse these initial assumptions. Without explicitly detailing all the factors, the public was evidently passive, disorganised and—or inattentive, except in a very individualised, atomistic sense. (That is, one worries about one's own aches and pains or those of near kin, but rapidly loses interest in the ills of others.) A seeming exception to this generalisation would be the activities of disease-specific groups, which promote special services for the afflicted or urge more research; but over time, the same self-centred behaviour emerged in that disease-specific groups quarrel with one another over resources more than they cooperate with each other to extract more resources from the external environment. The same observation can be made, *mutatis mutandis*, about the primary actors in the health system as a whole.

Another assumption that fell by the empirical wayside was the public-enhancing nature of decentralisation of decision-making over health care. Participant-observation as well as indepth interviews indicated that the more decentralised the decision-making system, the more power health professionals wield over their lay colleagues. Status and expertise are professional resources which the lay participant finds hard to counter – even given the obvious argument that only the wearer knows where the shoe pinches.

The emergent model then is one where health professionals hold pride of place in decision-making. Political leaders still retain the function of legitimating decisions that are made, and indeed raising the resources whose allocations are then largely determined by health professionals. Professionals supply the advice and information on which politicians to a large extent base their decisions; and not surprisingly the information and advice rarely run counter to the interests of the professionals. The primary source of dispute, within the community of 'helping professionals', is how the resources are to be divided among specialities. Frequently political leaders delegate authority for these decisions to committees, which rely on advice from medical professionals.

In the emergent revised model, the roles of the public and the politicians become less central. One suspects that the issue of 'participation' is but a fad which may leave behind some residual rituals and (on a more optimistic note) provide some additional market information about health care preferences on a regular basis. But power-wielding in an overt sense by the political sectors (whether mass or elite) will be routinised into formulae. At the same time however, the influence and indeed power of the bureaucrats will rise. The reasons for the augmented power of bureaucrats are at least two-fold.

First, as government expands by taking on new responsibilities and functions, and passes the laws which legitimate such activities, the state bureaucracy is charged with implementing these mandates. The actual applications of these activities are via the rules and regulations that bureaucrats devise. The amount of discretion left to these bureaucrats grows in direct proportion to the inattentiveness of the political sectors (which are distracted by other issues, by crisis management, and the general attention cycle). Hence the relative size of the bureaucracy to the whole population grows.

Second, organisations which provide health services are themselves becoming bureaucratised. As size increases along with an elaborated division of labour and function, the clinics and hospitals and other health service agencies (including those for planning) become internally differentiated. Despite the power of health professionals, derived from their expertise and centrality, these same providers are countered by bureaucrats who aspire to professional status. The administrative bureaucrat has become as ubiquitous as the medical professional in the health system, and supplies the most pervasive immediate challenge to the latter's power and influence.

In its clearest form then, the explanatory model emphasises decentralisation of authority (both political and administrative) and professional penetration of administrative and decision structures as the two primary independent variables determining resource allocation in the health sector. The model assumes a neo-institutional perspective in that the structured patterns of health care practices, as well as the agencies of government, channel and constrain behavioural dynamics among the categories of actors. Changes (or the lack of them) in allocations over a specific period can thus be noticed and measured against initial institutional conditions. Between the independent variables (decentralisation and professional penetration) and the dependent variable (resource allocation) lie such process-channeling variables as the nature and extent of governmental regulation of health care services, and the prevailing political culture.

SUBSTANTIVE FINDINGS

During the fifteen years prior to 1990, I conducted several different research projects on the politics of the health sector. The initial projects – not reported here – dealt with the impacts of intergovernmental relations on health care in the United States, and with the political context of comparative health planning. The former examined the effects (direct, indirect, and reciprocal) of changes in child health policies at federal and state levels over forty years; and the latter examined problems of effectively implementing health planning programmes in Europe and the United States. A second undertaking investigated who governs the health sector in Western industrialised states. A third project examined how health resources are allocated in Third World countries. I will report briefly on the second and third of these studies, then discuss methodological issues in the conduct of comparative health policy research.

The question of 'who governs' in the health sector has been pursued through a 'most similar design' method by examining health politics in Britain, Sweden, and the United States. These societies provide appropriate systems for comparison because they are very much alike in shared culture, health status, democratic institutions, and industrial economy. Yet along the dimension of how authority over health services is distributed, these nation-states differ sharply. Therefore, as Table 11.1 indicates, these three nation-states can be arrayed along a continuum of policies for allocating decision-making authority over health care. Britain is highly centralised and its National Health Service is directly financed by the central government from general tax revenues. Sweden, although a unitary state, has granted important financial and organisational roles to regional levels. In contrast, although recently marked by a dramatic experiment in capping federal payments for Medicare costs, organisational and financial arrangements for health care in the United States remain fragmented and pluralistic.

Table 11.1 Comparative health expenditures by source of funding (by approximate percentage of national total)

	Britain	*Sweden*	*United States*
Total public (central government)			
1950	85 (79)	78 (26)	28 (13)
1970	85 (80)	85 (31)	38 (25)
1985	93 (87)	92 (27)	43 (28)
Total private (patient derived)			
1950	15 (15)	22 (16)	72 (57)
1970	15 (15)	15 (15)	62 (35)
1985	7 (6)	8 (8)	57 (27)

Furthermore Sweden, Britain and the United States differ in the degree to which various constituencies are represented on decision-making and–or advisory bodies, and at what levels, as well as differing in methods of selecting representatives at various levels of activity and function. Some modes of selection emphasise a descriptive representation of the surrounding community. Others stress the substantive representation of selected 'natural' or 'deserving' interests, while other interests are ignored or excluded. And still other selection modes experiment with novel forms of 'mediated' participation. The field studies investigated what difference it makes for planning, financing and operating health services as to who is represented and who participates in the decision-making process; and what difference different mixes of participants make at various levels of decision-making.

In order to research the question of 'who governs', three successive case-studies were conducted in subnational health regions, which were also selected through the 'most similar design' method. Each multi-county region had similar geographic and population size, broad historical continuity, similar levels of morbidity and mortality, and a single major medical school plus teaching hospital. The regions differed primarily in terms of relative autonomy or dependency along the dimension of decentralisation discussed above. Fieldwork focused on participants at the regional level, but inquiries and interviews necessarily extended up to central authority and down to local units.

Current goals of the health systems in Britain, Sweden and the United States are very similar, as indeed they are (at least in terms of lip-service) throughout the world. These goals include the expeditious provision at reasonable cost of good quality medical care for every citizen when needed. Against such as ideational consensus however, different organisational and financial arrangements have been developed throughout the world for approximating these ends. And such alternative arrangements generate political questions that underpin the delivery of health (specifically medical) services. The basic questions are broad but simple: who decides and enforces health policy? Who makes binding decisions in the health sector, especially during provision of medical services? Once decision-makers in health policy and operations are identified, one enquires why they have such power? What are the sources of their ability to make binding decisions? Thirdly, do perceptions about power vary among those who plan, finance, and operate health services? If so, how and why? Finally, is there a preferred state-of-affairs which at present is not being achieved? If so, what alternative arrangements should be made and how might they be attained?

The problem of how health resources are allocated in Third World states has been examined through a 'most different design' method at two distinct levels. First, the countries of South Asia, East Asia, and subsaharan Africa have distinctly different political systems even though they all broadly share similar resource constraints. And second, the experiences of India, Sri Lanka, Pakistan, China, Kenya, Senegal, Tanzania and Zaïre over the past decade are contrasted with the advanced Western systems. Admittedly, this second 'most different design' method was not initially intentional but when retrospectively applied it illuminated patterns of resource allocation and highlighted problems of comparative research even within the 'most similar design' method.

As background to research on health resource allocations in the Third World, a campaign launched in 1978 by the World Health Organisation and its 134 member governments seeks to achieve 'Health for All by the Year 2000'. The vehicle for attaining this worldwide goal is primary health care provided by community health workers, and the campaign seeks to increase the political commitment of member countries to meeting the health needs of the rural and urban poor. Primary health care is not merely front-line or first-contact care, but rather includes a package of principles which distinguish it from the narrower, more medically-exacting understanding of primary health care. These principles are: equitable distribution, community involvement, focus on prevention, appropriate technology, and the involvement of other sectors of the economy. Obviously the 'primary health care approach' has a thoroughly political theme in redesigning decision-making.

The magnitude of this undertaking to meet health care needs and to redesign decision-making in the health sector is evident from Table 11.2. In low-income countries life expectancy at birth averages only 51 years while mortality rates for infants and children are ten to twenty times higher than in developed countries. Yet for those who reach the age of five, life expectancy is only eight or nine years less than the average elsewhere.

Table 11.2 Health related indicators (1979) by income-grouping

	Low-income countries		Middle-income countries	Industrialised countries
	(N = 34)	< $370 <	*(N = 60)*	*(N = 18)*
Per capita GNP	$240		$1420	$9440
Crude birth rate/1000	42		34	15
Crude death rate/1000	16		10	10
Life expectancy (years)	51		61	74
Infant mortality rate	49–237		12–157	13
Child mortality rate (per 1000 aged 1–4 years)	18		10	1

National statistics in the aggregate of course disguise wide disparities between the conditions of the rural and urban poor on the one hand, and the conditions of the more affluent city dwellers on the other. The latter not only have higher incomes but tend to be better educated and have better access to health services. Consequently their health status closely resembles the general average profile of industrialised countries. As economic development proceeds in Third World countries, the more prosperous regions of a country gain advantages not only of greater individual and collective wealth but also of greater political leverage. National policies therefore give priority to their needs so that the limited health resources available are concentrated in urban areas, and the gap between urban and rural populations widens.

Furthermore, in the quest for economic development, protective measures for occupational health and safety as well as for the environment tend to lag behind. Such measures are often initially expensive and only enforceable by firm legislation followed by competent inspection procedures with meaningful sanctions. Rapid development thus produces new personal health problems as well as environmental pollution. Most probably urban health problems will increasingly dominate health patterns in the developing world, even though at present its needs are predominantly rural. It is estimated that by the year 2000, the urban population in developing countries will average 43 per cent of the total Third World, so the primary health care approach for rural health problems will need to be modified to address the emerging problems of the urban setting as well.

The overwhelming problem of developing countries is that they must meet the range of urban *and* rural health needs with just a fraction of the financial and human resources available in the developed world. Expensive new technologies that are (disputably) appropriate for the developed North will not serve the purposes of the South. Yet the latter's health systems remain dominated by physicians and medical associations whose training, aspirations, and psychological (not to mention financial) rewards are drawn from their counterparts in the North. At times the pervasiveness of communications in this global village leads to counterproductive reference systems and pernicious results.

Consequently health services in the Third World are maldistributed both in terms of need and appropriate technology. Access to health services is uneven, and large segments of the rural population are not reached. Health facilities and skilled personnel are concentrated in urban areas, where their services are further biased toward the middle- and upper-income city dwellers. Both the urban and rural poor are neglected and, unless there is sustained political commitment to apply resources where the need is greatest, little progress can be expected.

Good health is of course a product of many factors, which include adequate nutrition, a supportive unpolluted environment, quality housing, education to practice self-care, access to personal medical services, and an organisational system to deliver these factors when and where needed. But in the shorthand of common usage, 'the politics of health are the politics of medicine', and the role of medical care providers centrally influences all developments in health care. The medical profession is of special importance because clinical decisions by its individual members have great impact on the demand for health facilities and the consumption of resources for diagnosis and treatment. In particular the model of medical care preferred by these providers is very important for determining outputs (from both the private and public sectors of medicine) and ultimately for influencing outcomes in health.

If a medical model emphasises high quality, capital-intensive, sophisticated technology which is oriented towards curative medicine, the results will be quite different from a medical model which emphasises adequate quality, labour-intensive, appropriate technology oriented towards preventive medicine. Usually the standard rhetoric by government officials, politicians, and medical spokespersons advocates a health care system which is rural and preventive in its biases, and based on community-level workers using simple techniques. Yet the end results in outputs (in health services), which determine ultimate outcomes (in health status), are to the contrary. Empirical patterns of distribution of medical manpower are skewed toward the urban areas; training in medical schools is oriented towards high-quality, highly specialised medical care; local health centres are under-staffed, under-resourced, and over-worked.

A political analysis of the relationship between health and development in South Asia alone begins to explain this persistent paradox between rhetoric and reality. First, at a macro-level of policy-making, the relevant governments have other goals that take precedence over health services. If we look past the rhetorical claims of politicians and instead examine actual investment patterns, we find much greater emphases on such items as defence, industrial development, and agriculture. Indeed the primary imperative for development in South Asian countries has been argued (Nayar, 1972) to be the quest for strong defence capability rather than the quest for social welfare.

Second, there are plausible political explanations for why the governments in South Asia – with the exception of Sri Lanka – have neglected basic investments in health services. For one thing the locus of authority over health care is diffuse; health is constitutionally a state subject, not a central subject, and even at state level it is administratively malcoordinated. Also governments defer to the role of the 'professional expert' in the health care system. Although spokesmen for private medical interests like the Pakistan, Sri Lankan, or Indian Medical Associations are not as powerful as their counterparts in Western countries, publicly financed medical schools generate much of the problem. Governments have basically written blank cheques (within limits) to medical schools, which in turn promote medical training based on a Western-derived curriculum. Indeed, while medical colleges in South Asia have expanded very rapidly and educated large numbers of physicians, these physicians are often alienated and embittered. They concentrate in urban areas (where ironically a literal surplus of MDs can be found); or they migrate to greener pastures, which leads to the problem of foreign medical graduates elsewhere.

Third, South Asian countries – again with the exception of Sri Lanka – neglected their poor, rural majorities in the early stage of national development efforts. Their primary development strategy has been to emphasise investments in large-scale industrial and agro-industrial projects rather than in social services. However some Third World countries have attained significant social goals in spite of poverty. In particular birth rates in Taiwan, Korea, and Sri Lanka started to decline sharply as the condition of the poor majority improved *well before* the introduction of effective national family planning programmes. Health and education statistics in these three countries are far more favourable than in other poor countries – and these accomplishments are due to effective, low-cost, mass delivery systems for education and health care. In per capita terms alone, Sri Lanka spends nearly three times as much on government expenditures for social services as do either India or Pakistan.

Furthermore, as a fourth explanation, it might be added that South Asian governments were excused from hard thinking about investment strategies and health services because, on many occasions, public attention was diverted from the need for a comprehensive system of primary, secondary, and tertiary units for delivering health services. Those diversions of attention have occured because governments set aside relatively huge sums of money – or obtained the money from outside sources – in order to run mass campaigns against specific diseases such as malaria, smallpox, leprosy, filaria, and the like. While the intrinsic value of such campaigns *per se* cannot be gainsaid, some argue that such campaigns have hindered the development of a permanent, easily accessible health services system in the rural areas of South Asia where most people live.

Money alone of course cannot ensure good health in the developing world. But the extreme poverty of most of the population in the South is the primary constraint on improving health status. Within the already low per capita GNP which yields little tax revenue, health services must compete with other pressing developmental needs. Likewise the analysis of health expenditures in developing countries is hampered by an abysmal lack of financial information on programmes operated by different levels of government as well as by the private sector. In some extreme cases, like Bangladesh and Zaïre, annual public health expenditures are less than one dollar per capita. Since recurrent expenditures are concentrated in urban areas where hospitals and medical personnel are located, it may be inferred that resources to operate health services for the rural population are very limited indeed. Furthermore, given organisational problems as well as pervasive poverty, the capacity of local government to generate tax revenues is severely limited. This situation would be unbearable were it not for the popular self-help movements (such as Sarvodaya in Sri Lanka and India) where community participation mobilises voluntary labour (*shramdan*) and materials for constructing health facilities plus some in-kind support for community health workers.

Even such voluntary activities are however inadequate to meet pressing health needs. As elsewhere, out-of-pocket payments plus access to nonWestern health systems help to alleviate (although not solve) the problem. Private spending on health care in many developing countries is estimated to be three or four times greater than government expenditures on health, so the share of GNP devoted to health services logically approximates 4–5 per cent. But the efficacy of this private spending (other than for psychological support) is questionable, and research into alternative systems of indigenous health practices is needed.

There are a number of obvious divergencies between my studies of the developed North and underdeveloped South but, considering health policies and politics in all the countries examined, one finding repeatedly emerged: no matter what the organisational arrangements or modes of financing or economic background, professionals dominate decision-making in the health sector. Not that they ever admit as much. Like everyone else, physicians insist they have no power and are the victims of circumstances and inertia. At times one wonders whether anyone is in charge at all. But the protestations of medical professionals are less convincing than those of other players; their exaggerations of powerlessness are less pronounced. Many other participants admit that they defer to physicians in matters of judgement over health policies – including trade-offs among financially expensive items; but physicians rarely acknowledge deference to anyone else, including other professionals. In India, to take the major Third World example, physicians have dominated every major health commission since independence. The regulations in the rule-books and the social codes that govern behaviour were devised, or at least greatly influenced, by medical personnel; they have already provided the precedents on which subsequent adminis- trators make their binding decisions. Only under conditions of economic scarcity in otherwise well-organised countries, such as in Britain, are the decision–making powers of medical professionals weakened; but even there they are not eliminated.

There remains then a 'private' government of medicine even in the public sector, comprised of physicians and administrators, who rule those who pay (insurers, government agencies, and ultimately the citizenry). The medical professionals are dominant, although periodi- cally they must repel challenges from the administrative 'professio- nals' while the public continues to pay. Efforts by the public sector – whether politicians, planners, or nonmedical interest groups – are spasmodic, unsustained, and generally unsuccessful in shaping the closed deliberations of this private government. The health sector throughout the world remains governed from within, not from without; and expectations of rapid, frequent public leverage over health services delivery systems are misplaced.

METHODOLOGICAL ISSUES

Given this broad and judgemental conclusion from several research projects on the politics of health policy, a series of methodological issues come to the fore. How valid, how replicable is this finding? Is it an artifact of one's method of enquiry? Does one find what one (perhaps subconsciously) looks for, despite the use of both most-similar and least-similar designs? All enquiries, but particularly comparative enquiries, are subject to problems of control and inference; to problems of operationalisation and measurement; to problems of data within variable cultural contexts.

There is, of course, no particular rank order to this series of problems. But the problems of control and inference are classic and cannot be wished away. No matter how well thought out one's research design may be, there are always exogenous variables that another can cite which could contaminate one's study and obviate one's conclusions. These variables may be ideational, in the sense of either an overriding, internalised ideology (for example, 'scientism' or the authority of expertise and knowledge) or just a common or garden-variety sense of prevailing culture (for example, 'doctor knows best') in matters of health care. Alternatively these exogenous variables may be physical in the sense of resource constraints; even given the pump-priming nature of Keynesian economics and–or the ability to borrow from future generations for today's expenditures, there are limits to how much money or other material resources are available. A vast, complicated agenda of other needs competes with allocations for health services (in either the narrow sense of medical care, or the broader sense of infrastructural investments in sanitation, water-supply, housing, education, and so on).

One of the devices to manage, at least in part, these problems of control and inference is to employ discriminant function analysis. If one knows that a dependent variable (say, the proportion of GNP devoted to health care; or, the allocation of health monies to inpatient care) obtains different values in relatively similar contexts during the same period of time, then one traces back the sequence of antecedent conditions and intervening variables in order to account for these variations. Hence the fact that for 30 years Sri Lanka has spent more than three times as much as India on per capita education and health is not due to natural resource constraints; both countries have had similar per capita incomes, although always about a 5:4 ratio to Sri Lanka's advantage. Rather one looks to (a) political history, since Sri Lanka gained universal sufferage in 1931 – sixteen years before India and only two years after the United Kingdom itself – that provided the basis for competitive party politics over *domestic* policy issues; (b) structure of the economy, since Sri Lanka's plantation sector provided more easily-monitored resources for extracting taxes to allocate elsewhere; (c) compact geographic size which makes medical communications – such as clinic placements and referral networks – easier in rural areas; and (d) competing claims on resources, since India maintains a relatively impressive defence establishment that annually consumes 20–22 per cent of central government revenues – or about four per cent of its GNP – whereas Sri Lanka is virtually demilitarised. Nevertheless in both countries the allocation of health monies (at the 3:1 ratio, respectively) have gone to 'allopathic' (that is, Western) medical facilities rather than to the indigenous systems of medicine (such as, Ayurvedic, Siddhi, Unani Tibbi) because the government commissions as well as health departments were staffed almost exclusively by Western-trained physicians. Even after independence, both countries established and–or expanded medical schools that reproduced large numbers of allopathic doctors – many of whom ironically migrated to the North to work as foreign medical graduates in American and European health systems. But that is another story to illustrate the international context within which so-called domestic health policies and programmes operate.

A similar set of arguments can be adduced to explain why Sweden spends almost twice as much of its GNP on health as does Britain – and even more on a per capita basis. But the methodological issue is the same; one looks for antecedent conditions to account for the known variations and then discovers that within the respective pools of allocated health monies, the medical professionals determine the pattern of their utilisation. In each case however, one can sense (at least psychologically if not quantitatively) that the explanatory agenda is incomplete and almost infinitely expandable.

A second and more familiar set of methodological problems deals with operationalisation and measurement. In terms of the concept of health care itself, its nature, content and context are constantly changing. There are disputes about the definition of health *per se*, ranging from the all-inclusive perfectionist ideal of the World Health Organisation, to various mechanistic, environmental, and socio-culturally determinative conceptions. As time passes the content of health care also shifts from treatments for and precautions against infectious diseases, to coping with the occupational diseases of industrial and postindustrial development and the degenerative diseases of affluence and old age. The North – both its First and Second Worlds of development – has largely eliminated the earlier conceptualisation of health care as infectious disease and now struggles with the successor stages. But due to both geographical location and economic system, the South has yet to contain, much less vanquish the astonishing range of pernicious tropical diseases (malaria, filaria, schistosomiasis, onchoceriasis, trypanosomiasis, leprosy, and so on) while simultaneously trying to anticipate the emergent health problems of accelerated economic development. In a very direct sense, comparing health policies between North and South is like the proverbial apples and bananas; the units for comparison are quite dissimilar. Yet when the issues are (a) political control and (b) proportionate resource allocations, a strong case can be made for the least-similar-design. If a similar pattern appears in these relational concepts across such diverse contexts, then one feels justified in claiming some reasonable explanatory power for the independent variable(s). Professional penetration has occurred in all these contexts; intra-sector allocations are made according to the preferences of medical professionals.

At the same time, one begins to question the other independent variable (the decentralisation of authority) for its impact on proportions of GNP allocated to health care. Given the 'most similar design' study, it appears that unitary states (like Britain and France) spend less on health services because they can 'cap' and control finances, whereas decentralised or federal systems (like Sweden on the one hand, and the United States and Germany on the other) spend more because they haemorrhage through a variety of financial conduits. But when applying the 'most similar design' to South Asia, one finds that the unitary state of Sri Lanka spends much more on health care than the federal state of India, where responsibility for health is consigned constitutionally to the component states as well as to a reasonably lively private sector. Each of these 'most similar design' projects would lead to a conclusion directly contradicting the other. So the 'least similar design' (even when applied *ex post facto*) makes one question the explanatory importance of government structures as a determinative independent variable.

Concepts *per se* are not of course meaningfully comparable for they are only conveyors (containers) of data or information. Rather the indicators of the concepts must be functionally equivalent in order to compare one nation-state or system with another. So a central methodological problem concerns the measured data. Are they valid? Are they comparable? Are they reliable over time as well as at any given point in time?

The dimension of time in particular needs to be emphasised, for no causation can occur without its passage. In a strict sense, cross-sectional deployment and analysis of variance can only show

association and correlation. One may impute causal relationships on
the basis of common sense but epistemiologically such causation is
assumed, not demonstrated. Only a series of observations over two
or more points of time can provide an adequate basis for causation.
Of course, despite such scientific language as 'cause and effect', it is
understood that comparative research seldom allows for anything
approaching really scientific experimentation.

In countries with stable traditions of accounting and empiricism,
data are arguably more reliable than in those where record-keeping
has only recently commenced. Indeed for many subsaharan African
countries one senses a great skepticism about the adequacy of even
government statistics, much less other sources of data. The concepts
are available; the categorical entries exist to be filled; but the
validation of reported data is suspect. Even in statistics reported to
and published by agencies of the United Nations, the 'trend-line' of
growth in certain indicators is so smooth and perfect that it could only
be derived by a careful, systematic annual multiplication of the
(putative) baseline by some constant (and politically palatable)
increment. At times one also finds more vaccinations reported for a
specific disease than the number of denizens of a district would merit;
and one concludes either that some people have received multiple
vaccinations, or that the reported data are fictitious. (A few
repetitions of such questionable data rapidly erode one's confidence
in *all* government documents and data of a particular country.)

Fortunately (although this observation undoubtedly reveals a
cultural bias on my part, which in turn can raise yet another
methodological issue – that is, how to detect, account for, and then
correct personal bias) the tradition of 19th century British empiricism
has not only been shared by its Anglo–American successors in the
North but also has penetrated its erstwhile Afro–Asian colonies in
the South. Given the indeterminacy of all evidence within the
philosophical confines of Heisenberg and Hempel, on a sliding scale
of intersubjective validity this author tends to trust South Asian as
well as European data. At the same time, previous collaborative
research efforts in both North America and Western Europe have
demonstrated pitfalls and problems with data under the 'best' of
conditions. For example, the categories for recording public health
data and expenditure are periodically redefined, expanded or
subdivided; except for overall aggregates, it is very difficult to
establish unambiguous trend lines. This difficulty is not surprising
since knowledge about health care (not to mention its shifting

conceptualisation mentioned above) is constantly changing; new discoveries and old achievements need to be reconciled and at least thus far – unlike Big Brother's dicta in *1984* – we do not go back to correct the historical record in order to get previous 'facts' in line with current events.

More pessimistically, this problem of shifting data-bases can be partly traced to efforts by bureaucrats, politicians, and even professionals to evade accountability. That is to say, just as reorganisation of an administrative agency can temporarily distract and confuse participants about who is responsible for what functions until a new routine settles in, so also the reorganisation and reconceptualisation of categories for data collection makes it difficult if not impossible to trace trends accurately and assign responsibility (particularly blame, but also conceivably credit) for the developments or changes. Since few actors are intentionally self-liquidating, a little persiflage can help protect one's security. Whether one is a politician, bureaucrat, or professional, one's first aim is to survive.

Empirical data come through several media which raise additional methodological issues. In comparative health research, types of data can be arrayed along a continuum in terms of how 'hard, medium, or soft' they are. That is to say (to reiterate the old saw of the spending-services cliché), financial records and accounts of money (both revenue and expenditures) are palpably 'hard' because they can be metrically measured, cross-checked, audited, and quantitatively compared. Monies allocated to health services in national plans, government budgets, institutional accounts, and post-audit records do indeed give one a fairly secure (at least psychologically speaking) basis for intra-country comparisons. Inter-country and inter-sector comparisons are more questionable, for the reasons of data-categorisation mentioned above. But with appropriately acknowledged simplifying assumptions (like proportion of GNP; or conversion at international exchange-rates; or even functional-equivalency in terms of some third referent within a country), comparisons and inferences can be made.

The classic problem with expenditure data however, is that they do not necessarily translate into health services *per se*; and they say even less about impacts on health status. Indeed one might quibble that over-spending reduces health by increasing chances for iatrogenic disease. Hence one needs to collect and compare some 'medium hard' sets of data – specifically morbidity rates and vital statistics. Like financial records, these body-counts are palpable in that they can be normalised against a base-population, and changes over time can be observed. The unit of analysis is also pragmatic in that (considering Alexander Pope's 'the measure of man is man') one compares human beings and their life-chances. The problem of such medium-data however is that they are subject to greater variation in initial reporting than even financial outlays. Vital statistics may go unreported, or misreported, and causes of illness or death can be wrongly – either purposely or accidentally – assigned. Furthermore, unlike the more or less metric or interchangeable nature of money, body-counts may mean different things in different contexts. To take an extreme example, in a hierarchically organised society, some 'bodies' count for less than other 'bodies' – either in being noticed or worthy of being reported. Ethnic minorities in many pluralistic nation-states go under-reported; and in some religions, women and children receive less recognition than men. The problems of cross-cultural reporting and cross-national comparisons are thus exacerbated, and the eventual plethora of exceptions, variations and cultural nuances leave a researcher somewhat skeptical of recorded evidence.

This problem becomes even worse when access to records is restricted, either for political reasons or because of simple incompetence. Fascinating as recent developments in the People's Republic of China may be, it has not been possible to piece together a complete picture of its health policy, practice, and performance. The same is true of many African states; and even in rural South Asia, non-allopathic practices are difficult to track and record with any overall precision. At best, estimates and guesstimates form the basis for comparisons – or, more appropriately, educated culturally-sensitive 'hunches'.

Finally, the 'soft' data required for comparative policy research are enough to cause scientific purists to throw up their hands in horror and utter despair. The reasons are similar to those afflicting attitudinal research ventures within a single culture or geographic entity. Interview data on what people believe, recall, predict, or assume are inevitably 'squishy soft'. The same respondent may – for various reasons – be open or closed to an interviewer; he or she may share truthfully his or her experiences and observations, or may deliberately distort the facts; or perhaps a respondent may not understand the context and content of the question, thus providing unintentionally misleading information. In conducting an analysis of 'head counts', one becomes painfully aware of the Roshomon Principle – and of the *Panchatantra* tale of blind men describing an elephant.

Furthermore the status or importance of an interviewee can vary across cultures so that, for example, a bureaucrat in country-A is considered to be beneath contempt while in country-B he or she is considered to be above reproach. The necessary corrective to this inherent cross-cultural problem is to poll a panel of area-experts about how to weight different categories of respondents' roles; simultaneously one should eschew any pretence of quantification other than simple direction and ordinal scale. In comparative research, one cannot assume equal weighting among survey respondents. At best one can compare respondents within specific role-positions, but always place their pooled responses within the larger social or institutional context.

In short, as one meditates on the variety of methodological issues and problems in comparative research, one begins to doubt the validity of any comparative research findings. Speaking for myself and several projects that try to employ discriminant function analysis, the problems of control and inference are legion. Exogenous factors crop up everywhere; data are chronically suspect; even countries and regions selected through a 'most similar design' method seem to become more and more unique as I delve into their respective histories and appreciate their nuanced developments. Certainly cross-national differences in the 'least similar design' studies would seem to overwhelm the relatively simple model that I had initially posited.

But oddly enough – if the reader will condone stream-of-consciousness – I feel even more certain that health policies and politics are determined in large part by the views and actions of medical professionals. It is difficult to demonstrate this dominance with a single integer or some unambiguous formula but, in case after case, interview after interview, and country after country, the medical professionals took (and take) precedence over the other actors – whether politicians, bureaucrats, public groups and and so on. Sometimes of course the medical profession 'loses a battle' and seems to say, 'see, we are no more powerful than anyone else'. But such losses are quickly turned to advantage, as with the 1965 passage of Medicare in the United States where doctors cried all the way to the bank; or in Sweden where salaried physicians suddenly found themselves with a lot more leisure time by earning the same income in fewer hours; or in South Asia, where the indigenous practitioners have been held at arm's length from the public coffers, or at best contained within a very narrow domain of publicly funded activity.

CROSS-POLICY COMPARISONS

Has this 'finding' about the health sector any parallels elsewhere? Is health a unique, unusual policy field – characterised at base-line by control over pain and suffering, over life and (sometimes deferable) death? Probably not. As one reads about other complex policies like energy-supply, defence, or even foreign affairs, one can observe how those who control 'expertise' dominate in their respective arenas. These fields also have professionals who share what John Stuart Mill once called 'received opinion', or the set of beliefs about preferred values, rules of evidence, and causal logic that collectively comprise a prevailing paradigm.

Such received opinion gives enormous advantage to the professionals because it is widely shared by the non-expert public as well. Through a long and fairly unconscious, almost unintentional process, laymen are socialised to accept the same paradigm *and* the notion that only an expert can and should wield decision-making power. It is psychologically comforting to think that 'doctor knows best' so one need only follow his or her advice to become well or avoid illness. Likewise it is comforting to believe that the generals and other military personnel who defend a nation are experts in their craft and competent in its exercise, and that diplomats know the niceties of promoting national interests while avoiding possible trouble, or that engineers and scientists have the potential knowledge to resolve chronic energy crises. Woe betide one's psychological well-being if such trust in the efficacy of experts is replaced by anxiety and insecurity.

This is not of course a recommendation that all submit to the dominion of sectoral experts and specialists. Rather it is just a cautionary recognition that often it is easier to 'go along to get along' through deference than to challenge a prevailing paradigm. While humans are quite clearly social and thinking animals, they are also more often than not subject to 'group think'. And political activities in the health field are no exception.

Technological complexity however has its own pitfalls and problems. Not only is such expert knowledge as involved in nuclear weaponry or in brain surgery beyond the ken and ability of most people, it is also often beyond the grasp of many so-called experts. While one may believe that somewhere, somehow, someone understands the whole edifice of scientific knowledge in a given field, usually each of the professional actors has only a partial grasp of the whole. At such points the technological complexity of a speciality eludes or overwhelms even those who putatively wield it. Out of control, the whole proceeds on its own inertia. No individual can be held directly and specifically accountable for the overall situation; only a series of partial, marginal adjustments can be made.

Even so, the professionals will defend their political turf, their influence over decision-making, because of their knowledge-base itself. Each has made considerable investments in time, resources and skills to obtain the basic expertise, as well as adequate information on which to ground activities. Such investments represent 'sunk capital costs' that cannot easily, if ever, be retrieved. Hence the expert professional has additional reasons to fend off any critics or, when at all possible, to block any proposals about sharing decision-making powers.

Finally, in each of these cross-policy comparisons questions of ethics arise. In an era of rapidly expanding knowledge and interdependent relationships, who judges the judges, guards the guardians, or even defines the good? These are classical problems of normative political theory, which affect complex policy areas just as much as the Greek pursuit of the good life. There are no answers to these reiterative dilemmas; only a process of sifting and sorting options, in which it is desirable that as many as possible take part in order to understand the problems and thereby cope with the inherent limitations of all proffered solutions.

What then can one conclude about the methodological issues raised in comparative studies of health policy? Are there any lessons to be learned from this discursive enquiry into comparative health policies on a North–South continuum? Probably the most salient political finding is the evident limitation of leverage over policy choices and implementation. There are of course some parameters within which policy choices can be made and effected. And there are some conditions necessary and others sufficient in order to achieve even a modicum of change from the status quo. But the range of change is restricted and viable options narrow to a few. At best a pragmatic idealist can only confront reality with successive approximations of solutions and thereby adopt a mode of satisfactory behaviour in order to get on with the job.

As for the 'scientific' dimensions of comparative enquiries into national health policies and their concommitant politics, potential lessons depend on one's judgemental perspective on the virtues of epistemiological purity as well as where one's objectives fall on a continuum from the elegantly theoretical to the mundanely pragmatic. Objectives may be defined as theoretical if, when, and to what extent the researcher aims at formulating, falsifying and–or modifying 'hypotheses, that is propositions stated in terms of universally defined variables . . .' (Wiatr 1977b, p.356). But objectives may also simply try to establish 'patterns of similarity and–or dissimilarity between countries, when the analysis does not intend to extend beyond description of these patterns. . . . Any study, even the most descriptive one, can bring very useful material for theory, and most theoretically oriented studies produce also descriptive analyses' (*ibid*, p. 357). Indeed Wiatr later elaborates the argument that 'existing dissimilarities, large as they may be, do not exclude the possibility of a general theory. General theory does not imply that all cases it refers to are identical or even similar; it only implies that they are comparable in the sense that they share certain common dimensions' (*ibid*, p. 367).

Hence cross-national research is not necessarily useless if it fails to test general hypotheses. Often the data alone are sufficient justification for a descriptive enterprise, because the study of comparative health policy badly needs facts set in cultural context – particularly on countries where little, if any, research has been done to date. Of course the data collected should be of a standardised character so that base-lines are laid for systematic comparisons as well as simple replications. Against such considerations, a partial but adequate foundation has now been laid for future in-depth and more rigorous studies of comparative health politics – all within the clear advance understanding that a certain amount of imprecision, not to say sloppiness, is inevitable. To revert to the egregious world of horticultural metaphor, neither the apples of the North nor the bananas of the South may be polished to perfection such that one's own image reflects back in their surfaces, but both remain types of fruit that are eminently palatable and in fact quite tasty.

Bibliography

Alford, R.R. (1975) *Health Care Politics: Ideological and Interest Group Barriers to Reform* (University of Chicago Press).

Altenstetter, C. (1974) *Health Policy Making and Administration in West Germany and the United States* (Beverly Hills, California: Sage Publications).

Altenstetter, C. (1980) 'Hospital Planning in France and the Federal Republic of Germany', *Journal of Health Politics, Policy and Law*, no. 5, pp. 309–32.

Altenstetter, C. and J.W. Björkman, (1983) *Federal-State Health Policies and Impacts: The Politics of Implementation* (Washington, DC: University Press of America, 1978).

Altenstetter, C. and J.W. Björkman, 'Planning and Implementation: A Comparative Perspective on Health Policy', *International Political Science Review*, no. 13, pp. 73–91.

Aluwihare, A.P.R. (1982) 'Traditional and Western Medicine Working in Tandem', *World Health Forum*, vol. 3, no. 4, pp. 450–1.

Ameline, C.E. (1984) 'Philosophy and Cost of Health Care in France', in Virgo, *loc. cit.*, pp. 17–29.

Anderson, O.W. (1972) *Health Care: Can There Be Equity? The United States, Sweden, and England* (New York: John Wiley and Sons).

Anderson, O.W. and J.W. Björkman, (1980) 'Equity and Health Services: Sweden, Britain, and the United States', in Heidenheimer and Elvander, *loc. cit.*, pp. 223–37.

Ashford, D. (ed.) (1980) *Comparative Public Policies: New Concepts and Methods* (Beverly Hills, California: Sage Publications).

Banerji, D. (1972) 'Social and Cultural Foundations of Health Services Systems', Economic and Political Weekly (Special August Number) pp. 1333–45.

Barnard, K. and K. Lee (eds) (1977) *Conflicts in the National Health Service* (London: Croom Helm).

Bausell, R.B. and A.J. Rinkus, (1979) 'A Comparison of Written Versus Oral Interviews'. *Evaluation and the Health Professions*, vol. 2, no. 4, pp. 477–86.

Berki, S.S. (1985) 'DRGs, Incentives, Hospitals, and Physicians', *Health Affairs*, vol. 4, no. 4, pp. 70–76.

Berlant, J.L. (1975) *Profession and Monopoly: A Study of Medicine in the United States and Great Britain* (Berkeley: University of California Press).

Björkman, J.W. (1977) 'Political-Administrative Relationships in Development: Contributions and Constraints', in Sharma, *loc. cit.*, pp. 601–616.

Björkman, J.W. (1979) *The Politics of Administrative Alienation* (Delhi: Ajanta Publications).

Björkman, J.W. (1982) 'Professionalism in the Welfare State: Sociological Saviour or Political Pariah?' *European Journal of Political Research*, no. 10, pp. 407–28.

Björkman, J.W. (1984) 'Health Policy and Politics in Sri Lanka: Developments in the South Asian Welfare State'. *Asian Survey*, vol. 34, no. 5, pp. 211–40.

310   *Conclusion*

Björkman, J.W. (1985) 'Who Governs the Health Sector? Comparative European and American Experiences with Representation, Participation and Decentralisation', *Comparative Politics*, no. 17, pp. 399–420.

Björkman, J.W. (ed.) (1986) *The Changing Division of Labour in South Asia: Women and Men in Politics, Economics, Society* (Riverdale, Maryland: The Riverdale Company).

Björkman, J.W. (1987) 'Health Policies and Human Capital: The Case of Pakistan', *Pakistan Development Review*, no. 11, pp. 411–30.

Björkman, J.W. (ed.), (1988) *Fundamentalism, Revivalists, and Violence in South Asia* (New Delhi: Manohar Publishers).

Björkman, J.W. (1989) 'Politicising Medicine and Medicalising Politics: Physician Power in the United States', in Freddi and Björkman, *loc. cit.*, pp. 28–73.

Björkman, J.W. and C. Altenstetter, (1979) 'Accountability in Health Care: An Essay on Mechanisms, Muddles, and Mires', *Journal of Health Politics, Policy, and Law*, no. 4, pp. 360–81.

Björkman, J.W. and B.W. Coyer, (1980) 'Comparative Policy Research and Discriminant Function Analysis', *Political Change* (Jaipur, India) no. 3, pp. 26–46.

Björkman, J.W. and G.A. Silver (1978) 'Citizen Control of Health Services: An International Perspective on Participation, Representation, and Social Policy', *Proceedings of the Ninth World Congress of Sociology* (Uppsala, Sweden, 12–19 August).

Bornstein, S. *et al.* (eds), (1984) *The State in Capitalist Europe* (London: Allen and Unwin).

Brown, L.D. (1982) *The Political Structure of the Federal Health Planning Program*, (Washington, DC: The Brookings Institution).

Carder, M. and B. Klingeberg, (1980) 'Towards a Salaried Medical Profession? How "Swedish" Was the Seven Crowns Reform?', in Heidenheimer and Elvander, *loc. cit.*, pp. 143–72.

Charles, C.A. (1976) 'The Medical Profession and Health Insurance: An Ontario Case Study', *Social Science and Medicine*, no. 10, pp. 33–8.

Cleverly, W. (ed), (1982) *Handbook of Health Care Accounting and Finance* (Maryland: Aspen Publishing).

Cochrane, A.C. (1972) *Effective Uses and Efficiency: Random Reflections on Health Services* (London: The Nuffield Provincial Hospitals Trust).

Cohen, S.S. and C. Goldfinger, (1975) 'From Permacrisis to Real Crisis in French Social Security: The Limits to Normal Politics', in Lindberg *et al.*, *loc. cit.*, pp. 57–98.

Commonwealth Secretariat, (1982) *The Contribution of Medical Schools to National Health Development* (Report of a Commonwealth Workshop at Kandy, Sri Lanka) (London: Marlborough House).

Derber, C. (ed.), (1982) *Professionals as Workers: Mental Labour in Advanced Capitalism* (Boston: G.K. Hall).

Derber, C. (1983) 'Sponsership and Control of Physicians', *Theory and Society*, no. 12, pp. 561–601.

Döhler, M. (1989) 'Physicians' Professional Autonomy in the Welfare State: Endangered or Preserved?', in Freddi and Björkman, *loc. cit.*, pp. 178–97.

Dudley, A. (1984) 'The DRG Tug-of-War', *Medicine and Computers* (September–October) pp. 34–7.

Ehrenreich, J. (ed.), (1978) *The Cultural Crisis of Modern Medicine,* (New York: Evergreen Press).

Elling, R.H. (1980) *Cross-National Study of Health Services: Political Economies and Health Care* (New Brunswick, New Jersey: Transaction Books).

Elston, M.A. (1977) 'Medical Autonomy: Challenges and Responses', in Barnard and Lee, *op. cit.*, pp. 26–51.

Evans, J.R., K. Hall and J. Warford, (1981) 'Health Care in the Developing World: Problems of Scarcity and Choice', *New England Journal of Medicine*, no. 305, pp. 1117–27.

Field, M.G. (1980) 'The Health System and the Polity: A Contemporary American Dialectic', *Social Science and Medicine*, no. 14A, pp. 397–413.

Franda, M. (1983) *Voluntary Associations and Local Development in India* (New Delhi: Young Asia Publications).

Frazier, H.S. and H.H. Hiatt, (1978) 'Evaluation of Medical Practices', *Science*, no. 200, pp. 875–8.

Freddi, G. and J.W. Björkman (eds) (1898) *Controlling Medical Professionals: The Comparative Politics of Health Policies* (London: Sage Publications).

Freidson, E. (1970) *Professional Dominance* (Chicago: Aldine Publishing Company).

Freidson, E. (1975) *The Profession of Medicine: A Study of the Sociology of Applied Knowledge* (New York: Dodd, Mead and Company).

Freidson, E. (1985) 'Reorganisation of the Medical Profession', *Medical Care Review*, no. 42, pp. 11–35.

Fuchs, V.R. (1974) *Who Shall Live? Health, Economics, and Social Choice* (New York: Basic Books, Inc.).

Fuchs, V.R. (1981) 'The Coming Challenge to American Physicians', *New England Journal of Medicine*, no. 304, pp. 1487–90.

Fuchs, V.R. (1982) 'The Battle for Control of Health Care', *Health Affairs*, vol. 1, no. 2, pp. 5–13.

Giddens, A. and G. Mackenzie (eds), (1982) *Social Class and the Division of Labour* (Cambridge: Cambridge University Press).

Glaser, W.A. (1978) *Health Insurance Bargaining: Foreign Lessons for Americans* (New York: Gardner Press).

Godt, P.J. (1984) 'Doctors and Deficits: Regulating the Medical Profession in France', *Proceedings of the annual meeting of the American Political Science Association* (Washington, DC: September).

Golladay, F. and B. Liese, (1980) *Health Problems and Policies in the Developing Countries* (Washington, DC: The World Bank).

Goodman, J.C. (1980) *The Regulation of Medical Care: Is the Price Too High?* (San Francisco: Cato Institute).

Grant, J.P. (1976) 'A Fresh Approach to Meeting Basic Human Needs of the World's Poorest Billion: Implications of the Chinese and Other "Success" Models', *Proceedings of the annual meeting of the American Political Science Association* (Chicago: 2–4 September).

Gray, B. (ed.), (1983) *New Health Care for Profit* (Washington, DC:

312 *Conclusion*

National Academy Press).

Harrison, S. and R.I. Schulz, (1989) 'Clinical Autonomy in Britain and the United States: Contrasts and Convergences', in Freddi and Björkman, *op. cit.*, pp. 198–209.

Heidenheimer, A.J. (1980) 'Conflicts and Compromises Between Professional and Bureaucratic Health Interests, 1947–1972', in Heidenheimer and Elvander, *loc. cit.*, pp. 119–42.

Heidenheimer, A.J. and N. Elvander (eds), (1980) *The Shaping of the Swedish Health System* (London: Croom Helm).

Heller, T. (1978) *Restructuring the Health Service* (London: Croom Helm).

Herzlich, C. (1982) 'The Evolution of Relations Between French Physicians and the State from 1880 to 1980', *Sociology of Health and Illness*, no. 4, pp. 241–53.

Hessler, R.M. and A.C. Twaddle, (1982) 'Sweden's Crisis in Medical Care: Political and Legal Changes', *Journal of Health Politics, Policy, and Law*, no. 7, pp. 440–59.

Horowitz, I.L. (1965) *The Three Worlds of Development* (New Brunswick, New Jersey: Transaction Books).

Howard, L.M. (1981) 'What Are the Financial Resources for "Health 2000?"', *World Health Forum*, vol. 2, no. 1, pp. 23–9.

Hunt, K. (1983) 'DRG – What It Is, How It Works, and Why It Will Hurt', *Medical Economics*, 5 September pp. 264–5.

Illich, I. (1973) *Medical Nemesis* (Boston: Beacon Press).

Jaggi, O.P. (1976) *All About Allopathy, Homeopathy, Ayurveda, Unani, and Nature Cure* (New Delhi: Orient Paperbacks).

Jacques, E. (ed.), (1978) *Health Services: Their Nature and Organisation and the Role of Patients, Doctors, Nurses, and the Complementary Professions* (London: Heinemann).

Jeffrey, R. (1976) 'Health Care Delivery System: A Comment', *Economic and Political Weekly* (10 July) pp. 1046–7.

Johnson, R. (1982) 'The State and the Professions: Peculiarities of the British', in Giddins and Mackenzie, *op. cit.* , pp. 186–208.

Kearney, R.N. (1973) *The Politics of Ceylon (Sri Lanka)* (Ithaca, New York: Cornell University Press).

Kelman, S. (1977) 'The Social Basis of the Definition of Health', *International Journal of Health Services*, no. 6, pp. 217–47.

Klein, R. (1977) 'The Corporate State, Health Service, and the Professions', *New University Quarterly*, no. 31, pp. 161–80.

Klein, R. (1983) *The Politics of the National Health Service* (London: Longmans).

Klein, R. and J. Lewis, (1976) *The Politics of Consumer Representation* (London: Centre for Studies in Social Policy).

Kohn, R. and K.L. White (eds), (1976) *Health Care: An International Study* (London: Oxford University Press).

Krause, E. (1977) *Power and Illness: The Political Sociology of Medical Care* (New York: Elsevier).

Lagergren, M. and K.E. Wictorsson, (1977) *Case Study on Health Planning Organisation and Process in Sweden* (Stockholm: Sjukvårdens och Socialvårdens Planerings och Rationaliserings Institut).

Lebish, D.J. (1982) 'PSROs and Utilisation Review: Life, Death, and Rebirth', in Cleverly, *op. cit.*

Leichter, H. (1979) *A Comparative Approach to Policy Analysis: Health Care Policy in Four Nations* (New York: Cambridge University Press).

Leslie, C. (ed.) (1976) *Asian Medical Systems: A Comparative Study* (Berkeley: University of California Press).

Levitt, R. (1977) *The Reorganised National Health Service*, 2nd edition (London: Croom Helm).

Lindberg, L. *et al.* (eds), (1975) *Stress and Contradiction in Modern Capitalism* (Lexington, Massachusetts: Lexington Books).

Luft, H.D. (1983) 'Economic Incentives and Clinical Decisions', in Gray, *op. cit.*, pp. 103–23.

McKinlay, J.B. (1982) 'Toward the Proletarianisation of Physicians', in Derber, *op. cit.*, pp. 37–65.

McLachlan, G. and A. Maynard (eds) (1982) *The Public/Private Mix for Health* (London: Nuffield Provincial Hospitals Trust).

Mahler, H. (1977) 'Blueprint for Health for All', *WHO Chronical*, no. 31, pp. 491–8.

Marmor, T.R. (1973) *The Politics of Medicare* (Chicago: Aldine Publishing Company).

Marmor, T.R., (1980) A. Bridges and W. Hoffman, 'Comparative Politics and Health Policies: Notes on Benefits, Costs, Limits', in Ashford, *op. cit.*, pp. 59–80.

Marmor, T.R. and J.A. Morone, (1980) 'Representing Consumer Interests: Imbalanced Markets, Health Planning, and the HSAs', *Health and Society: Milbank Memorial Fund Quarterly*, no. 58, pp. 125–65.

Marmor, T.R. and D. Thomas, (1972) 'Doctors, Politics, and Pay Disputes: "Pressure Group Politics" Revisited', *British Journal of Political Science*, no. 2, pp. 422–42.

Maxwell, R. (1975) *Health Care: The Growing Dilemma: Needs v. Resources in Western Europe, the US, and the USSR*, 2nd edition (New York: McKinsey).

Maxwell, R. (1981) *Health and Wealth: An International Study of Health Care Spending* (Lexington, Massachusetts: Lexington Books).

Mechanic, D. (1976) *The Growth of Bureaucratic Medicine* (New York: John Wiley and Sons).

Mechanic, D. (1984) 'The Transformation of Health Providers', *Health Affairs*, no. 4, pp. 65–74.

Morone, J.A. and A.B. Dunham, (1984) 'DRGs and the Waning of Professional Dominance', *Health Affairs*, no. 3, pp. 73–86.

Mosher, F. (1978) 'Professions in Public Service', *Public Administration Review*, no. 38, pp. 144–50.

Moskop, J.C. (1981) 'The Nature and Limits of the Physicians' Authority', in Staum and Larson, *loc. cit.*, pp. 29–43.

Nayar, B.R. (1972) *The Modernisation Imperative* (New Delhi: Vikas Publications).

Niessen, M. and J. Peschar (eds), (1982) *International Comparative Research: Problems of Theory, Methodology, and Organisation in Eastern and Western Europe* (Oxford: Pergamon Press, Ltd.).

Poullier, J.J. (ed.) (1977) *Public Expenditures on Health* (Paris: OECD Studies in Resource Allocation, no. 4,).

Przeworski, A. and H. Teune, (1970) *The Logic of Comparative Social Inquiry* (New York: Wiley-Interscience, John Wiley and Sons).

Robson, J. (1973) 'The NHS Company, Inc.? The Social Consequences of Professional Dominance in the National Health Service', *International Journal of Health Services*, no. 3, pp. 413–26.

Rodwin, V.G. (1981) 'The Marriage of National Health Insurance and "La Médicine Libérale" in France: A Costly Union', *Health and Society: Milbank Memorial Quarterly* no. 59, pp. 16–43.

Rodwin, V.G. (1982) 'Management Without Objectives: The French Health Policy Gamble', in McLachlan and Maynard, *op. cit.*, pp. 289–325.

Sharma, S.K. (ed.) (1977) *Dynamics of Development: An International Perspective* (New Delhi: Concept Publishing Company).

Shenkin, B.N. (1973) 'Politics and Medical Care in Sweden: The Seven Crowns Reform', *New England Journal of Medicine*, no. 288, pp. 555–9.

Sidel, R. and V.W. Sidel, (1982) *The Health of China: Current Conflicts in Medical and Human Services for One Billion People* (Boston: Beacon Press).

Silver, G.A. (1976) *et al.*, *Impact of Federal Health Policies in the States of Connecticut and Vermont* (Springfield, Virginia: National Technical Information Service) (PB–262–959).

Silvard, R.L. (1979) *World Military and Social Expenditures 1979* (Leesburg, Virginia: World Priorities).

Silvard, R.L. (1982) *World Military and Social Expenditures 1982* (Leesburg, Virginia: World Priorities).

Silvard, R.L. (1986) *World Military and Social Expenditures 1986* (Leesburg, Virginia: World Priorities).

Starr, P. (1982) *The Social Transformation of American Medicine* (New York: Basic Books).

Staum, M.S. and D.E. Larson (eds), (1981) *Doctors, Patients, and Society* (Waterloo, Ontario: Wilfried Laurier University Press).

Steffen, M. (1983) 'Régulation Politique et Stratégiés Professionnelles: Médicine Libérale et Émergence des Centres de Santé' (Grénoble: manuscript).

Steudler, F. (1977) 'Médicine Libérale et Conventionnement', *Sociologie du Travail*, no. 17, pp. 176–98.

Steudler, F. (1984) 'State and Health in France' (Paris: manuscript).

Stone, D.A. (1980) *The Limits of Professional Power: National Health Insurance in the Federal Republic of Germany* (Chicago: University of Chicago Press).

Szalai, A. and R. Petrella (eds), (1977) *Cross-National Comparative Survey Research: Theory and Practice* (Oxford: Pergamon Press, Ltd.).

Taylor, R.C.R. (1984) 'State Intervention in Postwar Western European Health Care: The Case of Prevention in Britain and Italy', in Bornstein *et al.*, *op. cit.*, pp. 91–117.

Tolliday, H. (1978) 'Clinical Autonomy', in Jacques, *op. cit.*, pp. 32–52.

Virgo, J.M. (ed.) (1984) *Health Care: An International Perspective* (Edwardsville, Illinois: International Health Economics and Management Institute).

Walt, G. and P. Vaughn, (1981) *An Introduction to the Primary Health Care Approach in Developing Countries* (London: Ross Institute of Tropical Hygiene).

Weller, G. and P. Manga, (1983) 'The Push for Reprivatisation of Health Care Services in Canada, Britain, and the United States', *Journal of Health Politics, Policy, and Law*, no. 8, pp. 495–518.

Wiatr, J. (1977) 'The Role of Theory in the Process of Cross-National Survey Research', in Szalai and Petrella, *op. cit.*, pp. 347–72.

Wilsford, D. (1989) 'Physicians and the State in France', in Freddi and Björkman, *op. cit.*, pp. 130–56.

Index

Index